RECOVERY OF MOTOR FUNCTION FOLLOWING SPINAL CORD INJURY

Edited by **Heidi Fuller** and **Monte Gates**

Recovery of Motor Function Following Spinal Cord Injury
http://dx.doi.org/10.5772/61539
Edited by Heidi Fuller and Monte Gates

Contributors
Mokhtar Arazpour, Sherif Amr, Juan Moreno, Diego Torricelli, Filipe Oliveira Barroso, Christina Francisca Vogelaar, Veronica Estrada, Lucia Slovinska, Juraj Blasko, Dasa Cizkova, Eva Szekiova, Miriam Nagyova, Antonio Ibarra, Salvatore Cuzzocrea, Emanuela Esposito, Irene Paterniti, Mengliang Zhang, Aimee Nelson, Aaron Bailey, Hunter Fassett, Tea Lulic, Jenin El Sayes, John V. Priestley, Adina Michael-Titus, Juan Larrain, Victor S Tapia, Giles Plant, Laura Marquardt, Bhavaani Jayaram, Vanessa Doulames, Christine Plant

Published by InTech
Janeza Trdine 9, 51000 Rijeka, Croatia

Publishing Process Manager Romina Rovan
Technical Editor SPi Global
Cover InTech Design team

First published July, 2016
Printed in Croatia

Additional hard copies can be obtained from orders@intechopen.com

Recovery of Motor Function Following Spinal Cord Injury, Edited by Heidi Fuller and Monte Gates
p. cm.
Print ISBN 978-953-51-2497-9
Online ISBN 978-953-51-2498-6

For EU product safety concerns:
IN TECH d.o.o., Prolaz Marije Krucifikse Kozulić 3, 51000 Rijeka, Croatia,
info@intechopen.com or visit our website at intechopen.com.

Meet the editors

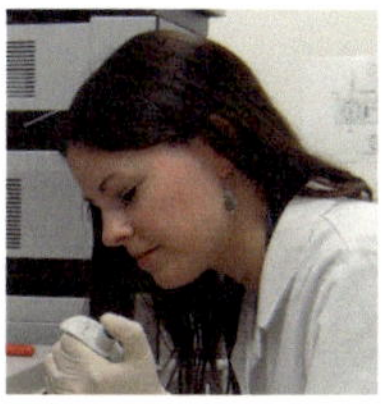

Dr. Fuller received a BSc honours degree in Biomolecular Science at Bangor University, UK, and went on to undertake a PhD studentship, based at the Robert Jones and Agnes Hunt Orthopaedic Hospital in Oswestry, UK. Following several years of postdoctoral studies in which she developed an interest in applying proteomics technologies to study neurological injury and disease, Dr. Fuller was recently appointed as a Lecturer in Medical Education at Keele University and Principle Investigator at the Keele Institute for Science and Technology in Medicine. Together with her research team, she aims to identify molecular and cellular targets for neurological regeneration and repair.

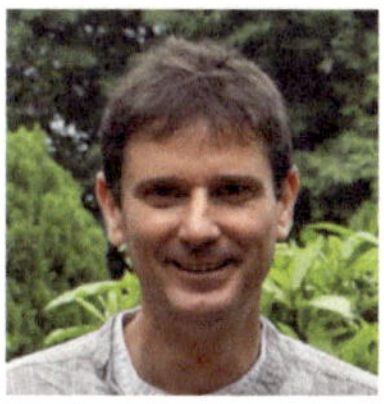

Dr. Gates graduated with a BS in Experimental Psychology and a BA in Philosophy from Austin Peay State University in the United States. From there, he went on to complete a PhD in Anatomy and Neurobiology at the University of Tennessee (UT), where he researched how glial cells affect the development and repair of neural circuits in the central nervous system. After postdoctoral studies in the laboratory of Dr. Anders Bjorklund at Lund University, Dr. Jeffrey Macklis at Harvard University, and Professor Stephen Dunnett at Cardiff University, he took up a lectureship position at Keele University. Here, his research focuses on the use of in vivo and in vitro models to understand how neuronal cells develop and find appropriate targets in the central nervous system, and how these processes may be manipulated as a strategy to repair motor circuitry defects.

Contents

Preface

Restoring motor function after a spinal cord injury (SCI) is one of the most challenging tasks medicine is facing today. To address this problem, and to translate research from the bench to the bedside, experimental models are required, which faithfully recapitulate the molecular, cellular and physiological responses to the injury. From there, researchers can begin to characterize and manipulate the complex mechanisms to facilitate repair and regeneration of motor circuitry. In addition to modulating the body's own cellular responses to SCI, surgical approaches continue to explore how grafting and cell replacement strategies may enhance endogenous repair mechanisms. Beyond these biological interventions, precision in assessing the degree of spinal cord injury and prognostic outlook, as well as tailoring rehabilitative-based interventions, are evolving to enhance mobility following spinal cord injury.

This book seeks to give the reader insight into the current understanding of each of these approaches to restoring motor recovery following SCI. What should become obvious to the reader is the large diversity, in terms of the number of specialized areas of the science involved in attempting to address this issue, as well as the complexity of the biological factors that play a role in regeneration and repair of SCI.

We are grateful to the authors who have contributed a rich diversity of articles to this book and to our publishing process manager, Ms. Romina Rovan, for her indefatigable organization and support.

Dr Heidi Fuller
Postgraduate Medicine and Institute for Science and Technology in Medicine,
Keele University, UK

Dr Monte Gates
School of Medicine and Institute for Science and Technology in Medicine,
Keele University, UK

Section 1

Models of Spinal Cord Injury

Experimental Spinal Cord Injury Models in Rodents: Anatomical Correlations and Assessment of Motor Recovery

Christina F. Vogelaar and Veronica Estrada

Additional information is available at the end of the chapter

http://dx.doi.org/10.5772/62947

Abstract

Human traumatic spinal cord injury (SCI) causes disruption of descending motor and ascending sensory tracts, which leads to severe disturbances in motor functions. To date, no standard therapy for the regeneration of severed spinal cord axons in humans exists. Experimental SCI in rodents is essential for the development of new treatment strategies and for understanding the underlying mechanisms leading to motor recovery. Here, we provide an overview of the main rodent models and techniques available for the investigation of neuronal regeneration and motor recovery after experimental SCI.

Keywords: spinal cord injury, regeneration, plasticity, rodent, motor recovery

1. Introduction

The challenge of spinal cord injury (SCI) research is to find the right model for testing new treatment strategies. Although rodents differ from humans in many aspects, the research on primates is prohibited in many countries, and there are very strict regulations on experimenting with nonhuman primates [1]. Therefore, rodent models are the first choice for testing the effectiveness and mechanisms of new potential treatments for SCI. Rodents, especially mice, provide the additional advantage of transgenic technologies (knock out and knock in) that can be helpful in SCI research. In this chapter, an extensive description is provided on the currently available rodent SCI models, methods of treatment application, histological analysis of regenerating axons, and functional analysis of motor recovery.

2. Anatomy of the longitudinal axon tracts in rodents and humans

In order to understand the impact of SCI, it is important to have some basic knowledge about the long axon tracts that are interrupted by the lesion. Descending tracts control various motor functions. Sensory information from ascending tracts is also essential for posture, balance, and coordination of movements. Here, the main projections from the brain to the spinal cord and vice versa are summarized.

2.1. Descending motor tracts

The descending tracts in the spinal cord (**Figure 1**, left-hand side) run from the brain and brainstem to the spinal cord and are all involved in motor control [2].

2.1.1. Corticospinal tract (CST)

The corticospinal tract (CST) is variable between species. The motor cortex in rodents, generally referred to as the sensorimotor cortex (a rostrocaudal gradient of motor and sensory areas), is not as well defined as it is in humans, who have separate areas for sensory and motor cortex. The CST is responsible for the control of fine movements of distal musculature (e.g., fingers). Pyramidal neurons in layer V of the motor area give rise to the corticospinal axons that run via the internal capsule to the brainstem pyramids where they cross. It then depends on the species which path the majority of CST axons follow. In primates, almost all crossed fibers run in the lateral CST, located in the dorsolateral part of the lateral column. In rodents, most fibers are located in the dorsal CST (dCST), running in the ventral part of the dorsal columns. In some species, a ventral CST (vCST) is also observed. The CST axons terminate mainly in lamina 3–6 of the grey matter. In humans, up to 20% of CST axons terminate directly on motoneurons in lamina 9. CST terminals are glutamatergic.

2.1.2. Rubrospinal tract (RST)

The rubrospinal tract (RST) plays a role in general locomotion and in some species controls more skilled motor tasks together with the CST. It arises from the caudal magnocellular part of the red nucleus and crosses in the ventral tegmental decussation. The RST descends in the dorsal part of the spinal cord lateral column. The axons terminate in laminae 5 and 6 (sometimes 7) in the cervical and lumbosacral enlargements corresponding to the limbs. In rats, direct termination on lamina 9 motoneurons has been reported. The RST is prominent in rodents, whereas in animals with a large lateral CST (e.g., primates and humans), the RST is smaller. RST axons use glutamate as neurotransmitter.

2.1.3. Reticulospinal tracts (ReST)

The reticular formation in the brainstem plays a role in the preparation of movements and postural control. Reticulospinal tracts run medially and laterally in the ventral part of the spinal cord white matter. Whereas the medial reticulospinal tract (ReST) remains uncrossed, part of the lateral ReST fibers cross to the contralateral side. The ReST does not form a clear bundle

http://dx.doi.org/10.5772/62947

but intermingles with fibers from other tracts, for example, the vestibulospinal and spinothalamic tracts. The axons terminate in laminae 5–9 and can be either glutamatergic or GABAergic [3].

2.1.4. Vestibulospinal tracts (VeST)

The medial and lateral vestibulospinal tracts (VeSTs) are responsible for the initiation of limb and trunk extensor activity, which is important for posture. The lateral VeST arises from the lateral vestibular nucleus and does not cross, whereas the medial VeST originates from both the medial and the spinal vestibular nuclei and partially crosses to the contralateral side. Both run in the ventral white matter and terminate in laminae 7–8, providing glutamatergic input [3].

2.1.5. Raphespinal and coeruleospinal tracts

The Raphe nuclei give rise to the raphespinal projections, which together with the coeruleospinal projections (from the locus coeruleus) modulate (among others) motor functions. The raphespinal projections include a non-serotonergic component that runs in the dorsolateral funiculus and is involved in gating pain, as well as a serotonergic component that runs in the ventrolateral white matter, terminating in the intermediate grey and on motoneurons in the ventral horn. The noradrenergic coeruleospinal fibers run without crossing in the ventral funiculus and project throughout the grey matter.

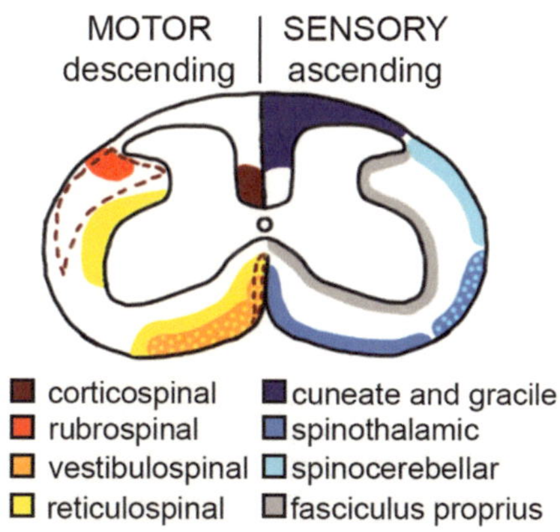

Figure 1. Spinal cord anatomy: schematic representation of the main ascending sensory tracts (right) and descending motor tracts (left) in a transverse section of the rodent spinal cord. Dotted areas represent locations where tracts are intermingled. Dashed lines indicate the location of the corticospinal tract in humans.

2.2. Ascending sensory tracts

The ascending tracts in the spinal cord (**Figure 1**, right-hand side) convey sensory information from the periphery to central nervous system (CNS) areas involved in walking, posture, and information processing about noxious stimuli [4].

2.2.1. Gracile and cuneate tracts

These two large ascending pathways contain axons from the dorsal root ganglia (DRGs) and provide sensory information from the limbs and trunk. In rodents, an additional dorsal column nucleus contains afferent axons from the tail. The tracts synapse in the gracile and cuneate nuclei located in the medulla oblongata. The second-order axons then cross the midline and run through the medial lemniscus to the thalamus. A subpopulation of DRG neurons synapses locally on dorsal horn neurons, whose axons also project to the gracile and cuneate nuclei. This is called the post-synaptic dorsal column pathway, whereas those DRG axons that do not synapse locally constitute the direct dorsal column pathway.

2.2.2. Spinothalamic, spinoreticular, and spinovestibular tracts

Several sensory tracts run in the ventrolateral funiculus of the spinal cord. These include the spinothalamic tract that conveys nociceptive, thermal, crude touch, and pressure information from the DRGs to the thalamus. The spinoreticular tract provides pain information to brain-stem nuclei of the reticular formation. The spinovestibular tract is important for bringing proprioceptive signals to the vestibular nuclei. Several other tracts are present in the ventro-lateral funiculus, such as the spinomesencephalic, spinoparabrachial, spinohypothalamic, and spinocervical tracts, each providing information to specific brain regions, that is, mesence-phalon, parabrachial nuclei, hypothalamus, and lateral cervical nucleus in the upper cervical cord, respectively.

2.2.3. Spinocerebellar tracts

Projection axons from the spinal cord to the cerebellum are located in the dorsolateral and ventrolateral funiculi (**Figure 1** right-hand side). They carry proprioceptive information from the muscles and tendons to the cerebellum, so that adjustments of posture and coordination of movements can take place.

2.3. The propriospinal system

The spinal cord's "own" projection system refers to neurons that are located in the spinal cord, whose axons interconnect various spinal cord levels [5]. This so-called propriospinal system constitutes a large part of the white matter. It comprises interneurons that are connected to either other interneurons or directly to motoneurons. With respect to locomotor control, short-axon propriospinal neurons are also called premotoneurons, because they modulate cortico-spinal and sensory input to motoneuron pools controlling fore- and hindlimb activity. The long-axon propriospinal neurons form connections between the cervical and lumbosacral enlargements and are responsible for coordination of fore- and hindlimbs. These axons run in the fasciculus proprius (**Figure 1**, right-hand side).

The propriospinal neurons also modulate input to the lumbar central pattern generator (CPG), a local system involved in reflexive stepping in total absence of supraspinal input [5]. Serotonin from brainstem neurons has been shown to play a major role in CPG activation [6, 7].

http://dx.doi.org/10.5772/62947

3. Rodent spinal cord injury models

The choice of SCI models is important in view of comparability with human SCI, but practical issues should also be considered. Although human lesions are usually compressions (but some may be sharp wounds as well or a mixture of both), from the experimental point of view it might be important to have a more "clean" and reproducible cut. Treatment strategies that fail to cause regeneration through a spinal cord transection lesion will probably have equally small effects after contusion lesions. On the contrary, treatments that induce regeneration in a transection model should then be tested and optimized in a contusion model. Partial injury models are useful for the investigation of the locomotor recovery over time, since not only regeneration but also sprouting from spared axon tracts can occur (see Section 5). Models of complete transection are used to study regeneration without the possibility of plasticity processes bypassing the lesion. While the complete transection of the spinal cord is a very reproducible injury, disadvantages of this lesion model are the poor degree of regenerative

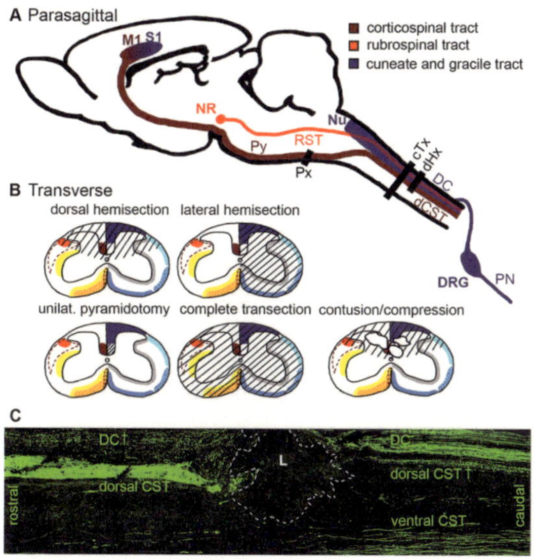

Abbreviations:
comTx: complete transection,
DC: dorsal columns,
dCST: dorsal corticospinal tract,
dorsHx: dorsal hemisection,
DRG: dorsal root ganglion,
M1: primary motor cortex,
Nu: nucleus (gracilis and cuneatus),
NR: nucleus ruber,
PN: peripheral nerve,
Px: pyramidotomy,
Py: pyramids,
RST: rubrospinal tract,
S1: primary sensory cortex,
YFP-H: yellow fluorescent protein – H (mouse line),
†: degenerated tract

Figure 2 Spinal cord lesions in rodent models of SCI: (A) schematic representation of a parasagittal section through the brain and spinal cord (modified from Paxinos & Watson, The Rat Brain in Stereotaxic Coordinates, 6th Edition). Tracts with clear localizations are indicated. It should be noted that these do not run in the same spinal cord section, with the RST (red) running more laterally than the CST (brown) and the cuneate and gracile tracts (blue). The dorsal hemisection, complete transection, and the pyramidotomy lesions are represented as black bars. (B) Schematic drawings of transverse sections through the spinal cord with bilateral motor tracts depicted left and bilateral sensory tracts depicted right (for exact description of the tracts see **Figure 1**). Dashed areas represent the extent of tissue damage produced by the different injury paradigms. Note that motor and sensory tracts run in both spinal cord hemispheres but are depicted separately for better understanding. (C) Histological parasagittal section through the spinal cord of YFP-H mice (The Jackson Laboratory) 7 days after a dorsal hemisection (compilation of 2 sagittal sections). Descending CST axons are intact rostrally and have degenerated caudally from the lesion site (dashed white line). Ventral CST fibers are not lesioned (plane of section causes apparent lack rostrally). Ascending dorsal column axons are intact caudally and have degenerated rostrally.

growth of the severed axons and the general inadequacy for most motor tests. In this section, the technical principles of each model in rats and mice are described.

3.1. Dorsal hemisection (Hx)

Spinal cord transection lesions are generally applied using scissors, scalpel blades, or fine retractable wire knives. The advantage of wire knives (McHugh Millieux) is that a SCI can be performed with high precision, because they can be attached to a stereotactic frame. The dorsal Hx (Figure 2A–C) is the most used SCI paradigm for the investigation of the regeneration of CST and, depending on the extent of lateral lesion, it also includes the RST. It is mostly performed at thoracic level 8 (T8) and involves the laminectomy at T8-9, opening of the dura mater and subsequent lesioning of the spinal cord [8, 9]. For mice, microdissection spring scissors (Fine Science Tools) are used to hemisect the spinal cord. Since this procedure is inherently variable, the experimenter needs to test various depths to determine the desired extension of the lesion. A more controlled technique for dorsal Hx in mice was described by Hill et al. (2009) who used a so-called Vibraknife (LISA-Vibraknife; Louisville, KY) [10, 11]. Dorsal hemisection lesions are usually applied at thoracic spinal cord levels and result in the formation of a dense inhibitory scar [12, 13]. Depending on the severity of the lesion, the animals spontaneously recover a certain degree of walking that can be further ameliorated by regeneration promoting treatments.

3.2. Lateral Hx

For lateral Hx, the lateral half of the spinal cord is transected in mostly the same technical procedure as the dorsal Hx, with the difference that the tracts on one side are left intact (Figure 2B). These lesions provide the advantage of an internal control situation [14], which is also reflected in the behavioral testing, where paw preferences are often scored (see Section 7.5.). Lateral Hx experiments are usually performed at cervical levels, allowing the analysis of both fore- and hindlimb recovery. Mostly, a lesion at cervical level C5 is produced, but some groups have specialized on the analysis of breathing musculature after a lesion at C2 [15].

3.3. Complete transection (Tx)

For a complete transection (Figure 2B), small scissors are generally used to transect the spinal cord after having cut the meninges. Alternatively, the dura mater is opened just enough to allow the insertion of a spinal cord hook (Fine Science Tools) between dura and spinal cord. The hook is then used to lift the cord in order to completely cut the spinal cord. The dura mater can be closed with fine sutures (10-O) after the procedure. The complete Tx model is useful to investigate the effect of treatments on the axonal regeneration, and on (limited) recovery of locomotor function. After a complete SCI in rats, there is usually the development of fluid-filled cavities, whereas in mice this is generally not the case [16].

http://dx.doi.org/10.5772/62947

3.4. Contusion and compression injury

Contusion injuries are the most widely used lesion type in SCI research, since the majority of human SCI involves a contusion or compression pathology. Several commercially available systems can be used to inflict standardized graded contusion injuries. These include the NYU MASCIS impactor (New York University Multicenter Animal SCI Study) [17], the OSU impactor (Ohio State University electromagnetic SCI device) [18, 19], the IH impactor (Infinite Horizon) [20], and the spinal cord compression device (Kopf Instruments). In general, a controlled pressure is exerted on the spinal cord after laminectomy by either dropping or placing a weight onto the cord, controlling the force and/or velocity [21]. Depending on the species (in rats more than in mice), contusion injury leads to cyst formation (Figure 2B), a feature also displayed by human SCI patients [19, 21]. Thoracic contusions are usually performed to induce dorsal bilateral lesions, whereas contusions at the cervical level are performed unilaterally [20].

Compression/decompression models are frequently used to investigate the occlusion of the central canal, another common symptom of SCI in human patients. To perform an experimental compression, injury clips, balloons, or forceps are widely used [21]. Vascular clips and calibrated forceps can be used to create graded and reproducible injuries. The clip compression model and the contusion injury model show some resemblances as they both inflict the injury via pressure to the outer surface of the spinal cord. These models can be fine-tuned so that injuries of varying degrees can be created. They lead to the formation of fluid-filled cysts which are surrounded by spared tissue. The remaining tissue continuity and axon sparing makes them also a suitable model for locomotor functional tests. For the same reason, however, SCI contusion and compression models are not as well suited as transection models to investigate the neuronal and axonal regeneration.

3.5. Pyramidotomy

An exclusive CST-only lesion can be achieved by pyramidotomy, a transection at the height of the pyramids [22] (Figure 2A–B). The injury of the CST by pyramidotomy does not greatly affect locomotion in rodents. Rats and mice use the CST primarily for fine finger movements, which is greatly relevant for human patients. For the study of motor recovery, specific forepaw tests are used (see Section 7.5.). Since this lesion is usually performed unilaterally, the intact side serves as an internal control and is also used for studying plasticity-related regeneration mechanisms [23].

3.6. New SCI models

Scientists are continuously looking for models that resemble the human injuries more closely. For example, two recent studies focused on lumbosacral SCI, a type of injury affecting an estimated one-third of patients [24, 25]. A model combining SCI and traumatic brain injury was recently introduced, because a proportion of SCI patients additionally suffer from head injuries, for example, due to traffic or diving accidents [26]. Finally, a recent publication on a closed-body SCI by applying a high-pressure air blast in mice provides a model resembling human traumatic SCI [27].

4. The application of treatments

After the choice of the appropriate lesion model for therapy development, the next decision in experimental SCI is the technique to use to apply a treatment. The application method determines the timing, frequency, and duration of the treatment. This section provides technical details of current methods for applying treatments in the various SCI models.

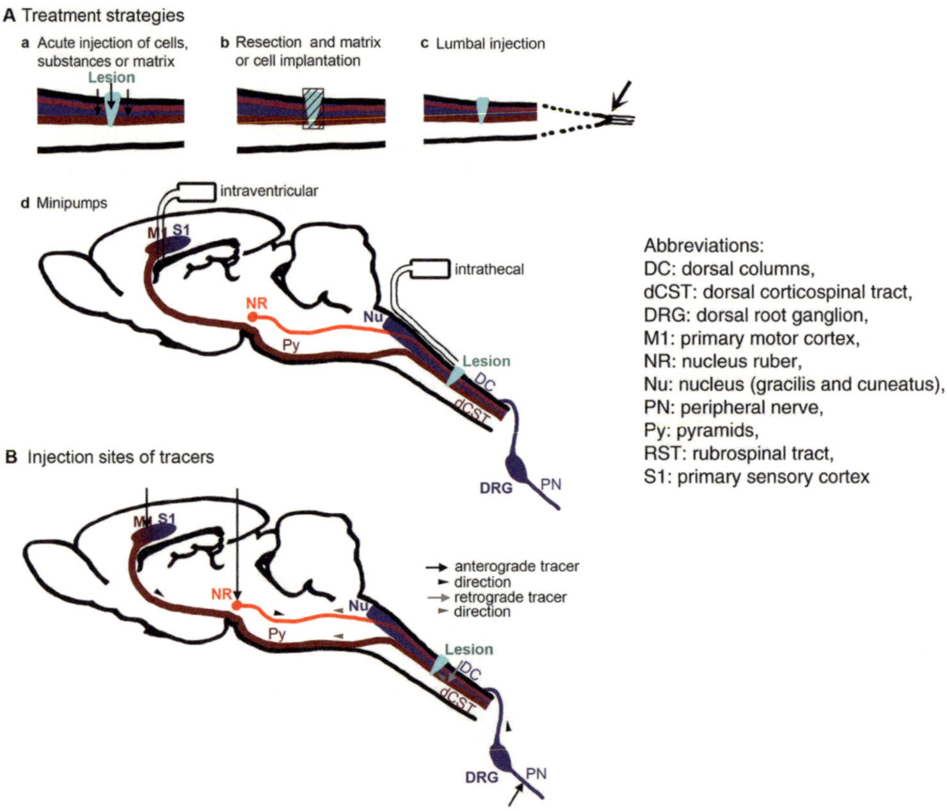

Figure 3 Strategies for the application of treatments and tracers exemplified in a schematic drawing of a dorsal Hx lesion: (A) treatments can be applied by (a) injection into the lesion site and/or adjacent tissue, (b) resection of the chronic lesion scar and subsequent matrix or cell implantation, (c) intrathecal lumbar injection, and (d) infusion over prolonged periods with minipumps and catheters either intraventricularly, intrathecally, or epidurally. The epidural catheter can be guided not only from rostral direction through the cisterna magna but also from the caudal side by performing an additional laminectomy [9, 28]. (B) Anterograde tracers are injected into the motor cortex and nucleus ruber in order to label CST and RST, respectively, and in the peripheral nerve to label the dorsal column axons. Injection of a retrograde tracer caudally to the lesion site is applied in order to visualize the cell bodies corresponding to regenerated axons or local interneuron circuits.

http://dx.doi.org/10.5772/62947

4.1. Injection into the spinal cord parenchyma

The simplest method for acutely applying a therapy is the (single) injection of a substance at the time of surgery. In some models, such as the dorsal Hx, the lesion site is open, so the treatment might potentially diffuse too quickly out of the area. Therefore, treatments are often injected in the intact tissue immediately adjacent to the lesion (Figure 3Aa). The injection volume should not be too high (<1 μl), and the injection should be performed slowly so that additional damage to the tissue is avoided. Controlled injection is achieved either by using a pump (e.g., the Pump 11 Elite Nanomite, Harvard Sachs Elektronik) or by introducing a delay of several minutes between injection and retraction of the needle. The injection method is most suitable for single acute treatments, because any additional doses will require additional surgery.

4.2. Lumbar injection into the CSF

A therapeutic can be applied to the CSF by lumbar intrathecal injection (Figure 3Ac), described in detail for mice by Lu et al, 2013. Shortly, the animal is subjected to a brief inhalation narcosis and kept in half-sleep by keeping its head in a dark environment. The L5 vertebra can be localized between the iliac crests of the hip bones. A 30-gauge needle is used to puncture the skin and enter the spine between the L5 and L6 spinous process. When the dura mater is punctured, a reflective flick of the tail is induced and up to 5 μl liquid can be applied [29]. This method is useful for renewing treatments multiple times after the initial injection.

4.3. Intrathecal application via minipumps

For continuous long-term application of liquid therapeutics, the use of minipumps is a standard delivery method (Figure 3Ad). Pumps can be implanted subcutaneously and attached to a catheter for intrathecal delivery. Minipumps either release the liquid via osmosis (Alzet®) or they use a programmable microprocessor (iPrecio®). They are commercially available in different sizes and with varying pumping rates and time periods. The subcutaneously placed minipumps can be removed after the required delivery period. The minipumps are connected to a catheter which can be inserted in the brain for intraventricular infusion [30], or the catheter can be guided through the epidural space underneath the vertebrae toward the lesion site [19, 28]. It is important to consider that the catheter by itself can produce a compression of the spinal cord. This is especially problematic in mice, because of their size, although special mouse catheters are available commercially (Alzet®).

4.4. Cellular transplantation strategies

Cell therapy is generally the focus in neurodegenerative diseases such as Alzheimer's or Parkinson's disease where the common goal is to replace degenerated neurons. In contrast, SCI is characterized by damage of the neuronal processes, whereas the corresponding cell bodies are located in various areas of the brain, brainstem, and DRGs, thus complicating cell replacement. Moreover, the projection neurons are thought to undergo atrophy in contrast to dying [31]. Therefore, cellular therapeutic approaches for experimental SCI concentrate on the spinal cord, where local cells are affected by the primary and secondary injury events. The therapies on the one hand aim to replace glial cells or local neurons. Peripheral nerve grafts or Schwann cell cables have been used to bridge the lesion [32, 33]. Transplanted oligodendrocyte precursor cells or Schwann cells have been shown to remyelinate axons, whereas olfactory ensheathing or mucosal cells may provide axon guidance and trophic support [34–36]. Cell therapies using embryonic stem cells, neural stem/progenitor cells, or induced pluripotent stem (iPS) cells mostly aim to provide local pools of neurons that might serve as relay stations, analogue to propriospinal neurons [37–40]. Stem cells might also differentiate into glial cells that can remyelinate axons. On the other hand, stem cells can bridge the lesion gap and promote regeneration by the secretion of trophic factors, the support of angiogenic events, or the inhibition of glutamate toxicity. These effects have been reported for mesenchymal stem cells, bone marrow mesenchymal stromal cells, or unrestricted somatic stem cells from umbilical cord blood [41–43].

The transplantation of (stem) cells is usually performed by injection of cell suspensions into the spinal cord parenchyma (Figure 3Aa). This can be performed acutely by injecting cells into the intact tissue adjacent to the lesion. Alternatively, the lesion is allowed to form over a certain time period (usually 7 days, also called subacute), and a new surgery is performed to inject the cells directly into the lesion site. Factors to consider are cell survival, migration, differentiation into neural/glial cell types, axon outgrowth, and synaptic contacts in the case of neuronal transplants and secretion of regeneration-supportive factors in the case of nonneural transplants.

4.5. Implantation of matrices

Although many studies have proven the beneficial effects of autologous or heterologous cellular grafts in acute and chronic SCI models in animals [44, 45], the use of cell transplantation in human patients often remains a controversial issue [46, 47]. The search for artificial biomaterials for the implantation into the injured spinal cord has been prompted due to the limited access to autologous donor material and immunological problems associated with allograft rejection.

Cavities or cysts that often form after SCI are a major obstacle impeding axonal regeneration. Therefore, the reconnection across the trauma cavity by means of scaffolds or matrices is a major focus in SCI research. In order to provide a favorable growth substrate for regenerating axons, a bridging material should provide and combine several structural, physicochemical, and molecular properties [48]. Materials should ideally be easily modifiable, serve as a scaffold for matrix molecules and/or cellular transplants, and further be immunologically inert and absorbable [49]. Positive results with acellular matrices have been obtained in numerous studies [45, 49–55]. Important advances have recently been reported in the development of biosynthetic conduits for spinal cord repair. Biosynthetic conduits equipped with ECM molecules and different cell lines, and supplemented with neurotrophic growth factors, have been shown to yield encouraging results in the treatment of experimental SCI [51].

In chronic SCI, cavity formation has occurred and a lesion scar has formed, which presents a stable physical and molecular barrier to axonal regeneration. Cavities and sites of scar resection

http://dx.doi.org/10.5772/62947

can be treated with bridging or scaffolding materials. Interesting effects were achieved with a polyethylene glycol (PEG) treatment in a chronic SCI paradigm [56]. PEG was used to fill the cavity that was created by resection of the 5-week-old lesion scar in spinal cord-injured rats (Figure 3Ab). After 8 months, long-distance axonal regeneration through and beyond the graft was observed. The PEG matrix was repopulated by blood vessels, astrocytes, and Schwann cells, the latter remyelinating bundles of regenerating axons. These histological parameters were accompanied by long-lasting functional motor improvement. This study suggests that the chronically lesioned tracts are still able to regenerate when provided with the right extracellular environment [56].

4.6. Implantation of a mechanical microconnector system

Complete transections result in a gap between the two spinal cord stumps. Recently, a novel and unique connector device was described [57]. The purpose of this mechanical microconnector system is to reconnect severed spinal cord tissue stumps in the submillimeter range. The microconnector consists of two elliptical discs lined with numerous honeycombed holes. After implantation into the injured rat spinal cord, the device is connected to a vacuum pump, and the tissue stumps are brought into close apposition via the application of negative pressure. The connector discs have a rough surface, allowing the adherence of the spinal cord tissue. Additional features of the mechanical microconnector system are an internal canal system and an inlet tube, which can be connected either to a syringe or to an osmotic minipump to achieve application of therapeutics into the lesion area. Even the implantation of the device alone was sufficient for axon regeneration and led to a significant improvement of locomotor function following complete transection of the thoracic spinal cord [57].

4.7. Electrical stimulation and neuroprothesis

Electric field stimulation has been shown to promote enhanced and/or oriented neurite outgrowth, thereby offering potential additional treatment strategies after PNS but also CNS injury [58–60]. For SCI treatment, epidural stimulation has been used to create electric fields to restore motor functions [61, 62]. Electrical current is applied at varying frequencies and intensities to the areas of the lumbosacral spinal cord, activating the CPG. The CPG can initiate stepping function even without any input from the brain. The lab of Grégoire Courtine developed a neuroprosthetic that achieves a high-fidelity control of leg kinematics. A closed-loop system, using muscle activity and other kinematic parameters in real-time to feed back into the system, allowed neuromodulation during walking [63]. Another study used neuroprosthetic intervention in the form of a Neurochip 2 recurrent brain-computer interface in a cervical hemisection model. The neurochip delivered electrical stimulation and measured in parallel the electromyographic (EMG) activity of the muscles, thus adjusting the stimulation according to the muscle activity. Animals that received this so-called targeted, activity-dependent stimulation displayed increased skilled forepaw reaching as compared to animals receiving non-targeted stimulations or physical training [64].

Although it has no direct effect on the regeneration of axons after SCI, epidural stimulation is a very promising approach already used for the rehabilitation of SCI patients with promising results [65].

4.8. Exercise and training

The first studies suggesting that exercise might stimulate motor recovery were performed using environment enrichment [66, 67]. During the last decades, several investigators developed new experimental settings to perform motor training of animals. For example, forced walking on treadmills, training either bipedal or quadrupedal stepping, has been shown to improve locomotor recovery after SCI [68–70]. The combination of treadmill training with epidural stimulation and the administration of serotonergic and dopaminergic agonists seemed to be especially effective in restoring motor activity. Extensive plasticity of corticospinal, brainstem, and intraspinal connectivity was shown to underlie the observed functional recovery [61].

Recently, Starkey et al. (2015) developed a new type of cage with enriched environment over three floors with different types of training possibilities (e.g., grasping tasks, ladder walking, and climbing). This so-called "natural habitat cage" was combined with a new three-dimensional animal tracking system to allow high-impact, self-motivated training. Interestingly, differences were observed between the animals' overall activity and preference for certain tasks. Healthy as well as SCI animals trained in these cages performed better in experimental tests for fine motor control of fore- and hindlimb [71]. For forelimb training, a robotic rehabilitation system was recently developed, in which the animal has to pull a bar to receive food. This setup could also be used to measure forelimb strength [72].

4.9. Other types of treatments

Systemic treatments (intravenous, intraperitoneal, subcutaneous) are not discussed above, although they are clinically relevant. For treatments outside the spinal column, it should in general be known whether the applied therapeutic can cross the blood-brain barrier. A much higher concentration must be applied peripherally to achieve an effective concentration centrally. Since human SCI almost invariably involves surgery, the possibility of local treatment is given.

4.10. Combination treatments

It has become more and more apparent that combination therapies will be necessary to successfully treat SCI. The above described matrices, cell transplantations, electrical stimulation, and training paradigms all offer possibilities of combination with trophic factors, pharmacological treatments, agonists or antagonists of neurotransmitters, anti-inhibitory treatments, and so forth. It seems likely that holistic treatments combining several regeneration mechanisms will be clinically more successful to target the multitude of SCI systems.

5. Possible treatment effects on neurons

5.1. Regeneration versus sprouting

For researchers, the "holy grail" is the regeneration of the injured fibers through the lesion scar and the subsequent reinnervation of their targets. After an initial retraction phase, the axons of the above-described tracts usually start regrowing toward the lesion site. Treatments can increase the regenerative growth of various tracts through and beyond the lesion site [73]. Although this process could be called "sprouting," it is important to distinguish between regenerative sprouting of the severed tract with the goal of regrowth toward the original connections and plastic sprouting, with the goal to find alternatives routes (**Figure 4**). Functional recovery of locomotion can also be achieved through plasticity of intact fibers that may form contralateral sprouts or make new synapses with local propriospinal neurons (**Figure 4**). In the last decade, the propriospinal system became a major focus for SCI. It can serve as a detour for bypassing the scar. Injured descending axons have been shown to sprout and rewire to propriospinal neurons, whose axons are located in the spared tissue and project into the lower denervated spinal cord [69, 74]. Also, the propriospinal interneurons can sprout to innervate new targets below the lesion. In addition, these neurons might regenerate better than the projection neurons, because of the shorter distance of the axon stump to the cell body. They have been shown to upregulate growth-associated proteins and have a high intrinsic capacity for plasticity [75]. In partial injury models, such as dorsal or lateral transection or contusion,

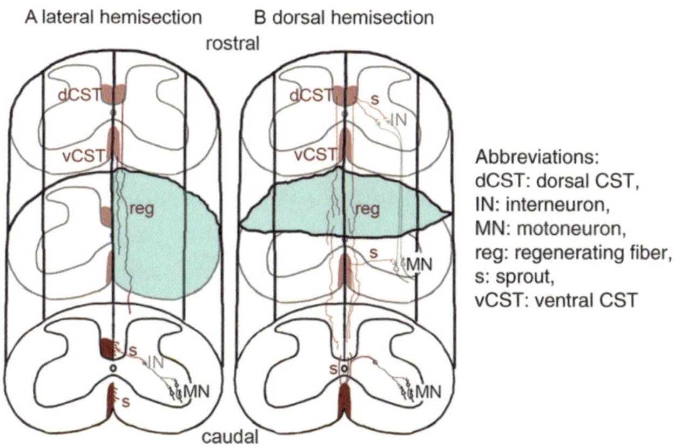

Figure 4 Axonal mechanisms leading to motor recovery exemplified for the dCST in two lesion models: (A) in the case of lateral Hx lesions, the contralateral intact dCST axons caudal to the lesion can sprout (s) and synapse with propriospinal interneurons (IN) connected to motoneurons (not necessarily at the same rostrocaudal level). The vCST on the intact side can also sprout to the ipsilateral side. Regeneration of the CST through the lesion is depicted by irregular lines since regenerating axons generally display a meandering and less straight course than the original tracts. (B) In the dorsal Hx model axons of the dCST can regenerate either through the lesion (irregular lines) or to form sprouts to make local connections with propriospinal interneurons whose axons run ventrally below the lesion and are connected to caudal motoneurons. The intact vCST can sprout and extend to the degenerated dCST tract or form new connections with interneurons that contact local motoneurons. Abbreviations: dCST: dorsal CST, IN: interneuron, MN: motoneuron, reg: regenerating fiber, s: sprout, vCST: ventral CST.

both regeneration from injured tracts and sprouting from spared tracts can be studied. It may be of importance to note that sprouting can be undirected, so that aberrant neuronal circuits may be formed [76]. Treatments can enhance sprouting and direct the sprouts to establish functional circuits.

5.2. Neuroprotection

After the primary insult, secondary damage due to, among others, inflammation, oxidative stress, and blood-brain barrier dysfunction causes the death of neurons (and glia) in the tissue surrounding the lesion [77]. The loss of local motor neurons leads to more extensive motor deficits in addition to the impairments caused by the injury to the descending motor tracts. The loss of spinal interneurons may disrupt intraspinal connections between motor centers. Therefore, a neuroprotective action of a treatment might, first, reduce functional impairments and, second, increase the possibility of local plasticity via interneurons (see Section 5.1.). For the analysis of neuroprotection, quantification of (moto-) neurons is performed at various distances rostrally and caudally from the lesion center [78]. A treatment could also lead to the protection of the brain and brainstem projection neurons from death or atrophy [8, 31, 79]. Quantification of the lesion size and spared white matter in standardized lesion models might also provide information about the protective effects of a treatment strategy.

6. Tracing and/or immunohistochemical (IHC) staining of motor and sensory tracts

The next step in SCI research is the histological analysis of regenerated axons. Short-term studies (up to several weeks after the injury) give information about early injury events, whereas long-term studies (up to several months or even years after the injury) are useful to investigate long-term effects and behavioral outcomes with a treatment compared to a control. In order to visualize regenerating axons from the specific spinal cord tracts, these can be marked via axonal tracing (Figure 3B) or detected by immunohistochemistry (IHC). In this section, the main techniques used in experimental SCI in rodents are summarized.

6.1. Tracing methods

6.1.1. Conventional tracing

Axonal tracing is an important tool for the investigation of regeneration after SCI (Figure 3B), holding the advantage that specific axonal populations are precisely marked. Conventional tracers label axons and neurons via the axonal transport [80]. Neuronal tracers can label the axons anterogradely (toward the axon terminal) which is the preferred method for analyzing their sprouting and regeneration. Retrogradely transported tracers (towards the cell body) are injected at the distal side of a lesion, in order to quantify the number of neurons with regenerated (distal) fibers and to visualize propriospinal neurons (see Section 6.4.).

http://dx.doi.org/10.5772/62947

Preferred application methods are pressure injection (liquid tracers), iontophoretic injection of electrically charged tracer molecules, or the insertion of dye crystals (carbocyanine dyes) [80]. The tracer can be detected via confocal microscopy using either its own fluorescence or IHC. The ideal survival time after the tracing depends on the tracer used, the distance between the site of tracer application and the area of interest, and the rate of its transport in the axons. A drawback of conventional tracing techniques is that in most cases not all axons of a neuronal population take up and transport the tracer substance. Many classical retrograde tracers are only, or more efficiently, taken up by injured axons and axon terminals, whereas the rate of the uptake by uninjured axons of passage is rather small. This can lead to nonspecific results [81].

Some examples for widely used monosynaptic neuronal tracers are the enzyme horseradish peroxidase, biotinylated dextran amine (BDA), and Fluoro Gold™. Examples of nonviral polysynaptic tracers are bacterial toxins, such as cholera toxin B. The drawback of nonviral polysynaptic tracers is, however, the dilution of signal after each synaptic step [82]. For the purpose of multisynaptic tracing, viral tracings are more suitable.

6.1.2. Viral tracings

When transneuronal tracing is desired, viral tracings are the method of choice. Transneuronal tracing is useful for the investigation of multisynaptic pathways and circuits [82]. The virus, which expresses a reporter gene in order to achieve the tracing, can replicate in the neurons and then infect other neurons which are connected via synapses. The virus replication further amplifies the signal, thereby avoiding the problem of signal dilution [8]. Very importantly, viral vector systems are very effective tools for gene therapeutic approaches. Frequently used viral systems used for axon tracing are adeno-associated viral vectors [83], lentiviral vectors [84], rabies virus [82], and herpes simplex virus [85]. The combination of viral tracings and gene therapy further offers the possibility to deliver a vector into specific areas.

A very elegant approach to investigate axonal pathways and their regeneration is the combination of viral tracing with optical tissue clearing and light sheet laser scanning microscopy [86–88].

6.2. Anterograde tracing of defined tracts

6.2.1. Motor cortex—CST tracing

In SCI research, the CST is the most established model tract for the investigation of regeneration and the associated locomotor functional outcome. Its origin in the sensorimotor cortex and its course through the pyramidal decussations and, in rodents, the dorsal center part of the spinal cord allow a very precise labeling and localization of the tract. By using a stereotactic frame, precise injections of the tracer of choice are applied into the sensorimotor cortex [8, 89]. In general, tracing is performed 2 (mice) to 3 (rats) weeks before sacrifice of the animals for histological analysis. In the case of BDA, tissue sections need to be stained with streptavidin coupled to a fluorescent marker. Fluorescently labeled BDA is available, but the signal is usually still enhanced by post-staining. Analysis is performed by confocal microscopy, counting regenerating axon profiles in and beyond the lesion site.

6.2.2. Nucleus ruber—RST tracing

The nucleus ruber can be traced in the same way as the CST; however, it is much smaller in size and therefore easier to miss [73].

6.2.3. Ascending sensory tracts: CTB tracing or CGRP staining

Cholera toxin β (CTB) is a tracer that is transported anterogradely, retrogradely and, as a recent study suggested, even transneuronally [90]. This tracer is used frequently to label the ascending sensory tracts in the dorsal column of the spinal cord. For this purpose, CTB is injected into the sciatic nerve that is crushed to achieve maximum uptake of the tracer [90]. This allows the specific analysis of the regeneration of ascending axons corresponding to the hindlimbs. In contrast, IHC staining for the marker calcitonin gene-related peptide CGRP allows the detection of axon profiles entering the spinal cord at all spinal segments. This, however, compromises the analysis of CGRP axons beyond the lesion, since axons from intact spinal levels above the lesion will also stain positively.

6.3. Raphespinal and coeruleospinal tracts

Because of their neurotransmitters serotonin (5-HT) and noradrenaline (NA), whose key synthesizing enzyme is tyrosine hydroxylase (TH), the tracts descending from the Raphe nuclei and locus coeruleus can be investigated by IHC using 5-HT- and TH-specific antibodies [73]. Since their fibers run both ventrally and dorsally, care should be taken to analyze only areas that are relevant to the localization of the lesion, for example, only the dorsal funiculus in case of a dorsal hemisection, with respect to regeneration. The possibility of sprouting from ventral axons cannot be ruled out, and some types of interneurons also express 5-HT.

6.4. Retrograde tracing

A very valuable tool for tracing regenerating neurons is retrograde tracing. When a tracer injected distally from the lesion site marks neurons proximally from the lesion site, these neurons have regenerated their fibers (provided the tracer is precisely located to the lesioned and not the spared region, and tracer diffusion can be ruled out). It can also answer the question whether axons from the intact side sprouted to the lesioned side. This technique was applied to show which brainstem nuclei were projecting into the distal cord [14] and to trace propriospinal interneuron networks [70]. If a retrograde tracer is applied to the spinal cord proximal to the lesion site, it can also be used to quantify the neurons "associated" with the lesion, for studying cell death or atrophy of neuronal populations [8].

http://dx.doi.org/10.5772/62947

7. Assessment of motor function

In order to assess motor recovery after experimental SCI and putative regenerative treatments, several functional tests are available. The choice of the tests depends not only on the lesion model but also on the costs, because some tests require specific commercial systems.

7.1. Basso, Beattie, and Bresnahan (BBB) locomotor score and subscore (rat) and Basso Mouse Scale (BMS, mouse)

The BBB open-field test, developed by Basso, Beattie, and Bresnahan [91], is an established test for the evaluation of hindlimb locomotor function of SCI rats. It is suitable for thoracic SCI models where it has become the first choice test to evaluate locomotor function [92]. The BBB score is based on the classification of hindlimb locomotor function using a scale which ranges from 0 (no spontaneous movement of the hindlimbs) to 21 (normal movement, coordinated walking pattern). For the evaluation procedure, the rats are placed in a defined open field where they are observed and evaluated by two trained observers. The animal's movements in the open field are scored over 4 minutes according to the criteria of the BBB locomotor rating scale [91]. The evaluation of coordination, an important parameter of the intermediate and late phases of the BBB, is not always clear without any doubt. This entails ratings in the medium-range scale intervals often leading to an artificial plateau. Therefore, and because usually not all aspects of locomotion are influenced by a treatment, the determination of a BBB subscore can be helpful to improve the sensitivity of the test [93]. Furthermore, additional automatic gait analysis helps to avoid potential subjective evaluation of coordination [94]. An advantage of the BBB locomotor rating scale is that preoperative training—which is a general requirement for many locomotor behavioral tests—is not necessary. However, as is generally the case for behavioral tests, preoperative handling of the experimental animals and their familiarization with the test surroundings are useful. Additionally, adaptations of the original BBB locomotor scale have been described also for severe thoracic injuries such as complete spinal cord transection [56, 95]. Since such severe lesions result in maximum BBB scores of 8–10, the spreading of the low and intermediate BBB values (BBB 1–10) allows a distinct evaluation of less prominent locomotor behavioral improvements.

The small size and rapid speed of mice caused investigators to develop a mouse-specific scale, the BMS [96]. The procedure of the animal walking in an open field is basically the same as described above, but parameters like coordination, paw position, and trunk instability are evaluated in a slightly different way than for rats. Similarly, for unilateral cervical SCI new locomotor rating scales have been developed, such as the forelimb locomotor assessment scale (FLAS) [97] or the forelimb locomotor scale (FLS) [98].

7.2. Horizontal ladder rung test and Gridwalk

The horizontal ladder walking test is used for the evaluation of fine motor control, coordination, and foot placing accuracy, all of which require certain degrees of sensory feedback. Therefore, this test is particularly useful for the investigation of locomotion after a thoracic CST injury. Video analyses of the runs allow the assessment of multiple parameters [99]. The mistakes the animals make during walking are evaluated and classified into predefined categories. The test apparatus consists of metal rungs (3 mm in diameter) placed between Plexiglas walls in predefined intervals (1–5 cm for rats). The spacing patterns should be regularly alternated to make sure that the animals' locomotor function and not their cognitive functions are evaluated. Care should be taken to provide gaps between the rungs that are neither too narrow (mistakes being made by an animal might not be observable) nor too large (the animal cannot walk across without fear of falling, or without having to jump between rungs). During pretraining, the animals learn to cross the horizontal ladder without interruption. Post-injury runs are recorded with a (high-speed) video camera from an angle slightly below the rod plane. This ensures the possibility to detect precise movements of all four paws and their digits. For evaluation, the predefined foot placing mistakes are counted. For mice, the procedure is similar, with smaller spacing (approximately 15 mm). For both species, several parameters of skilled walking can be observed, including correct placement, slight and deep slip, total miss, (partial) replacement, and correction [22, 99]. Alternative to the ladder test, the Gridwalk test makes use of grids to asses skilled walking.

7.3. Automated gait analysis methods

7.3.1. CatWalk™

The CatWalk™ system for automated quantitative gait analysis in SCI rats was developed by Hamers et al (2001). Classically, gait analysis in the form of footprint analyses has been (and still is by some groups) performed by painting the animal's paws with ink and letting it run on paper (or, an elegant variation, with developer and photographic paper) [100]. Static measures such as the distance between paws and toes could be measured, but no spatiotemporal resolution was achieved. The Catwalk™ system consists of a glass plate through which fluorescent light is internally reflected. When a mouse or rat places its paw on the glass, the light is deflected from the glass and the paw print lights up. The intensity is related to the pressure or weight support, which provides additional information about the functionality of the paw. A high-speed camera placed below the glass plate records all the runs (originally, a mirror projected the light toward the camera, but the commercial version (Noldus) images directly). A narrow walkway corridor on top of the glass plate ensures that the animals walk in a straight line. After a few days of habituation training, the animals walk steadily through the corridor. Recording is performed in the dark, but the commercial setup has a lid with red light above the walkway, so that the outline of the animal is visualized. After analysis, main parameters of interest are the stride length (step size), the base of support (distance between left and right paws), the walking speed, the duration of the swing and stand phase, the regularity index as a measure of coordination, and the intensity of the prints. Many more parameters can be studied, the choice of which can be based on the animal model [101, 102]. The CatWalk™ system has been used in the following SCI models: thoracic CST Tx, RST Tx, and dorsal Hx [8, 103]; thoracic contusion [101, 102]; pyramidotomy models [22]; and lateral cervical spinal cord contusion [104, 105], and in recent studies assessing the effects of training and gene therapy [106, 107]. The CatWalk™ can furthermore be combined with the horizontal

http://dx.doi.org/10.5772/62947

ladder test by placing the ladder above the glass plate, so that footslips light up because the animal touches the glass plate [108].

7.3.2. *Automated gait analysis using treadmill*

The CatWalk™ is semi-automated, because the animals must voluntarily walk across the walkway and need pretraining. Again, scientists are striving to improve the existing systems (Neckel, 2015). New fully automated gait analysis platforms have been developed, including the DigiGait™ (Mouse Specifics, Inc.) [109–111] and the TreadScan™ (Clever Sys Incorporated) systems [112]. These two systems use transparent treadmills allowing the animals' gait analysis at constant speed, including the possibility to measure at different speeds.

7.3.3. *MotoRater and kinematic analysis*

The growing number of SCI models is accompanied by the need to modify the test systems. Recently, a new method for profiling locomotor recovery was developed in the lab of Martin Schwab [113]. This setup, now commercially available as the so-called MotoRater (TSE Systems), makes use of mirrors to image the mouse or rat that is walking in a Plexiglas basin from three sides (left, right, and below). The animals are tattooed on anatomical landmarks such as ilias crest, trochanter major of the hip, condylus lateralis of the knee, malleolus lateralis of the ankle, and the tip of the fifth toe. This way the walking is precisely monitored as stick diagrams and followed in time. As with the CatWalk™, the kinetics of even-ground walking patterns are analyzed. In contrast to the Catwalk, the researchers included new levels of difficulty in this system. A horizontal ladder is introduced to monitor precise paw placement and forelimb-hindlimb coordination. Alternatively, the basin is filled with water, either at levels where animals are wading (3 cm for rats, 1 cm for mice) or at levels where the animals have to swim. Wading brings the advantage that the water provides weight support. Furthermore, the animal's strength can be measured, because of the desire of the animal to raise its body as much as possible out of the water. In the original article, three types of SCI were compared (dorsal Hx, ventral Hx, and lateral Hx). For each lesion model, various aspects of the test revealed to be suitable in different ways. For example, skilled walking and overground locomotion are most suitable for the evaluation of thoracic dorsal Hx. For thoracic ventral Hx, wading was described to be the better test and for cervical lateral Hx, the authors observed improvement of hindlimb movements during wading and swimming. Due to the forepaw impairment, cervical Hx animals can hardly perform the ladder test and are poor at normal even-ground locomotion. Further studies of the same group made use of the MotoRater to assess the contribution of the brain stem nuclei to locomotor recovery [14] and the effects of training on motor skills after SCI [71].

Another kinematic gait analysis system makes use of reflective markers at essentially the same hallmarks as the MotoRater system (iliac crest, hip, knee, ankle, metatarsophalangeal joint, and toe). A motion capture system (SIMI Reality Motion Systems) is used to analyze gait parameters combined with electromyogram recording (EMG) [69, 70].

7.4. Sensory testing

Although less relevant than motor recovery, the recovery of sensory functions has a potential impact on locomotion. Furthermore, lesioned animals can develop neuropathic pain [114] which may be attenuated or, worse, aggravated by a treatment. Sensory tests performed after SCI include mechanical and nociceptive tests.

Sensorimotor reflexes can be tested by light touch to the paw, causing contact placing of the paw. Proprioceptive placing is elicited by stretching a tendon or joint [21]. Von Frey filaments are used to assess the animal's sensitivity to sub-threshold mechanical stimuli. For this purpose, filaments of increasing thickness are applied to the foot sole, exerting a defined force. This is normally not painful to the animal, so that only animals that suffer from mechanical allodynia (pain reaction from a normally non-painful stimulus) withdraw their paw from the filament. The minimum force eliciting a pain response is scored as paw withdrawal threshold [115]. Electronic versions of this test are available commercially (e.g., IITC Life Science, Ugo Basile). For the assessment of cutaneous hyperalgesia (increased pain from a pain-provoking stimulus), a hot plate or a commercial Plantar Test setup (e.g., Hargreaves Apparatus, Ugo Basil) [116] is used. The paw of interest is placed on a source of radiant heat or, in the case of the Planar Test, an infrared beam is precisely aimed at the central part of the animal's sole. The paw withdrawal time is recorded. Each paw is tested three times since the animal can also withdraw the paw spontaneously. Compared to the traditional hot plate test setup, the Plantar Test has the advantage of an automated, and therefore, accurate end-point detection [116].

For the majority of the sensory tests, the animal has to be able to move (withdraw) the paw. They can, therefore, generally not be performed with severely and completely spinal cord-injured animals that often lack the ability to perform limb movements below the level of the injury. For severely injured animals, the tail-flick test, a modification of the plantar hot plate test where the base of the tail is heated, can be applied [92].

7.5. Forelimb tests

For cervical hemisection lesions and for pyramidotomy, specific tests to analyze forelimb motor recovery have been developed [21]. Since these lesions are usually one-sided, the healthy side serves as an internal control. First, new locomotor rating scales (alternatives for the BBB) have been developed, such as the forelimb locomotor assessment scale (FLAS) [97] or the forelimb locomotor scale (FLS) [98]. Second, broad tests for paw preference are applied, such as the cylinder test, where the choice of the weight-bearing forelimb is monitored [22], and the grooming test, where the preferred paw for grooming is scored. Popular tests assessing dexterity include pasta eating or the Irvine, Beatti, Bresneham (IBB) forelimb rating scale, where the forelimb function is assessed, while the rat is eating a round-shaped cereal [117]. Furthermore, tests for the assessment of fine finger movements include the single pellet-grasping test or the staircase test [21, 71]. In these skilled forepaw tests, mice or rats have to reach for and grasp sugar pellets through a slit in a Plexiglas wall or from wells in a staircase setup (Lafayette Instruments (rat), Campden Instruments (mouse)). Video analyses of the sessions allow the assessment of multiple parameters. Some groups use the horizontal ladder as well to score forepaw locomotion, but the animals are usually poor at performing this test.

To further quantify grip a commercial grip strength meter is available (TSE Systems, Ugo Basile, Columbus Instruments), or the ability of the animal to keep its balance and hold on stably to an inclined plane (or cage grid) is measured.

7.6. Important considerations for functional testing

Several studies indicate that the choice of the motor tests should be based on the type of injury and the degree of impairment [113, 118]. For thoracic dorsal Hx, the horizontal ladder test and CatWalk™ gait analysis systems are suitable since even-ground walking and skilled walking are impaired, but display recovery over time. In the case of ventral Hx, the wading and swimming paradigms in the MotoRater provide more useful information on impairment and recovery. Cervical lateral Hx animals also perform better during wading and swimming. With regard to swimming, an assessment tool was developed in Sweden, where parameters like fore- and hindlimb usage, hindlimb alternation and position, trunk instability, body angle, and tail movements are precisely scored [119].

Care should, however, always be taken with the evaluation of the results. Animals can develop compensation strategies to perform a task in a different way than before the injury [118]. For example, animals primarily use their hindlimbs for swimming, but after a thoracic injury, they utilize their forelimbs. Therefore, distance or speed may recover, but the actual functional recovery of the hindlimbs might be still impaired. Another example is the grasping of food pellets that animals with forelimb impairment cannot do. Some animals tend to successfully develop a scooping strategy to retrieve pellets [118]. Investigators should be aware of this and monitor the strategies the animals use. The use of video equipment to accompany a test is therefore advisable.

The strain of the animals (and even the substrain produced by different suppliers) also plays an important role. Some animal strains perform better than others in tests which require the acquisition of certain skills [118, 120]. For example, in the staircase-skilled forepaw reaching test, Lister-hooded and Long-Evans rats perform much better than Lewis rats and Fischer rats [121, 122]. Housing is also of importance, since the amount of motor activity in the cage can provide training effects. This might mask a treatment effect, because the spontaneous recovery due to training may be too prominent. A popular cage enrichment in the form of sunflower seeds might compromise skilled grasping tests [118]. On the contrary, if the chosen test is too difficult for the animals in view of their impairment, recovery of function might be missed too. Other variables like circadian rhythms and stress can introduce variability. Therefore, it is vital to habituate the animals to the experimenters, to perform pre-injury recordings of the basal performance of the animals in the tests and to perform testing always at the same time of day under the same circumstances.

8. Discussion and conclusions

This chapter provides an overview of the main rodent models, experimental treatment strategies, histological analysis methods, and motor tests that are available for the investigation of neuronal regeneration and locomotor function after experimental SCI. The choice of the appropriate model depends on the research question and on the type of human injury which the investigation is based on. There is ongoing controversy regarding the comparability of experimental blunt versus sharp lesions to the clinical situation of human patients. Contusion/compression injuries are very suitable for studying human traumatic SCI. These types of injury maintain tissue continuity even in the most severe cases, which is also observed in the vast majority of human spinal cord traumata. However, spared tissue bridges might compromise the analysis of treatment effects in experimental SCI. Moreover, blunt force spinal cord traumata are often accompanied by sharp lesions like maceration, laceration, or transection, for example by bone splinters. Therefore, sharp transections are also valid models, not least because they are easier to control and reproduce.

SCI experiments in rodents are essential for the development of new treatment strategies. They aim to extensively test treatment effects on multiple nerve tracts, to elucidate their mechanisms of action and, using multiple motor and sensory tests, to shed light on their ability to restore function. It is highly important to know whether a treatment is effective via neuroprotection, spared axon sprouting, or axon regeneration, since this will influence the choice of treatment that suits the patient best. Patients with incomplete lesions may benefit from plasticity-inducing treatments, whereas patients suffering from complete injuries require therapeutic strategies that induce regeneration. Patients with contusion lesions or complete injuries might further benefit from matrix or stem cell implantation to fill up cavities. When a treatment strategy displays promising effects in rodent SCI models, the next step will be to test it in a model system that is more close to human patients. In primates, the CST projects mainly dorsolaterally and originates from both left and right motor cortex, because a number of CST axons decussate along the spinal cord midline. These axons are capable of forming detour circuits reconnecting the motor cortex with denervated spinal cord areas in monkeys with lateral cervical Hx [123–125]. Due to the comparability with the anatomy of humans, the nonhuman primate cervical Hx model has been proposed to be a suitable model to test the recovery of forelimb skills after SCI [126].

Rodent research provided numerous important insights into the SCI field. To name a few, the regeneration and/or sprouting responses of tracts involved in locomotion, the involvement of the propriospinal system, the CPG circuits, and the ability to stimulate these without supraspinal input all contributed to a better understanding of human spinal cord pathophysiology. Numerous treatments have been tested and have provided even more insights into how the various systems can be manipulated. However, to date, despite many years of extensive research, there are no clinical standard therapies for SCI which significantly increase the regenerative response to such a degree that they achieve strong (locomotor) improvements in human patients. This reflects the complexity of SCI. Although many treatments did not reach the clinic, they have been of enormous value to understanding the mechanisms of regeneration leading to functional motor recovery.

http://dx.doi.org/10.5772/62947

Author details

Christina F. Vogelaar[1*] and Veronica Estrada[2]

*Address all correspondence to: tineke.vogelaar@unimedizin-mainz.de

1 Institute of Microanatomy and Neurobiology, Johannes Gutenberg-University, Mainz, Germany

2 Molecular Neurobiology Laboratory, Department of Neurology, Heinrich-Heine-University, Duesseldorf, Germany

References

[1] Abbott A. Biomedicine: the changing face of primate research. Nature. 2014;506(7486): 24–6.

[2] Watson C, Harvey AR. Projections from the brain to the spinal cord 168. In: Watson C, Paxinos G, Kayalioglu G, editors. The Spinal Cord. A Christopher and Dana Reeve Foundation Text and Atlas. 1st ed. London: Academic Press; 2009. pp. 168–74.

[3] Du Beau A, Shakya Shrestha S, Bannatyne BA, Jalicy SM, Linnen S, Maxwell DJ. Neurotransmitter phenotypes of descending systems in the rat lumbar spinal cord. Neuroscience. 2012;227:67–79.

[4] Kayalioglu G. Projections from the spinal cord to the brain. In: Watson C, Paxinos G, Kayalioglu G, editors. The Spinal Cord. A Christopher and Dana Reeve Foundation Text and Atlas. 1st ed. London: Academic Press; 2009. pp. 148–58.

[5] Conta AC, Stelzner DJ. The propriospinal system. In: Watson C, Paxinos G, Kayalioglu G, editors. The Spinal Cord. A Christopher and Dana Reeve Foundation Text and Atlas. 1st ed. London: Academic Press; 2009. pp. 180–6.

[6] Slawinska U, Miazga K, Jordan LM. The role of serotonin in the control of locomotor movements and strategies for restoring locomotion after spinal cord injury. Acta Neurobiologiae Experimentalis. 2014;74(2):172–87.

[7] Ghosh M, Pearse DD. The role of the serotonergic system in locomotor recovery after spinal cord injury. Front Neural Circuits. 2014;8:151.

[8] Klapka N, Hermanns S, Straten G, Masanneck C, Duis S, Hamers FP, et al. Suppression of fibrous scarring in spinal cord injury of rat promotes long-distance regeneration of corticospinal tract axons, rescue of primary motoneurons in somatosensory cortex and significant functional recovery. The European Journal of Neuroscience. 2005;22(12): 3047–58.

[9] Vogelaar CF, Konig B, Krafft S, Estrada V, Brazda N, Ziegler B, et al. Pharmacological suppression of CNS scarring by deferoxamine reduces lesion volume and increases regeneration in an in vitro model for astroglial-fibrotic scarring and in rat spinal cord injury in vivo. PLoS One. 2015;10(7):e0134371.

[10] Hill RL, Zhang YP, Burke DA, Devries WH, Zhang Y, Magnuson DS, et al. Anatomical and functional outcomes following a precise, graded, dorsal laceration spinal cord injury in C57BL/6 mice. Journal of Neurotrauma. 2009;26(1):1–15.

[11] Zhang YP, Walker MJ, Shields LB, Wang X, Walker CL, Xu XM, et al. Controlled cervical laceration injury in mice. Journal of Visualized Experiments: JoVE. 2013;75:e50030.

[12] Hermanns S, Klapka N, Muller HW. The collagenous lesion scar—an obstacle for axonal regeneration in brain and spinal cord injury. Restorative Neurology and Neuroscience. 2001;19(1–2):139–48.

[13] Silver J, Miller JH. Regeneration beyond the glial scar. Nature Reviews Neuroscience. 2004;5(2):146–56.

[14] Zörner B, Bachmann LC, Filli L, Kapitza S, Gullo M, Bolliger M, et al. Chasing central nervous system plasticity: the brainstem's contribution to locomotor recovery in rats with spinal cord injury. Brain. 2014;137(Pt 6):1716–32.

[15] Mantilla CB, Greising SM, Stowe JM, Zhan WZ, Sieck GC. TrkB kinase activity is critical for recovery of respiratory function after cervical spinal cord hemisection. Experimental Neurology. 2014;261:190–5.

[16] Surey S, Berry M, Logan A, Bicknell R, Ahmed Z. Differential cavitation, angiogenesis and wound-healing responses in injured mouse and rat spinal cords. Neuroscience. 2014;275:62–80.

[17] Young W. Spinal cord contusion models. Progress in Brain Research. 2002;137:231–55.

[18] Jakeman LB, Guan Z, Wei P, Ponnappan R, Dzwonczyk R, Popovich PG, et al. Traumatic spinal cord injury produced by controlled contusion in mouse. Journal of Neurotrauma. 2000;17(4):299–319.

[19] Stokes BT, Jakeman LB. Experimental modelling of human spinal cord injury: a model that crosses the species barrier and mimics the spectrum of human cytopathology. Spinal Cord. 2002;40(3):101–9.

[20] Lee JH, Streijger F, Tigchelaar S, Maloon M, Liu J, Tetzlaff W, et al. A contusive model of unilateral cervical spinal cord injury using the infinite horizon impactor. Journal of Visualized Experiments: JoVE. 2012;65.

[21] Geissler SA, Schmidt CE, Schallert T. Rodent models and behavioral outcomes of cervical spinal cord injury. Journal of Spine. 2013;Suppl. 4. DOI: 10.4172/2165-7939.S4-001

[22] Starkey ML, Barritt AW, Yip PK, Davies M, Hamers FP, McMahon SB, et al. Assessing behavioural function following a pyramidotomy lesion of the corticospinal tract in adult mice. Experimental Neurology. 2005;195(2):524–39.

[23] Lang C, Bradley PM, Jacobi A, Kerschensteiner M, Bareyre FM. STAT3 promotes corticospinal remodelling and functional recovery after spinal cord injury. EMBO Reports. 2013;14(10):931–7.

[24] Moonen G, Satkunendrarajah K, Wilcox JT, Badner A, Mothe A, Foltz W, et al. A new acute impact-compression lumbar spinal cord injury model in the rodent. Journal of Neurotrauma. 2016;33(3):278–89.

[25] Wen J, Sun D, Tan J, Young W. A consistent, quantifiable, and graded rat lumbosacral spinal cord injury model. Journal of Neurotrauma. 2015;32(12):875–92.

[26] Inoue T, Lin A, Ma X, McKenna SL, Creasey GH, Manley GT, et al. Combined SCI and TBI: recovery of forelimb function after unilateral cervical spinal cord injury (SCI) is retarded by contralateral traumatic brain injury (TBI), and ipsilateral TBI balances the effects of SCI on paw placement. Experimental Neurology. 2013;248:136–47.

[27] del Mar N, von Buttlar X, Yu AS, Guley NH, Reiner A, Honig MG. A novel closed-body model of spinal cord injury caused by high-pressure air blasts produces extensive axonal injury and motor impairments. Experimental Neurology. 2015;271:53–71.

[28] Opatz J, Kury P, Schiwy N, Jarve A, Estrada V, Brazda N, et al. SDF-1 stimulates neurite growth on inhibitory CNS myelin. Molecular and Cellular Neuroscience. 2009;40(2): 293–300.

[29] Lu R, Schmidtko A. Direct intrathecal drug delivery in mice for detecting in vivo effects of cGMP on pain processing. In: Krieg T, Lukowski R, editors. Methods in Molecular Biology. Guanylate Cyclase and Cyclic GMP. Springer Link, Humana Press; 2013. pp. 215–21. DOI: 10.1007/978-1-62703-459-3_14

[30] DeVos SL, Miller TM. Direct intraventricular delivery of drugs to the rodent central nervous system. Journal of Visualized Experiments: JoVE. 2013;75:e50326.

[31] Carter LM, Starkey ML, Akrimi SF, Davies M, McMahon SB, Bradbury EJ. The yellow fluorescent protein (YFP-H) mouse reveals neuroprotection as a novel mechanism underlying chondroitinase ABC-mediated repair after spinal cord injury. The Journal of Neuroscience. 2008;28(52):14107–20.

[32] David S, Aguayo AJ. Axonal elongation into peripheral nervous system "bridges" after central nervous system injury in adult rats. Science. 1981;214(4523):931–3.

[33] Bunge MB. Bridging the transected or contused adult rat spinal cord with Schwann cell and olfactory ensheathing glia transplants. Progress in Brain Research. 2002;137:275–82.

[34] Tso D, McKinnon RD. Cell replacement therapy for central nervous system diseases. Neural Regeneration Research. 2015;10(9):1356–8.

[35] Papastefanaki F, Matsas R. From demyelination to remyelination: the road toward therapies for spinal cord injury. Glia. 2015;63(7):1101–25.

[36] Jin Y, Bouyer J, Shumsky JS, Haas C, Fischer I. Transplantation of neural progenitor cells in chronic spinal cord injury. Neuroscience. 2016;320:69–82.

[37] Slawinska U, Miazga K, Jordan LM. The role of serotonin in the control of locomotor movements and strategies for restoring locomotion after spinal cord injury. Acta Neurobiologiae Experimentalis. 2014;74(2):172–87.

[38] Sharp KG, Yee KM, Steward O. A re-assessment of long distance growth and connectivity of neural stem cells after severe spinal cord injury. Experimental Neurology. 2014;257:186–204.

[39] Lu P, Wang Y, Graham L, McHale K, Gao M, Wu D, et al. Long-distance growth and connectivity of neural stem cells after severe spinal cord injury. Cell. 2012;150(6):1264–73.

[40] Lu Y, Wang MY. Neural stem cell grafts for complete spinal cord injury. Neurosurgery. 2012;71(6):N13–5.

[41] Chen CT, Foo NH, Liu WS, Chen SH. Infusion of human umbilical cord blood cells ameliorates hind limb dysfunction in experimental spinal cord injury through anti-inflammatory, vasculogenic and neurotrophic mechanisms. Pediatrics and Neonatology. 2008;49(3):77–83.

[42] Schira J, Gasis M, Estrada V, Hendricks M, Schmitz C, Trapp T, et al. Significant clinical, neuropathological and behavioural recovery from acute spinal cord trauma by transplantation of a well-defined somatic stem cell from human umbilical cord blood. Brain. 2012;135(Pt 2):431–46.

[43] Schira J, Falkenberg H, Hendricks M, Waldera-Lupa DM, Kogler G, Meyer HE, et al. Characterization of regenerative phenotype of unrestricted somatic stem cells (USSC) from human umbilical cord blood (hUCB) by functional secretome analysis. Molecular and Cellular Proteomics. 2015;14(10):2630–43.

[44] Jones LL, Oudega M, Bunge MB, Tuszynski MH. Neurotrophic factors, cellular bridges and gene therapy for spinal cord injury. The Journal of Physiology. 2001;533(Pt 1):83–9.

[45] Samadikuchaksaraei A. An overview of tissue engineering approaches for management of spinal cord injuries. Journal of NeuroEngineering and Rehabilitation. 2007;4:15.

[46] Markakis EA, Redmond DE, Jr. Know thyself: autologous cell transplantation strategies for brain repair. Experimental Neurology. 2005;196(1):6–8.

http://dx.doi.org/10.5772/62947

[47] Ori S, Okada Y, Nishimura S, Sasaki T, Itakura G, Kobayashi Y, et al. Long-term safety issues of iPSC-based cell therapy in a spinal cord injury model: oncogenic transformation with epithelial-mesenchymal transition. Stem Cell Reports. 2015;4(3):360–73.

[48] Estrada V, Tekinay A, Muller HW. Neural ECM mimetics. Progress in Brain Research. 2014;214:391–413.

[49] Bakshi A, Fisher O, Dagci T, Himes BT, Fischer I, Lowman A. Mechanically engineered hydrogel scaffolds for axonal growth and angiogenesis after transplantation in spinal cord injury. Journal of Neurosurgery: Spine. 2004;1(3):322–9.

[50] Cai J, Ziemba KS, Smith GM, Jin Y. Evaluation of cellular organization and axonal regeneration through linear PLA foam implants in acute and chronic spinal cord injury. Journal of Biomedical Materials Research Part A. 2007;83(2):512–20.

[51] Novikova LN, Novikov LN, Kellerth JO. Biopolymers and biodegradable smart implants for tissue regeneration after spinal cord injury. Current Opinion in Neurology. 2003;16(6):711–5.

[52] Friedman JA, Windebank AJ, Moore MJ, Spinner RJ, Currier BL, Yaszemski MJ. Biodegradable polymer grafts for surgical repair of the injured spinal cord. Neurosurgery. 2002;51(3):742–51.

[53] Horn EM, Beaumont M, Shu XZ, Harvey A, Prestwich GD, Horn KM, et al. Influence of cross-linked hyaluronic acid hydrogels on neurite outgrowth and recovery from spinal cord injury. Journal of Neurosurgery: Spine. 2007;6(2):133–40.

[54] Prang P, Muller R, Eljaouhari A, Heckmann K, Kunz W, Weber T, et al. The promotion of oriented axonal regrowth in the injured spinal cord by alginate-based anisotropic capillary hydrogels. Biomaterials. 2006;27(19):3560–9.

[55] Tysseling-Mattiace VM, Sahni V, Niece KL, Birch D, Czeisler C, Fehlings MG, et al. Self-assembling nanofibers inhibit glial scar formation and promote axon elongation after spinal cord injury. The Journal of Neuroscience. 2008;28(14):3814–23.

[56] Estrada V, Brazda N, Schmitz C, Heller S, Blazyca H, Martini R, et al. Long-lasting significant functional improvement in chronic severe spinal cord injury following scar resection and polyethylene glycol implantation. Neurobiology of Disease. 2014;67:165–79.

[57] Brazda N, Voss C, Estrada V, Lodin H, Weinrich N, Seide K, et al. A mechanical microconnector system for restoration of tissue continuity and long-term drug application into the injured spinal cord. Biomaterials. 2013;34(38):10056–64.

[58] Haan N, Song B. Therapeutic application of electric fields in the injured nervous system. Advances in Skin and Wound Care (New Rochelle). 2014;3(2):156–65.

[59] Singh B, Xu QG, Franz CK, Zhang R, Dalton C, Gordon T, et al. Accelerated axon outgrowth, guidance, and target reinnervation across nerve transection gaps following a brief electrical stimulation paradigm. Journal of Neurosurgery. 2012;116(3):498–512.

[60] Young W. Electrical stimulation and motor recovery. Cell Transplant. 2015;24(3):429–46.

[61] van den Brand R, Heutschi J, Barraud Q, DiGiovanna J, Bartholdi K, Huerlimann M, et al. Restoring voluntary control of locomotion after paralyzing spinal cord injury. Science. 2012;336(6085):1182–5.

[62] Lavrov I, Gerasimenko Y, Burdick J, Zhong H, Roy RR, Edgerton VR. Integrating multiple sensory systems to modulate neural networks controlling posture. Journal of Neurophysiology. 2015;114(6):3306–14.

[63] Wenger N, Moraud EM, Gandar J, Musienko P, Capogrosso M, Baud L, et al. Spatiotemporal neuromodulation therapies engaging muscle synergies improve motor control after spinal cord injury. Nature Medicine. 2016;22(2):138–45.

[64] McPherson JG, Miller RR, Perlmutter SI. Targeted, activity-dependent spinal stimulation produces long-lasting motor recovery in chronic cervical spinal cord injury. Proceedings of the National Academy of Sciences U S A. 2015;112(39):12193–8.

[65] Angeli CA, Edgerton VR, Gerasimenko YP, Harkema SJ. Altering spinal cord excitability enables voluntary movements after chronic complete paralysis in humans. Brain. 2014;137(Pt 5):1394–409.

[66] Koopmans GC, Brans M, Gomez-Pinilla F, Duis S, Gispen WH, Torres-Aleman I, et al. Circulating insulin-like growth factor I and functional recovery from spinal cord injury under enriched housing conditions. The European Journal of Neuroscience. 2006;23(4): 1035–46.

[67] Lankhorst AJ, ter Laak MP, van Laar TJ, van Meeteren NL, de Groot JC, Schrama LH, et al. Effects of enriched housing on functional recovery after spinal cord contusive injury in the adult rat. Journal of Neurotrauma. 2001;18(2):203–15.

[68] Fouad K, Tetzlaff W. Rehabilitative training and plasticity following spinal cord injury. Experimental Neurology. 2012;235(1):91–9.

[69] Courtine G, Song B, Roy RR, Zhong H, Herrmann JE, Ao Y, et al. Recovery of supraspinal control of stepping via indirect propriospinal relay connections after spinal cord injury. Nature Medicine. 2008;14(1):69–74.

[70] Shah PK, Garcia-Alias G, Choe J, Gad P, Gerasimenko Y, Tillakaratne N, et al. Use of quadrupedal step training to re-engage spinal interneuronal networks and improve locomotor function after spinal cord injury. Brain. 2013;136(Pt 11):3362–77.

[71] Starkey ML, Bleul C, Kasper H, Mosberger AC, Zorner B, Giger S, et al. High-impact, self-motivated training within an enriched environment with single animal tracking

dose-dependently promotes motor skill acquisition and functional recovery. Neurorehabilitation and Neural Repair. 2014;28(6):594–605.

[72] Sharp KG, Duarte JE, Gebrekristos B, Perez S, Steward O, Reinkensmeyer DJ. Robotic rehabilitator of the rodent upper extremity: a system and method for assessing and training forelimb force production after neurological injury. Journal of Neurotrauma. 2016;33. DOI: 10.1089/neu.2015.3987

[73] Schiwy N, Brazda N, Muller HW. Enhanced regenerative axon growth of multiple fibre populations in traumatic spinal cord injury following scar-suppressing treatment. The European Journal of Neuroscience. 2009;30(8):1544–53.

[74] Filli L, Schwab ME. Structural and functional reorganization of propriospinal connections promotes functional recovery after spinal cord injury. Neural Regeneration Research. 2015;10(4):509–13.

[75] Siebert JR, Middelton FA, Stelzner DJ. Intrinsic response of thoracic propriospinal neurons to axotomy. BMC Neuroscience. 2010;11:69.

[76] Beauparlant J, van den Brand R, Barraud Q, Friedli L, Musienko P, Dietz V, et al. Undirected compensatory plasticity contributes to neuronal dysfunction after severe spinal cord injury. Brain. 2013;136(Pt 11):3347–61.

[77] Onose G, Anghelescu A, Muresanu DF, Padure L, Haras MA, Chendreanu CO, et al. A review of published reports on neuroprotection in spinal cord injury. Spinal Cord. 2009;47(10):716–26.

[78] Samano C, Kaur J, Nistri A. A study of methylprednisolone neuroprotection against acute injury to the rat spinal cord in vitro. Neuroscience. 2016;315:136–49.

[79] Carter LM, McMahon SB, Bradbury EJ. Delayed treatment with chondroitinase ABC reverses chronic atrophy of rubrospinal neurons following spinal cord injury. Experimental Neurology. 2011;228(1):149–56.

[80] Oztas E. Neuronal tracing. Neuroanatomy. 2003;2:2–5.

[81] Huh Y, Oh MS, Leblanc P, Kim KS. Gene transfer in the nervous system and implications for transsynaptic neuronal tracing. Expert Opinion on Biological Therapy. 2010;10(5):763–72.

[82] Ginger M, Haberl M, Conzelmann KK, Schwarz MK, Frick A. Revealing the secrets of neuronal circuits with recombinant rabies virus technology. Frontiers in Neural Circuits. 2013;7:2.

[83] Blits B, Derks S, Twisk J, Ehlert E, Prins J, Verhaagen J. Adeno-associated viral vector (AAV)-mediated gene transfer in the red nucleus of the adult rat brain: comparative analysis of the transduction properties of seven AAV serotypes and lentiviral vectors. The Journal of Neuroscience Methods. 2010;185(2):257–63.

[84] Parr-Brownlie LC, Bosch-Bouju C, Schoderboeck L, Sizemore RJ, Abraham WC, Hughes SM. Lentiviral vectors as tools to understand central nervous system biology in mammalian model organisms. Frontiers in Molecular Neuroscience. 2015;8:14.

[85] McGovern AE, Davis-Poynter N, Rakoczy J, Phipps S, Simmons DG, Mazzone SB. Anterograde neuronal circuit tracing using a genetically modified herpes simplex virus expressing EGFP. The Journal of Neuroscience Methods. 2012;209(1):158–67.

[86] Soderblom C, Lee DH, Dawood A, Carballosa M, Jimena Santamaria A, Benavides FD, et al. 3D imaging of axons in transparent spinal cords from rodents and nonhuman primates. eNeuro. 2015;2(2).

[87] Schwarz MK, Scherbarth A, Sprengel R, Engelhardt J, Theer P, Giese G. Fluorescent-protein stabilization and high-resolution imaging of cleared, intact mouse brains. PLoS One. 2015;10(5):e0124650.

[88] Ertürk A, Becker K, Jahrling N, Mauch CP, Hojer CD, Egen JG, et al. Three-dimensional imaging of solvent-cleared organs using 3DISCO. Nature Protocols. 2012;7(11):1983–95.

[89] Steward O, Zheng B, Ho C, Anderson K, Tessier-Lavigne M. The dorsolateral cortico-spinal tract in mice: an alternative route for corticospinal input to caudal segments following dorsal column lesions. The Journal of Comparative Neurology. 2004;472(4): 463–77.

[90] Lai BQ, Qiu XC, Zhang K, Zhang RY, Jin H, Li G, et al. Cholera toxin B subunit shows transneuronal tracing after injection in an injured sciatic nerve. PLoS One. 2015;10(12):e0144030.

[91] Basso DM, Beattie MS, Bresnahan JC. A sensitive and reliable locomotor rating scale for open field testing in rats. Journal of Neurotrauma. 1995;12(1):1–21.

[92] Sedy J, Urdzikova L, Jendelova P, Sykova E. Methods for behavioral testing of spinal cord injured rats. Neuroscience and Biobehavioral Reviews. 2008;32(3):550–80.

[93] Lankhorst AJ, Duis SE, ter Laak MP, Joosten EA, Hamers FP, Gispen WH. Functional recovery after central infusion of alpha-melanocyte-stimulating hormone in rats with spinal cord contusion injury. Journal of Neurotrauma. 1999;16(4):323–31.

[94] Koopmans GC, Deumens R, Honig WM, Hamers FP, Steinbusch HW, Joosten EA. The assessment of locomotor function in spinal cord injured rats: the importance of objective analysis of coordination. Journal of Neurotrauma. 2005;22(2):214–25.

[95] Antri M, Orsal D, Barthe JY. Locomotor recovery in the chronic spinal rat: effects of long-term treatment with a 5-HT2 agonist. The European Journal of Neuroscience. 2002;16(3):467–76.

[96] Basso DM, Fisher LC, Anderson AJ, Jakeman LB, McTigue DM, Popovich PG. Basso Mouse Scale for locomotion detects differences in recovery after spinal cord injury in five common mouse strains. Journal of Neurotrauma. 2006;23(5):635–59.

[97] Anderson KD, Sharp KG, Hofstadter M, Irvine KA, Murray M, Steward O. Forelimb locomotor assessment scale (FLAS): novel assessment of forelimb dysfunction after cervical spinal cord injury. Experimental Neurology. 2009;220(1):23–33.

[98] Singh A, Krisa L, Frederick KL, Sandrow-Feinberg H, Balasubramanian S, Stackhouse SK, et al. Forelimb locomotor rating scale for behavioral assessment of recovery after unilateral cervical spinal cord injury in rats. The Journal of Neuroscience Methods. 2014;226:124–31.

[99] Metz GA, Whishaw IQ. Cortical and subcortical lesions impair skilled walking in the ladder rung walking test: a new task to evaluate fore- and hindlimb stepping, placing, and co-ordination. The Journal of Neuroscience Methods. 2002;115(2):169–79.

[100] Vogelaar CF, Vrinten DH, Hoekman MF, Brakkee JH, Burbach JP, Hamers FP. Sciatic nerve regeneration in mice and rats: recovery of sensory innervation is followed by a slowly retreating neuropathic pain-like syndrome. Brain Research. 2004;1027(1–2):67–72.

[101] Hamers FP, Lankhorst AJ, van Laar TJ, Veldhuis WB, Gispen WH. Automated quantitative gait analysis during overground locomotion in the rat: its application to spinal cord contusion and transection injuries. Journal of Neurotrauma. 2001;18(2):187–201.

[102] Hamers FP, Koopmans GC, Joosten EA. CatWalk-assisted gait analysis in the assessment of spinal cord injury. Journal of Neurotrauma. 2006;23(3–4):537–48.

[103] Hendriks WT, Eggers R, Ruitenberg MJ, Blits B, Hamers FP, Verhaagen J, et al. Profound differences in spontaneous long-term functional recovery after defined spinal tract lesions in the rat. Journal of Neurotrauma. 2006;23(1):18–35.

[104] Gensel JC, Tovar CA, Hamers FP, Deibert RJ, Beattie MS, Bresnahan JC. Behavioral and histological characterization of unilateral cervical spinal cord contusion injury in rats. Journal of Neurotrauma. 2006;23(1):36–54.

[105] Cao Y, Shumsky JS, Sabol MA, Kushner RA, Strittmatter S, Hamers FP, et al. Nogo-66 receptor antagonist peptide (NEP1-40) administration promotes functional recovery and axonal growth after lateral funiculus injury in the adult rat. Neurorehabilitation and Neural Repair. 2008;22(3):262–78.

[106] Hou J, Nelson R, Nissim N, Parmer R, Thompson FJ, Bose P. Effect of combined treadmill training and magnetic stimulation on spasticity and gait impairments after cervical spinal cord injury. Journal of Neurotrauma. 2014;31(12):1088–106.

[107] Hayakawa K, Uchida S, Ogata T, Tanaka S, Kataoka K, Itaka K. Intrathecal injection of a therapeutic gene-containing polyplex to treat spinal cord injury. Journal of Controlled Release. 2015;197:1–9.

[108] Smith JM, Lunga P, Story D, Harris N, Le Belle J, James MF, et al. Inosine promotes recovery of skilled motor function in a model of focal brain injury. Brain. 2007;130(Pt 4):915–25.

[109] Neckel ND. Methods to quantify the velocity dependence of common gait measurements from automated rodent gait analysis devices. The Journal of Neuroscience Methods. 2015;253:244–53.

[110] Ek CJ, Habgood MD, Callaway JK, Dennis R, Dziegielewska KM, Johansson PA, et al. Spatio-temporal progression of grey and white matter damage following contusion injury in rat spinal cord. PLoS One. 2010;5(8):e12021.

[111] Zhang B, Bailey WM, Braun KJ, Gensel JC. Age decreases macrophage IL-10 expression: implications for functional recovery and tissue repair in spinal cord injury. Experimental Neurology. 2015;273:83–91.

[112] Beare JE, Morehouse JR, DeVries WH, Enzmann GU, Burke DA, Magnuson DS, et al. Gait analysis in normal and spinal contused mice using the TreadScan system. Journal of Neurotrauma. 2009;26(11):2045–56.

[113] Zörner B, Filli L, Starkey ML, Gonzenbach R, Kasper H, Rothlisberger M, et al. Profiling locomotor recovery: comprehensive quantification of impairments after CNS damage in rodents. Nature Methods. 2010;7(9):701–8.

[114] Gwak YS, Kang J, Unabia GC, Hulsebosch CE. Spatial and temporal activation of spinal glial cells: role of gliopathy in central neuropathic pain following spinal cord injury in rats. Experimental Neurology. 2012;234(2):362–72.

[115] Detloff MR, Fisher LC, Deibert RJ, Basso DM. Acute and chronic tactile sensory testing after spinal cord injury in rats. Journal of Visualized Experiments: JoVE. 2012;62:e3247.

[116] Hargreaves K, Dubner R, Brown F, Flores C, Joris J. A new and sensitive method for measuring thermal nociception in cutaneous hyperalgesia. Pain. 1988;32(1):77–88.

[117] Irvine KA, Ferguson AR, Mitchell KD, Beattie SB, Lin A, Stuck ED, et al. The Irvine, Beatties, and Bresnahan (IBB) Forelimb Recovery Scale: an assessment of reliability and validity. Frontiers in Neurology. 2014;5:116.

[118] Fouad K, Hurd C, Magnuson DS. Functional testing in animal models of spinal cord injury: not as straight forward as one would think. Frontiers in Integrative Neuroscience. 2013;7:85.

[119] Xu N, Akesson E, Holmberg L, Sundstrom E. A sensitive and reliable test instrument to assess swimming in rats with spinal cord injury. Behavioural Brain Research. 2015;291:172–83.

[120] Kjell J, Sandor K, Josephson A, Svensson CI, Abrams MB. Rat substrains differ in the magnitude of spontaneous locomotor recovery and in the development of mechanical

hypersensitivity after experimental spinal cord injury. Journal of Neurotrauma. 2013;30(21):1805–11.

[121] Nikkhah G, Rosenthal C, Hedrich HJ, Samii M. Differences in acquisition and full performance in skilled forelimb use as measured by the 'staircase test' in five rat strains. Behavioural Brain Research. 1998;92(1):85–95.

[122] Galtrey CM, Fawcett JW. Characterization of tests of functional recovery after median and ulnar nerve injury and repair in the rat forelimb. Journal of the Peripheral Nervous System. 2007;12(1):11–27.

[123] Rosenzweig ES, Courtine G, Jindrich DL, Brock JH, Ferguson AR, Strand SC, et al. Extensive spontaneous plasticity of corticospinal projections after primate spinal cord injury. Nature Neuroscience. 2010;13(12):1505–10.

[124] Nout YS, Ferguson AR, Strand SC, Moseanko R, Hawbecker S, Zdunowski S, et al. Methods for functional assessment after C7 spinal cord hemisection in the rhesus monkey. Neurorehabilitation and Neural Repair. 2012;26(6):556–69.

[125] Nout YS, Rosenzweig ES, Brock JH, Strand SC, Moseanko R, Hawbecker S, et al. Animal models of neurologic disorders: a nonhuman primate model of spinal cord injury. Neurotherapeutics. 2012;9(2):380–92.

[126] Friedli L, Rosenzweig ES, Barraud Q, Schubert M, Dominici N, Awai L, et al. Pronounced species divergence in corticospinal tract reorganization and functional recovery after lateralized spinal cord injury favors primates. Science Translational Medicine. 2015;7(302):302ra134.

[127] Kuypers HG, Ugolini G. Viruses as transneuronal tracers. Trends in Neurosciences. 1990;13(2):71–5.

Chapter 2

In Vitro Models of Spinal Cord Injury

Lucia Slovinska, Juraj Blasko, Miriam Nagyova,
Eva Szekiova and Dasa Cizkova

Additional information is available at the end of the chapter

http://dx.doi.org/10.5772/63459

Abstract

Living organisms are extremely complex functional systems. At present, there are many *in vivo* models of spinal cord injury (SCI) that allow the modeling of any type of central nervous system (CNS) injury, however, with some disadvantages. The production of injury models can be a highly invasive and time-consuming process and requires high technical requirements, and costly financial issues should also be taken into account. Of course, a large number of animals have been used to obtain the relevant data of statistical significance. All of these aspects can be reduced by carrying out experiments in *in vitro* conditions. The primary advantage of *in vitro* method is that it simplifies the system under study. There are two major groups of *in vitro* model in use: cell culture and organotypic slice (OTS) culture. OTS is an intermediate system of the screening of *in vitro* cell culture and animal models and represents the *in vitro* system preserving the basic tissue architecture that able to closely mimic the cellular and physiological characteristics *in vivo*. *In vitro* models are the preferred methods for the study of acute or subacute pathophysiology after a trauma stimulus, enabling precise control on the extracellular environment, easy and repeatable access to the cells.

Keywords: *in vitro* model, spinal cord injury (SCI), cell culture, co-culture, organotypic slice (OTS) culture

1. Introduction

Spinal cord injury (SCI) is a critical incurable difficulty affecting the quality of life of patients and society equally. The spinal cord injury interferes predominantly with motor function defects, which substantially restrict normal daily activities, thus leading to serious psychological trauma. Today, the majority of patients are left paralyzed with unsuccessful treatment currently available. Many strategies, including surgical, transplantations, pharmacological, neurophysiological, and others approaches, have been used and examined in attempts to develop new and successful therapies that will allow patients to get the valuable life they lived before the injury [1].

First, before devising a new treatment for spinal cord injury, it is also important to know the processes of nerve tissue regeneration, neurogenesis, and gliogenesis, which can be influenced in many ways. The answer to these needs, a growing number of animal models have been introduced and utilized. The creation of *in vivo* injury models requires many invasive interventions and is time consuming. The financial costs of such models as well as technical equipment are often high. However, the biggest problem of the *in vivo* models is the utilization of large amounts of experimental animals. All of these facts can be reduced by carrying out experiments in *in vitro* conditions. *In vitro* experimental models are needed to understand the cellular mechanisms and pathophysiology of the injured spinal cord (SC) and to provide evidence for further treatment. This is also the right place to mention the principles of the 3Rs (Replacement, Reduction, and Refinement). The principles of the 3Rs were developed as a framework for humane animal research and became embedded in national and international legislation regulating the use of animals in scientific procedures in most world countries. There are two major groups of *in vitro* model in use: cell culture and organotypic slice (OTS) culture.

2. Cell cultures

After central nervous system (CNS) injury, the acute primary and the chronic secondary damage takes place. After initial mechanical insult, a rapid deformation of CNS tissue happens, causing an immediate cell death in the epicenter of injury site followed by a cascade of processes leading to the secondary damage. Traumatic injury disrupts spinal white matter tracts resulting in the loss of sensory and motor function. This loss of function is generally permanent due to the limited regenerative capacity of the CNS [2]. Cells used for *in vitro* modeling should have morphological, functional qualities, and relevant requirements depending on disease, injury, and ultimate goal of the proposed experiments. The commonly used *in vitro* cell culture models of SCI include:

i. Primary isolated cells, neurons, oligodendrocytes, astrocytes, or microglia cells [3, 4]. Primary cells are obtained from the dissociated neural tissues, spinal cord, or brain and are usually cultivated immediately after the isolation as "primo-cultures." The origin of these cells could be embryonal, fetal, neonatal, or adult [5, 6]. It is well known that younger cells are more potent according to their strong proliferative activity, in contrary to terminally differentiated poor proliferating capacity owning adult cells [6]. By using the primary cultures, we can investigate the behavior and intercommunication of the individual or mixed cell populations. These populations preserve the main characteristics similar to the *in vivo* examined types of cells [7]. Very often used are also the immortalized cell lines, which are in fact the primary cells with genetical modification.

ii. Co-culture of neuronal cells with different cell types, which are present in the glial scar [8, 9]. *In vitro* cultures offer simplified, high throughput systems to study disease, drug toxicity, and biological processes by controlling environmental factors and directly measuring cell responses [10].

2.1. *In vitro* model of glial scar

The characteristic manifestation of the secondary reactive phase is scar formation at the initial impact site, which represents the major obstruction to CNS regeneration. The glial scar is rich in different cells (microglia and reactive astrocytes), myelin-associated inhibitors, and it physically surrounds the damaged tissue. To study the components of the glial scar, many models of co-cultivation of neurons with others glial scar situated cells have been developed [8, 9, 11]. By combining two pivotal aspects of CNS damage, mechanical injury and co-cultivation with meningeal cells in *in vitro* scar formation model, it has been shown that astrocytes increase the expression of GFAP (glial fibrillary acidic protein), as well as the scar-associated markers, e.g., phosphacan, neurocan, and tenascin. Subsequent short-time co-cultivation with different developmental neuronal populations led to significantly reduced neurite growth in this scar-like model [9]. After spinal cord injury, demyelination of spared white matter significantly hinders spontaneous function recovery [12]. To understand the processes related to this phenomenon, a wide range of developed cultures in which the many stages of myelination can be followed over time are used [13–15]. These myelinating cultures involve plating dissociated rat spinal cord cells onto a confluent monolayer of neurosphere-derived astrocytes. Sorensen et al. [16] compared the different types of cells in the process of myelination promotion of CNS axons. The mixed cell population of dissociated embryonal spinal cord was cultivated on olfactory ensheathing cells (OECs), Schwann cells (SchCs), or neurosphere-derived astrocytes to study the mutual interactions in context to affect the myelination. Myelin internodes and nodes of Ranvier were often found only in the cells cultivated onto neurosphere-derived astrocytes. This model is very useful to investigate the CNS axonal myelination because it recapitulates the processes occurring in CNS *in vivo*. On the basis of these cultures, it has been shown that astrocytes have a direct role in promoting myelination either by releasing a soluble factor or by cell–cell contact [16]. Also, the phenotype of astrocytes has a crucial role in determining their effects on myelination. Myelination is poor when the myelinating cultures are plated on quiescent astrocytes but enhanced when they are plated on a more reactive/activated phenotype. Interestingly, quiescent astrocytes secreted CXCL10, which did not appear to directly affect the purified oligodendrocyte progenitor cell differentiation but had the effect on the ability of oligodendrocytes to ensheath axons [13]. Astrocytes exhibit dynamic cell process movement and changes in their membrane topography as they interact with axons and oligodendrocytes during the process of myelination [15]. These observations may have important implications with respect to the development of therapeutic strategies to promote CNS remyelination in demyelinating diseases. Also other models have been developed to investigate and to understand the molecular mechanisms of CNS axon regeneration. The process of axon regeneration can be monitored by neurite outgrowth assays, which often represent the phenotypic expression of regeneration progress. In neurite outgrowth assays, the neurons are cultivated on an adherent substrate, and the neurite growth is evaluated in specific medium conditions for extended periods of time, and then the overall length of the radial outgrowth is measured. Primary neurons (neurons derived from dorsal roots ganglion, cerebellum, cortex, or hippocampus) are considered more biologically relevant to neurons *in vivo* instead of induced pluripotent stem cells or any special cell lines [17].

2.2 *In vitro*

The majority of SCI occurring in human is due to the compression of spinal cord; therefore most *in vitro* models have been designed to mimic this type of injury. To simulate the spinal cord injury *in vitro*, the confluent layer of astrocytes and dissociated embryonic spinal cord cells plated onto them are cut with scalpel blade, the so-called scratch model. Such treatment creates an empty area without any cells—lesion. With an increasing time of cultivation, the situation around the injury becomes comparable to the SCI *in vivo*. The microglial cells and astrocytes start to migrate to the injury site. Conversely, the decrease in neurite density and the process of demyelination start as the consequences of disrupting confluent cell layer. The main purpose of this model is to find out, to recognize any factors, molecules, biomaterials, even cells that can contribute, may be, to accelerate the potential regeneration of remaining cells destroyed by injury. The closure of this lesion could be modified using different Rho/ROCK inhibitors [11] or by cAMP modulators, which promote neurite outgrowth and myelination [5]. *In vitro* models are the preferred methods for the study of acute or sub-acute pathophysiology after a trauma stimulus enabling the precise control of the extracellular environment, easy and repeatable access to the cells.

To imitate the SCI in our experimental model, the P1 rat spinal cord cells were mechanically scratched across the cell monolayer with a pipette tip. The result of this handling was the linear cell-free area/lesion which varied between 400 - 600 μm in width. After washing out the scraped cells with PBS (phosphate-buffered saline), cells were maintained for up to 10 days in culture. During the cultivation time, the cultures remained viable. Cell migration or wound closure of the scratched surface was observed and photographed at daily intervals. To investigate the potential stimulative effect of mesenchymal stem cells (MSCs) on the neural cells, we treated such injured cultures with conditioned medium obtained from rat bone marrow MSCs. In fact, MSCs cannot differentiate into fully functional neurons, or into others neural cells; the supporting effect of neuroregeneration and neuroprotection is mediated by specific neurotrophic factors and cytokines produced by MSCs [18]. All experiments conformed to the Slovak Law for Animal Protection No. 377/2012 and 436/2012 transposed from the European Communities Council Directive (2010/63/EU) and were approved by the Institutional Ethical Committee for animal research. Our preliminary data showed that the cell-free area in injured group treated with MSC conditioned medium became filled with reactive astrocytes, microglia cells, and oligodendrocyte in a shorter time when compared to untreated controls (**Figure 1**).

http://dx.doi.org/10.5772/63459

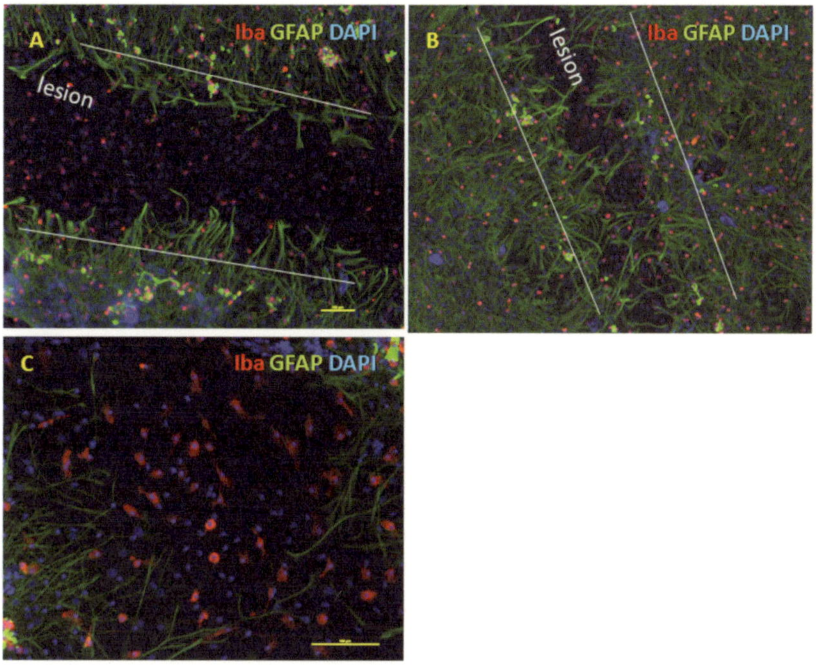

Figure 1. Fluorescent microscopy images of spinal cord culture injured by mechanical insult, control group (A) and group treated (B) with conditioned medium obtained from MSCs. The images were taken on day 2 after injury. Cells were stained with GFAP/astrocytes/green antibody, Iba/microglia cells/red antibody and DAPI/nuclear/blue marker, and (C) the detail of microglia cells infiltrating the lesion on day 2. Scale bar is 100 μm.

The cell culture approaches lack the complexity and physiological relevance of *in vivo* system. However, animal studies offer complexity, which cannot be modeled *in vitro* and which is also difficult to control and manipulate and therefore results in data that must be extrapolated to human systems [10].

3. Organotypic slices

Organotypic cultures are whole slices of tissue cultured without dissociation of the individual cells. Organotypic slices (OTSs) preserve the basic structural and connective organization of their original tissue (organotypic) and represent an interim system sharing the properties of the cell culture *in vitro* and an animal *in vivo* model. The OTS culture allows long-term maintenance of tissue architecture in "dish" [19].

OTS preparation is carried out according to the following steps. Briefly, after tissue removal under sterile conditions, the tissue is cut into 150–400 μm thick sections using a tissue chopper or vibratome. After washing, the slices are attached to a substrate and cultivated under appropriate conditions for several weeks. Today, we know many ways of OTS preparation depending on the final thickness of the slices and the survival time in culture. In *roller-tube cultures*, the slices embedded in plasma clot or collagen matrix on glass coverslips are placed in plastic culture tube containing a small amount of medium and undergo continuous slow rotation which allows the oxygenation of these slices by regular changing of the liquid–gas interface [20]. Because the slices become flattened to a quasi monolayer during cultivation procedure, this technique is appropriate when individual living nerve cells have to be observed by normal optical conditions for several weeks [21]. For obtaining quantitatively more pieces of OTSs, the modified roller method for organotypic cultivation of free-floating sections of postnatal rats can be used. This innovative procedure enables the simultaneous cultivation of multiple amount of OTS in one bottle (up to 50 and even more). For this reason, this method is advantageous for the investigation of cytotoxic injury of neural cells and appropriate immunocytochemical and molecular analysis [22]. Another, but not so frequently used, is the method, where the slices are placed either directly on collagen coated or embedded in collagen gels in Petri dishes and are totally covered by medium. These cultures survive only a few days and are mainly used for electrophysiology [21].

The most used and popular OTS-cultivating methods are the membrane cultures, where the slices are directly placed at the air–medium interface on semiporous membranes and kept stationary during the entire cultivation. Slices can collect the nutrients from an appropriate growth medium from below via capillary process and oxygen from above (**Figure 2**) [21, 23].

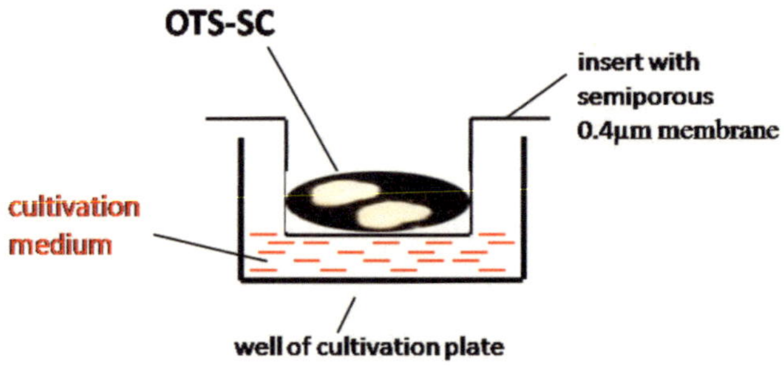

Figure 2. Schematic illustration of the most used OTS cultivating methods called "interface method". Organotypic spinal cord slice (OTS-SC) is placed on semiporous membrane through which OTS can obtain the nutrition from medium and oxygen from above.

At the beginning, experiments were carried out using hippocampal slices. However, cerebellar, cortical, and spinal cord explants have also been tested with positive results [23]. The advantage of this technique is that these OTSs are never covered with embedding materials or media which allow the study of the effect of a therapeutic agent added directly onto the OTSs during all stages of culturing longer time while maintaining semi-three-dimensional structure of tissue. Positioning of slices on the membrane is extremely easy and may represent an advantage also for co-culture experiments. This technique also has some limitations. The problem may concern the accessibility of individual neurons, because the cultured slices remain a few cell layers thick and are covered by fibers and glial processes. During OTS preparation and cultivation, we should avoid some troubles. Slices should be placed in the middle of the membrane without contacting one another. In this position, every slice can be easily reached to perform the impact injury. If any impact injury is performed, the uninjured and damaged sections have to be situated on individual insert; otherwise, excytotoxins released from damaged sections may induce injury in the controls. Sections with defective or lacking layers should be rejected from the examination. It is important to start the concrete experiments about 12–14 days after the beginning of OTS cultivation [24]. In some studies, the time of OTS culture before starting the actual experiment is shorter (1 week) [25, 26]; so the mechanical damage caused by slicing disappears, and the cells can reach a more advanced developmental stage. In addition, this time period will allow the slices to acclimatize to the culturing conditions and mature. Organotypic cultures survive from weeks to months, providing options for long-term studies, such as those studying different processes of neurodegeneration and recovery following excytotoxicity ischemia and traumatic injury.

Since the first description of organotypic hippocampal slice cultures based on the method of Gahwiler [20], the hippocampal regions are likely the most widely used organotypic slice culture model for the study of neural tissues [27]. Together with the accumulation of practical experiences and increased necessity to answer the questions dealing with nerve tissue regeneration after spinal cord injury (SCI), the development and entrenchment of organotypic spinal cord slice (OTS-SC) models became more actual. Today, there is a wide choice of methods and OTS models of both spinal cord and brain derived from different animals—mouse, rats, and rabbits [28], even the human too [29], which have been used to describe ways of monitoring spontaneous or induced neuronal degeneration in organotypic brain slice cultures [30], to study the different processes of neurodegeneration after tissue traumatic injury, and to investigate mechanisms and treatment strategies for the neurodegenerative disorders like stroke (ischemia) [31–33]. These models can simulate several pathological aspects of various neurological conditions depending on different factors, e.g., (i) the applied stimulus which causes damage, (ii) the age of OTS donor animal (iii) which parameter is the experiment focused on.

4. Insults

4.1. Ischemic insults

Damage of nerve tissue may be caused by a number of insults. Previously, organotypic slice preparations have been used in several injury models including ischemia (experimental models with oxygen-glucose deprivation) and cytotoxicity studies (exposure to glutamate receptor agonists) [24]. Ischemic insults can be generated by oxygen-glucose deprivation of the cultures by placing them for 1h in glucose-free medium saturated with 95% N_2, 5% CO_2 using standard interface method [34]. To induce stroke-like, energy failure conditions in slice cultures can be achieved in several other ways, like use of anoxic chambers or OTS submersion in glucose-free medium saturated with nitrogen [35]. In a study of free radical-induced damage in CNS using OTS exposed to H_2O_2 as a model of oxidative injury in the brain, the results provide evidence that glial cells in cultured slices are vulnerable to H_2O_2toxicity as pyramidal neurons, and that H_2O_2-mediated cell death was significantly alleviated by antioxidants and independent of calcium influx in both glial and neuronal populations [36].

The hypoxic environment in SCI has been shown to inhibit recovery. One of the promising treatments for hypoxic ischemia sustained during SCI is gene therapy. Vascular endothelial growth factor (VEGF) increasingly has gained attention as a potential factor in gene therapy to replace or improve damaged neurons in SCI because of its role in neurogenesis and neuroprotection, astrocyte proliferation, and neurite outgrowth. The controlled release of VEGF in hypoxia-inducible VEGF gene delivery system in the OTS-SC may prove to be useful for providing neuroprotection and in stimulating the neural growth in the hypoxic environment of the injured spinal cord [37]. The principal feature of acute SCI pathophysiology is excitotoxicity that is considered the main contributor to the clinical outcome. An established *in vitro* SCI model using excitotoxic damage evoked by transient kainate application to organotypic slice cultures (with predominant neuro- rather than glio-toxicity) closely mimics the *in vivo* pathophysiology of SCI. The results from such model indicate that, after an excitotoxic stimulus, extracellular S100b, a useful biomarker in serum or cerebrospinal fluid for brain or spinal cord injury, was significantly elevated in association with ongoing neuronal damage and unscathed glia [38]. The application of glutamate is believed to mimic excitotoxicity that occurs as a consequence of ischemic stroke. Also, glutamate-induced excitotoxicity is a major contributor to motor neuron (MN) degeneration in disorders such as amyotrophic lateral sclerosis, stroke, and spinal cord injury. On the basis of using OTS from different parts of SC (i.e., cervical, thoracic, and lumbar), it is found out that the MN susceptibility to glutamate-induced excitotoxicity differs within diverse populations of MNs. This sensitivity is in correlation to the segmental variable expression of glutamate receptor sub-types in MN populations. In the cervical and lumbar parts, the AMPA receptor is in dominance, whereas in thoracic segments, the NMDA receptors predominate. These results should be taken into account by devising a new drug screening experiment with cell culture system [39].

4.2. Mechanical insults

Adamchik et al. [24] described two original models of moderate mechanical trauma containing the induced primary and secondary traumatic damage in organotypic slice cultures. The primary trauma injury was achieved by quickly rolling a stainless steel cylinder (weight, 0.9 g; diameter, 5 mm; length, 7 mm) twice on the organotypic slice. To model the secondary trauma injury, a weight of 0.137 g was dropped from a height of 2 mm on a localized area of the organotypic slice. The primary damage delivered by rotating the steel cylinder on sections induces injury following the head accidents, while the damage caused in this model for secondary injury, limited initially to a small area of the section, enables to monitor the expansion of dying cells.

Almost all SCI occurring in human are due to the compression of spinal cord; therefore, most *in vitro* models have been designed to mimic this type of injury. For that reason, an *in vitro* model of neurotrauma was developed and assessed by using organotypic slice culture of adult mice spinal cord to facilitate the investigation of primary and secondary mechanisms of cell death that occur after mechanical SCI [25]. The mechanical trauma was achieved by using a weight drop model of injury, where an impactor (pin) with a weight of 0.2g was dropped from 1.7 cm onto the center of the culture slice. They modified previously described methods for generating murine spinal trauma in OTS [40]. In contrary to other models, where the OTS-SC from embryonic or neonatal mice was used, the modified model used the OTS from adult animals according to the different regenerative capabilities.

Organotypic slice cultures of spinal cord have been used in neuroscience research for a long time, but classically, these cultures were cut in the transverse plane. The transverse slices could be, however, obtained from only a single part of the spinal cord. In order to reflect the spinal cord microenvironment, the longitudinal cultures are required to maintain the basic cytoarchitectonic organization of the intact spinal cord. In contrary to the previous model, Bonnici and Kapfhammer [41] used the spinal cord slices for their study that were cut not in the transverse but in the sagittal longitudinal plane such that several spinal cord segments were included in the slide culture. This OTS-SC model is well suited for the study of axonal growth because the typical ventro-dorsal polarity of the SC is maintained after a culture period of 2 weeks, and intrinsic spinal cord axons formed a strong fiber tract extending along the longitudinal axis of the slice. The axons became myelinated during the culture period, and synaptic contacts were present in these cultures. After mechanical lesions originated by completely transecting the SC tissue with a scalpel blade, the remaining spinal cord neurons had a considerable capability to regenerate the axons. The amount of renewed axons infiltrating the wound site decreased with increasing cultivation time and maturation of the culture. This indicates that the cellular differentiation and cytoarchitectonic organization of the spinal cord neurons are similar to that of slice cultures of the transverse plane and reflects the *in vivo* situation well [41]. Some scientists use the OTS for the study of radiation effect on cell damage. By determining the time-dependent course of choline uptake in mature organotypic slice cultures of rabbit and assessing the effects of continuous and single high-dose irradiation on choline uptake, the results demonstrate that the delivery of continuous but relatively low-dose rate gamma irradiation is more efficacious than single high-dose external irradiation on high-affinity choline uptake in nervous tissues [28].

5. Age of donor animal

The age of the donor animal influences the viability of OTS, the degree of tissue organization, and the successfulness of experiment at all. Early postnatal periods (P0–P9) are ideally suited for culturing [26, 39, 42]. Since most diseases of the spinal cord concern the adults, some organotypic spinal cord slice culture models from grown rats were established [25, 26]. But the isolation of the cord from adult individuals is, however, much more problematic. The fully myelinated spinal cord is very sensitive to any damage, and cutting it with tissue chopper causes injury to about 60% of slices. The slice culture survives about 7 days maintaining proper parallel fiber tract architecture. Also, the constant high vitality and tissue organization are preserved up to 4–5 weeks in neonatal slices, while the vitality of adult slice cultures decreases significantly upon the first 5 days of cultivation [26]. On the contrary, spinal cord organotypic culture from adult mouse can be used to produce neurospheres that can be further differentiated into astrocytes and neuronal cells of different phenotypes. Although, it is not clear what exactly triggers the formation of neurospheres, one explanation could be, that neuronal loss and/or long-term culturing of spinal cord slices resets the internal cell program and stimulates proliferation and further specification of neuronal stem cells (NSCs) [43]. Most researchers did not use cultures from animals older then P6, because neuronal survival in such cultures was more variable and a longitudinal fiber tract did not develop consistently [41]. The same goes for the transverse spinal cord slice cultures, in which neuronal survival also appears to be declining in cultures derived from older postnatal animals [44].

6. Utilization of organotypic slices

Because the OTS system is accessible to experimental manipulations, OTSs represent a suitable model which may be used for different research projects not only for investigation of various parameters accompanying the CNS injury but also for the development of therapeutic application for such injury. Spinal cord injury leads to the death of various cell types, including neurons, oligodendrocytes, astrocytes, and precursor cells. A high percentage of astrocytes and oligodendrocytes in the white matter at the site of injury die within a short time after injury leading to axonal demyelination. Grafts of cells used as a treatment or as the source of supporting factors can be directly transplanted in the slices and in this way, the graft--host interaction, behavior, and fate of grafted cells can be analyzed. The injured spinal cord microenvironment is very inhospitable for survival and differentiation of transplanted or endogenous NSCs. To mimic NSC grafting into the spinal cord, NSCs were seeded on top of cultured spinal cord slices with the Hamilton syringe between 7 and 10 days after the initial culture. In such culture system, possible effects of environmental manipulation on biological behavior of either exogenous grafted NSCs or endogenous neural progenitor cells in a complex tissue environment similar to that of *in vivo* system were studied. The majority of focally applied exogenous NSCs survived up to 4 weeks, and dispersing cells did not show any preference to either the white or the gray mater. Cultured spinal cord slices retained the non-neurogenic characteristics of *in vivo* spinal cord tissue since they did not support neuronal differentiation of either exogenous NSCs or endogenous neural progenitors [42]. Also, it is very much preferred to use the OTS derived from animals with some genetic alteration, which is manifested in special disease features. For example, to study the process of the myelination and myelin support, the OTSs obtained from the cerebellum of shiverer mice were used. These mice are genetically modified in myelin basic protein (MBP) gene resulting in wide CNS dysmyelination. After the transplantation of oligodendrocyte precursors into such modified sections, the direct observation of myelin produced by grafted cells is possible. This system is more advantageous in comparison with neuron-oligodendrocyte cell co-cultures for its propinquity with *in vivo* system [45].

The impact of individual cells on the regeneration of damaged CNS tissue can be studied not only by direct transplantation of cells to OTS but also by the so-called co-culture system, where the exogenous populations are cultivated underneath the slice co-cultures without direct contact using a Transwell system. The cultured OTSs are then influenced by factors released from exogenous, co-cultured cells. Indirect co-cultivation of exogenous cells along with OTS-SC permits the analysis of the factors secreted into the medium by both cells and the spinal cord tissue and the determination of their mutual influence. For example, MSCs, the promising candidates for neuroregenerative cell therapies, promote neuronal regeneration by significantly enhanced fiber outgrowth, an effect that may be mediated by a higher expression of brain-derived neurotrophic factor (BDNF) and basic fibroblast growth factor [46]. So, the role of the MSCs is in establishing the microenvironment to be more favorable for tissue repair.

Cho et al. [47] demonstrated that the treatment of lumbar slices of spinal cord with lysolecithin caused an important degree of cell death and demyelination of nerve fibers. However, after the co-cultivation of lumbar sections with human MSCs (hMSCs), the earlier observed effects were elevated to a significant range. Since the spinal cord slice culture is totally isolated and does not have any circulating immune cells originated from the host, it excludes the possibility of any systemic immune response to transplanted human cells. The results demonstrated that direct hMSC transplantation into the demyelinated organotypic spinal cord slice culture alter the tissue microenvironment and clearly increased the survival of endogenous cells and promoted axonal outgrowth of nerves in this organotypic spinal cord slice culture. So, the OTS-SC cultures provide the opportunity to investigate the underlying mechanisms of nerve regeneration after injury in the adult nervous system and to identify the factors which enhance axonal outgrowth as well as cell survival. The ease by which organotypic slice cultures can be manipulated and inspected also make them interesting tools for studies of cell proliferation, chronic CNS astrogliosis [48] and migration [49].

The OTS could be applied also to study the neurons and glial damage during bacterial infection. In the course of pneumococcal meningitis, both spontaneous and antibiotic-induced lysis of bacteria occurs. During this process, not only cell wall constituents but also nucleic acids of the bacteria are liberated. Therefore, organotypic hippocampal slices were utilized for the investigation of possible toxic effects of complete bacteria causing meningitis or their components on neuronal and glial tissue in the absence of leukocytes. The neuronal tissue of an infected host is damaged as a result of the intense inflammatory response against the attacking bacteria. Though OTS closely mimics the *in vivo* system, during the actual cultivation, it represents only the part of more complex unit derived from, which is closed without any circulating immune cells. According to this, by the measurement of neuron-specific enolase in cultivation medium, as an additional indicator of neuronal damage, it was found out that not only heat-inactivated whole bacteria but also diverse bacterial elements were capable of inducing nervous tissue damage, such as bacterial walls and nucleic acids [50]. Also, the organotypic brain slice cultures of bovine origin are a suitable model to study aspects of host–pathogen interaction in listeric encephalitis and potentially in other neuroinfectious diseases [51]. To evaluate the effect of HIV-1 virus on neural cells, a method for culturing human fetal organotypic brain slices in the presence of live virus was developed. The brain--derived OTSs were maintained on membranes, and co-cultured with HIV-1–infected T-cells on the well bottom. Thus, OTSs were exposed to live virus during whole cultivation time, HIV-1 proteins, and other molecules produced by the infected T-cells. The results obtained from this model indicate the gliosis observed *in vivo*. This valuable method can be used to model the dynamics and the microenvironment of brain tissue exposed to HIV-1 and can eventually be used to test therapies directed at preventing HIV-1-induced neural damage in CNS [52].

Within the wide range of available OTSs derived from different CNS sections, the OTS-SC system represents an attractive model with some benefits, when compared to generally used *in vitro* and *in vivo* models. OTS-SC can be kept under cultivation conditions for a long time. During the whole cultivation time, this system enables quick and direct evaluation and identification of huge diapason of different cellular, molecular relations involved in regeneration processes. Moreover, OTS-SCs can be utilized to improve the *ex vivo* neurological disorders and thus represent an intermediate step between *in vitro* experiments and animal models [53].

7. Experimental study

The aim of our study was: (i) to imitate the spinal cord injury (SCI) in organotypic spinal cord slice (OTS-SC) and (ii) to treat these injured OTS-SCs (OTS-SCIs) in the presence of rat mesenchymal stem cells (rMSCs). We imitate the SCI in the OTS-SC not by direct mechanical impact, but the injury was induced by OTS-SC treated with conditioned medium obtained from injured spinal cord (CM-SCI). CM-SCI represents a cocktail of cytokines and chemokines released by central lesion segments of injured spinal cord. We examined the impact of CM-SCI, as well as rMSCs on behavior of microglia cells, astrocytes, and neurons in the organotypic spinal cord slice cultures.

7.1. Methods

The SCI was induced by modified balloon-compression technique in adult rats [54], and after 3 days of animal survival, the central lesion segments were dissected and cultured for 24 h *in vitro* to obtain CM-SCI used for OTS-SC treatment. Similarly, we obtained the conditioned medium from control-intact thoracic spinal cord (CM-SC), which in our experiment served as a source of control-conditioned medium. The OTS-SCs were prepared from lumbal SCs of naive adult male rats. The isolated SCs were transversely cut with a Mcllwain tissue chopper into 400 μm OTS-SC sections and cultivated for an adaptation for 5 days in 1ml/well of culture media containing DMEM, 10% fetal bovine serum, and 1% penicillin–streptomycin and incubated at 37°C in humidified atmosphere with 5% of CO_2 using standard interface method. The study was performed with the approval and guidelines of the Institutional Animal Care and Use Committee of the Slovak Academy of Sciences and with the European Communities Council Directive (2010/63/EU) regarding the use of animals in Research, Slovak Law for Animal Protection No. 377/2012 and 436/2012.

7.2. *In vitro* model of spinal cord injury and treatment

After adaptation, OTS-SCs were divided into four groups according to the treatment and cultivated for the next 3 days. (i) **OTS-SC** (OTS treated with CM-SC), (ii) **OTS-SCI** (OTS treated with CM-SCI) (iii) **OTS-SC + MSCs** (OTS co-cultured with rMSCs in CM-SC), and (iv) **OTS-SCI + MSCs** (OTS co-cultured with rMSCs in CM-SCI) (**Figure 3**).

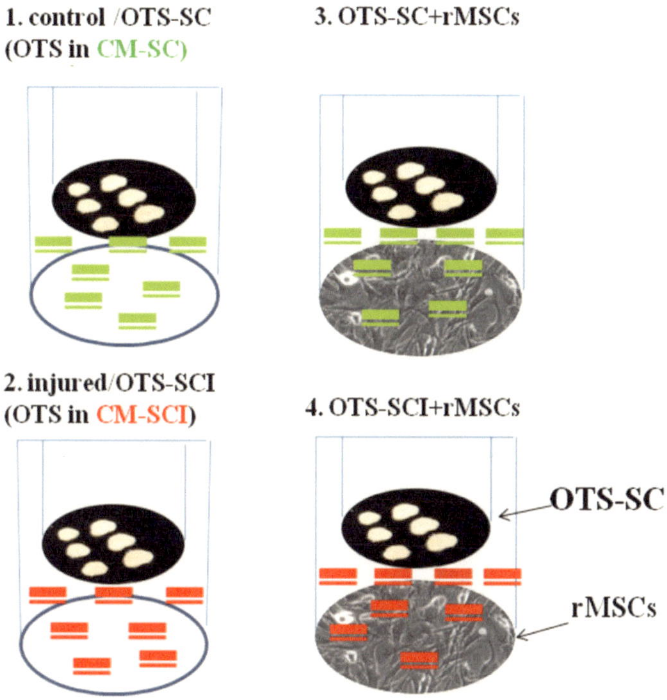

Figure 3. The design of the experiment. After adaptation, OTS-SCs were divided into four groups according to the treatment and cultivated for the next three days. Control group is represented by OTS-SCs treated with conditioned medium obtained from intact spinal cord. OTS-SCs treated with conditioned medium from injured spinal cord represent *in vitro* model of spinal cord injury. Both groups were co-cultured with mesenchymal stem cells to investigate the potential influence of these cells on behavior of different cell population in OTSs.

Rat MSCs were isolated from bone marrow of the long bones (femur, tibia) of adult male Wistar rats (290–320 g). To confirm the phenotypic characteristics of rMSC of the third passage, the surface markers (CD29, CD90, and CD45) were analyzed by flow cytometry [55]. The co-culture of rMSCs with OTS-SCs started at the same time with CM-SCI or CM-SC influence. On the basis of immunohistochemistry analyses for cell markers (Iba-microglial cells, GFAP-astrocytes, NeuN-neurons), after 3 days of treatment, OTS-SCs were analyzed using a Leica SP5X confocal microscope and an inverted Nikon ECLIPSE Ti fluorescence microscope. We examined the percentage of NeuN and Iba positive cells calculated from the total number of DAPI (4′,6-diamidino-2-phenylindole) - positive cells in 10 random visual fields (600 × 600 μm) in OTSs. The quantification of immunofluorescence intensity of GFAP positive cells was also analyzed by Image J software according to the previous protocol [56]. Data are presented as mean ± SEM. Statistical differences between groups were evaluated with ANOVA, and values of $*p < 0.05$ and $**p < 0.01$ were considered to be statistically significant.

7.3. Results

During the cultivation time, slices preserved their morphological and structural integrity with clear differentiation of white and gray matter. In response to injury induced by conditioned medium from injured spinal cord, both astrocytes and microglia were activated, while astrocytes served as a stimulus for microglial-mediated inflammation.

The highest positivity of the microglial populations was observed in the injured OTS-SCI group (3.98 ± 0.64%) when compared to control OTS-SC (1.36 ± 0.46%, $^{**}p < 0.01$) and OTS-SC + MSCs (1.22 ± 0.62%, $^{**}p < 0.01$) (**Figure 4**). OTS-SCI represents *in vitro* model of spinal cord injury. The treatment in *in vitro* model of spinal cord injury with MSCs, in OTS-SCI + MSCs group, caused a significant decrease of microglial cell population (2.9 ± 0.85%, $^{*}p < 0.05$) in comparison with the actual *in vitro* model of spinal cord injury. Astrocytes showed a similar pattern of behavior like microglia cells. The highest activation of astrocytes was observed in the OTS-SCI (density/25.26 ± 3.29) in comparison with the OTS-SC (density/14.31 ± 4.33, $^{*}p < 0.05$) and OTS-SCI + MSCs (density/19.52 ± 5.22, $^{*}p < 0.05$) groups (**Figure 5**). We observed an adverse impact of CM-SCI on the neuron presence in slices. The smallest number of the neurons (4.38 ± 1.77%) was found in the injured OTS-SCI slices. The co-culture with MSCs elevated the amount of the neurons (13.78 ± 4.51%, $^{**}p < 0.01$) in OTS-SC + MSCs when compared to actual *in vitro* model (**Figure 6**).

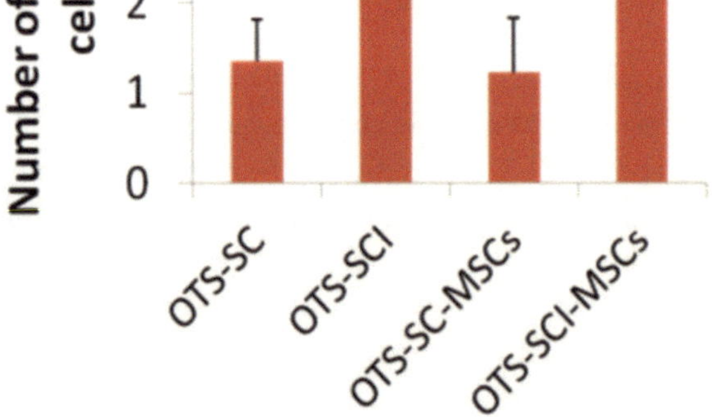

Figure 4. The number of Iba positive microglia cells observed in OTS-SCs treated with conditioned medium from intact/injured spinal cord OTS-SC/OTS-SCI and co-cultured with mesenchymal stem cells. Cultivation of spinal cord slices in CM-SCI caused a significant increase in number of microglial positive cells when compared to controls. Besides, co-cultivation of injured OTS with MSCs (OTS-SCI + MSCs) inhibits the activation of microglial cells causing a significant decrease of Iba positive cells in comparison to untreated *in vitro* model of spinal cord injury (OTS-SCI).

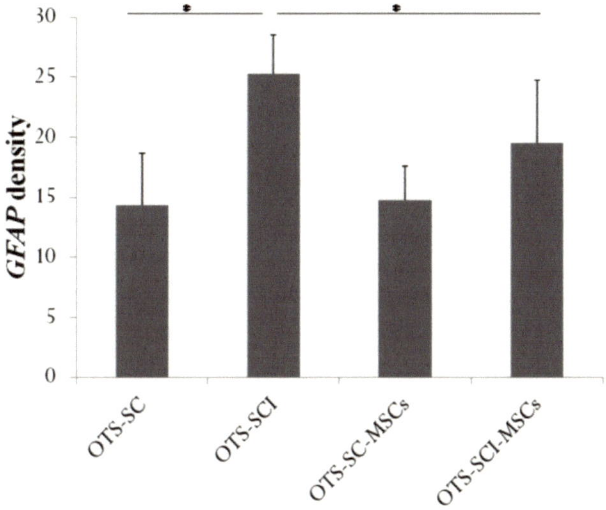

Figure 5. The GFAP density detected in OTS-SCs treated with conditioned medium from intact/injured spinal cord OTS-SC/OTS-SCI and co-cultured with mesenchymal stem cells. The highest activation of astrocytes was observed in the OTS-SCI and co-cultivation of injured OTS with MSCs (OTS-SCI + MSCs) caused a significant decrease of astrocytes when compared to untreated *in vitro* model of spinal cord injury (OTS-SCI).

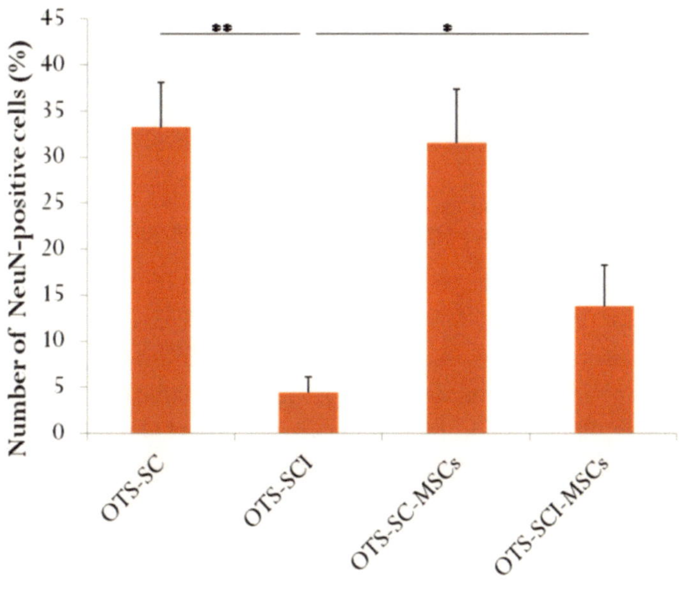

Figure 6. The number of NeuN positive cells noted in spinal cord slices treated with conditioned medium from intact/injured spinal cord OTS-SC/OTS-SCI and co-cultured with mesenchymal stem cells. Cultivation of spinal cord slices in CM-SCI caused a significant decrease in number of neuronal cells when compared to controls. MSCs have neurotrophic effects resulting in an increase of neuronal cells in *in vitro* model of spinal cord injury treated with MSCs (OTS-SCI + MSCs).

Our data revealed increased activity of microglia and astrocytes and elimination of neurons in experimental group treated with CM-SCI. We observed the presence of hypertrophied astrocytes with increased proliferation activity within the white matter of injured experimental group in contrary to controls. Astrocytes are one of the major glial cell types that maintain homeostasis in the undamaged CNS. After injury, astrocytes become reactive and prevent regeneration; however, it has also been suggested that astrocytes can become activated and promote regeneration. This indicated that reactive astrogliosis may exert both beneficial and detrimental effects in a context-specific manner determined by distinct molecular signaling cascades. Resident microglia in the control group OTS-SC was in the resting state and cells were few in number and smaller in size (**Figure 7A**). After inducing damage effects in the OTS-SCI with CM-SCI, quiescent microglial cells became activated, were bigger, and created ramified processes (**Figure 7B**).

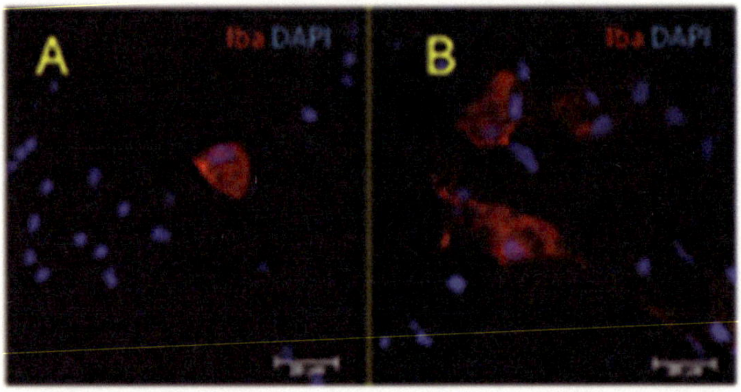

Figure 7. Fluorescent microscopy images of the residual microglia (red) in organotypic spinal cord slices (400 μm) stained with specific Iba antibody. The immunoreactive cells in control OTS-SC group (A) and injured OTS-SCI group (B). Scale bar is 10 μm.

Our study showed that (i) OTS-SC *in vitro* model closely mimics the post-injury microenvironment affecting the microglia and astrocytes cell response following secondary damage and is suitable for various pharmacy-therapeutic approaches, and that (ii) rMSCs are able to inhibit the activation of microglial cells and have neurotrophic effects on the neural cells. Thus, the effects shown in this study are directly mediated from various factors or proteins secreted from rMSCs. Our study represents the rMSC as a promising candidate for SCI treatment due to their potential to perform the immunomodulatory functions and to produce specific neurotrophic components and cytokines likewise to other results [57]. These techniques give us the possibility to achieve a moderate trauma in *in vitro* preparation, the organotypic slices that can be used to study short- and long-term effects and mechanisms of traumatic injury. Our study supports the recent hypothesis regarding the role of MSCs in establishing microenvironment more favorable for tissue repair. MSCs have a great potential in therapy for a range of neural insults.

http://dx.doi.org/10.5772/63459

8. Summary

Many *in vitro* models are invented, and others are still waiting for their further application, depending on the interest of researchers and key problems they are focused on. Many *in vitro* models are used in bright research field concerning the influence of any factor originated due to human activity we come into contact every day. For example, exposure of primary rat cortical neurons to extremely low-frequency electromagnetic fields has only limited (developmental) neurotoxic potential *in vitro* manifested by unchanged cell viability and neurite outgrowth [58]. Organotypic slice cultures have the potential to become powerful tools in the arsenal of drug discovery technology, lying at the interface between high-throughput screening and clinically relevant animal disease models. It has to be mentioned, however, that the cultured slices cannot represent all the *in vivo* properties. However, organotypic slices can model different histopathological aspects of neurological conditions and are a suitable *in vitro* system to address a wide range of questions concerning mechanisms of nerve regeneration after injury in the adult nervous system and to identify the factors supporting or preventing axonal outgrowth as well as cell survival that will ultimately add to the development of therapeutic application for spinal cord injury. Organotypic culture technique is easy, efficient, and practical and allows reduction of animal number and preserves the three-dimensional neuronal network. Although these *in vitro* organotypic slices have been able to model and reproduce many processes taking place after CNS injury with subsequent regeneration, some limitations exist, including the lack of any functioning vasculature, an incomplete immune system. Thus, OTSs have their own advantages and disadvantages with regard to stimulating *in vivo* conditions. Obviously, organotypic slices cannot replace *in vivo* models, which are still necessary and remain the only way to evaluate the functional outcome of a therapeutic strategy [59].

Acknowledgements

We acknowledge the financial support given by the Grant Agency of the Slovak Academy of Sciences: VEGA 2/0169/13, VEGA 2/0125/15, and VEGA 2/0145/16.

Author details

Lucia Slovinska*, Juraj Blasko, Miriam Nagyova, Eva Szekiova and Dasa Cizkova

*Address all correspondence to: slovinska@saske.sk

Institute of Neurobiology, Slovak Academy of Sciences, Kosice, Slovakia

References

[1] Rowland J, Hawryluk GW, Kwon B, Fehlings MG: Current status of acute spinal cord injury pathophysiology and emerging therapies: promise on the horizon. Neurosurg Focus 2008; 25: E2.

[2] Fawcett JW, Asher RA: The glial scar and central nervous system repair. Brain Res Bull 1999; 49: 377–391.

[3] Rudge JS, Silver J: Inhibition of neurite outgrowth on astroglial scars in vitro. J Neurosci 1990; 10: 3594–3603.

[4] Tom VJ, Steinmetz MP, Miller JH, Doller CM, Silver J: Studies on the development and behavior of the dystrophic growth cone, the hallmark of regeneration failure, in an in vitro model of the glial scar and after spinal cord injury. J Neurosci 2004; 24: 6531–6539.

[5] Boomkamp SD, McGrath MA, Houslay MD, Barnett SC: Epac and the high affinity rolipram binding conformer of PDE4 modulate neurite outgrowth and myelination using an in vitro spinal cord injury model. Br J Pharmacol 2014; 171: 2385–2398.

[6] Slovinska L, Szekiova E, Blasko J, Devaux S, Salzet M, Cizkova D: Comparison of dynamic behavior and maturation of neural multipotent cells derived from different spinal cord developmental stages: an in vitro study. Acta Neurobiol Exp (Wars) 2015; 75: 107–114.

[7] Morrison B, 3rd, Saatman KE, Meaney DF, McIntosh TK: In vitro central nervous system models of mechanically induced trauma: a review. J Neurotrauma 1998; 15: 911–928.

[8] Shearer MC, Niclou SP, Brown D, Asher RA, Holtmaat AJ, Levine JM, Verhaagen J, Fawcett JW: The astrocyte/meningeal cell interface is a barrier to neurite outgrowth which can be overcome by manipulation of inhibitory molecules or axonal signalling pathways. Mol Cell Neurosci 2003; 24: 913–925.

[9] Wanner IB, Deik A, Torres M, Rosendahl A, Neary JT, Lemmon VP, Bixby JL: A new in vitro model of the glial scar inhibits axon growth. Glia 2008; 56: 1691–1709.

[10] Hopkins AM, DeSimone E, Chwalek K, Kaplan DL: 3D in vitro modeling of the central nervous system. Prog Neurobiol 2015; 125: 1–25.

[11] Boomkamp SD, Riehle MO, Wood J, Olson MF, Barnett SC: The development of a rat in vitro model of spinal cord injury demonstrating the additive effects of Rho and ROCK inhibitors on neurite outgrowth and myelination. Glia 2012; 60: 441–456.

[12] Kim BG, Hwang DH, Lee SI, Kim EJ, Kim SU: Stem cell-based cell therapy for spinal cord injury. Cell Transplant 2007; 16: 355–364.

[13] Nash B, Thomson CE, Linington C, Arthur AT, McClure JD, McBride MW, Barnett SC: Functional duality of astrocytes in myelination. J Neurosci 2011; 31: 13028–13038.

http://dx.doi.org/10.5772/63459

[14] Ioannidou K, Edgar JM, Barnett SC: Time-lapse imaging of glial-axonal interactions. Curr Protoc Neurosci 2012; 72: 2.23.21–22.23.14.

[15] Ioannidou K, Anderson KI, Strachan D, Edgar JM, Barnett SC: Astroglial–axonal interactions during early stages of myelination in mixed cultures using in vitro and ex vivo imaging techniques. BMC Neurosci 2014; 15: 59.

[16] Sorensen A, Moffat K, Thomson C, Barnett SC: Astrocytes, but not olfactory ensheathing cells or Schwann cells, promote myelination of CNS axons in vitro. Glia 2008; 56: 750–763.

[17] Al-Ali H, Beckerman S, Bixby JL, Lemmon VP: In vitro models of axon regeneration. Exp Neurol 2016. In press - doi:10.1016/j.expneurol.2016.01.020

[18] Ribeiro C, Slgado AJ, Fraga JS, Silva NA, Reis RL, Sousa N: The secretome of bone marrow mesenchymal stem cells-conditioned media varies with time and drives a distinct effect on mature neurons and glial cells (primary cultures). J Tissue Eng Regen Med 2011; DOI: 10.1002/term.

[19] Gahwiler BH: Organotypic cultures of neural tissue. Trends Neurosci 1988; 11: 484–489.

[20] Gahwiler BH: Organotypic monolayer cultures of nervous tissue. J Neurosci Methods 1981; 4: 329–342.

[21] Gahwiler BH, Capogna M, Debanne D, McKinney RA, Thompson SM: Organotypic slice cultures: a technique has come of age. Trends Neurosci 1997; 20: 471–477.

[22] Victorov IV, Lyjin AA, Aleksandrova OP: A modified roller method for organotypic brain cultures: free-floating slices of postnatal rat hippocampus. Brain Res Protoc 2001; 7: 30–37.

[23] Stoppini L, Buchs PA, Muller D: A simple method for organotypic cultures of nervous tissue. J Neurosci Methods 1991; 37: 173–182.

[24] Adamchik Y, Frantseva MV, Weisspapir M, Carlen PL, Perez Velazquez JL: Methods to induce primary and secondary traumatic damage in organotypic hippocampal slice cultures. Brain Res Protoc 2000; 5: 153–158.

[25] Krassioukov AV, Ackery A, Schwartz G, Adamchik Y, Liu Y, Fehlings MG: An in vitro model of neurotrauma in organotypic spinal cord cultures from adult mice. Brain Res Protoc 2002; 10: 60–68.

[26] Sypecka J, Koniusz S, Kawalec M, Sarnowska A: The organotypic longitudinal spinal cord slice culture for stem cell study. Stem Cells Int 2015; 2015: 471216.

[27] Förster E, Bartos M, Zhao S: Hippocampal slice cultures. In: Poindron P, Piguet P, Förster E (eds.) New methods for culturing cells from nervous tissues. BioValley Monogr, vol. 1. Basel, Karger; 2005: p. 1–11.

[28] Savas A, Warnke PC, Ginap T, Feuerstein TJ, Ostertag CB: The effects of continuous and single-dose radiation on choline uptake in organotypic tissue slice cultures of rabbit hippocampus. Neurol Res 2001; 23: 669–675.

[29] Jeong D, Taghavi CE, Song KJ, Lee KB, Kang HW: Organotypic human spinal cord slice culture as an alternative to direct transplantation of human bone marrow precursor cells for treating spinal cord injury. World Neurosurg 2011; 75: 533–539.

[30] Noraberg J, Kristensen BW, Zimmer J: Markers for neuronal degeneration in organotypic slice cultures. Brain Res Protoc 1999; 3: 278–290.

[31] Morrison B, 3rd, Eberwine JH, Meaney DF, McIntosh TK: Traumatic injury induces differential expression of cell death genes in organotypic brain slice cultures determined by complementary DNA array hybridization. Neuroscience 2000; 96: 131–139.

[32] Ravikumar M, Jain S, Miller RH, Capadona JR, Selkirk SM: An organotypic spinal cord slice culture model to quantify neurodegeneration. J Neurosci Methods 2012; 211: 280–288.

[33] Noraberg J, Poulsen FR, Blaabjerg M, Kristensen BW, Bonde C, Montero M, Meyer M, Gramsbergen JB, Zimmer J: Organotypic hippocampal slice cultures for studies of brain damage, neuroprotection and neurorepair. Curr Drug Targets CNS Neurol Disord 2005; 4: 435–452.

[34] Sundstrom L, Morrison B, 3rd, Bradley M, Pringle A: Organotypic cultures as tools for functional screening in the CNS. Drug Discov Today 2005; 10: 993–1000.

[35] Frantseva MV, Carlen PL, El-Beheiry H: A submersion method to induce hypoxic damage in organotypic hippocampal cultures. J Neurosci Methods 1999; 89: 25–31.

[36] Feeney CJ, Frantseva MV, Carlen PL, Pennefather PS, Shulyakova N, Shniffer C, Mills LR: Vulnerability of glial cells to hydrogen peroxide in cultured hippocampal slices. Brain Res 2008; 1198: 1–15.

[37] An SS, Pennant WA, Ha Y, Oh JS, Kim HJ, Gwak SJ, Yoon DH, Kim KN: Hypoxia-induced expression of VEGF in the organotypic spinal cord slice culture. Neuroreport 2011; 22: 55–60.

[38] Mazzone GL, Nistri A: S100beta as an early biomarker of excitotoxic damage in spinal cord organotypic cultures. J Neurochem 2014; 130: 598–604.

[39] Nava J, Mayorenko II, Grehl T, Steinbuch HWM, Weis J, Brook GA: Differential pattern of neuroprotection in lumbar, cervical and thoracic spinal cord segments in an organotypic rat model of glutamate-induced excitotoxicity. J Chem Neuroanat 2013; 53: 11–17.

[40] Balentine JD, Greene WB, Bornstein M: In vitro spinal cord trauma. Lab Invest 1988; 58: 93–99.

[41] Bonnici B, Kapfhammer JP: Spontaneous regeneration of intrinsic spinal cord axons in a novel spinal cord slice culture model. Eur J Neurosci 2008; 27: 2483–2492.

[42] Kim HM, Lee HJ, Lee MY, Kim SU, Kim BG: Organotypic spinal cord slice culture to study neural stem/progenitor cell microenvironment in the injured spinal cord. Exp Neurobiol 2010; 19: 106–113.

[43] Glazova MV, Pak ES, Murashov AK: Neurogenic potential of spinal cord organotypic culture. Neurosci Lett 2015; 594: 60–65.

[44] Delfs J, Friend J, Ishimoto S, Saroff D: Ventral and dorsal horn acetylcholinesterase neurons are maintained in organotypic cultures of postnatal rat spinal cord explants. Brain Res 1989; 488: 31–42.

[45] Bin JM, Leong SY, Bull SJ, Antel JP, Kennedy TE: Oligodendrocyte precursor cell transplantation into organotypic cerebellar shiverer slices: a model to study myelination and myelin maintenance. PLoS One 2012; 7: e41237.

[46] Sygnecka K, Heider A, Scherf N, Alt R, Franke H, Heine C: Mesenchymal stem cells support neuronal fiber growth in an organotypic brain slice co-culture model. Stem Cells Dev 2014; 24: 824–835.

[47] Cho JS, Park HW, Park SK, Roh S, Kang SK, Paik KS, Chang MS: Transplantation of mesenchymal stem cells enhances axonal outgrowth and cell survival in an organotypic spinal cord slice culture. Neurosci Lett 2009; 454: 43–48.

[48] Dean JM, Riddle A, Maire J, Hansen KD, Preston M, Barnes AP, Sherman LS, Back SA: An organotypic slice culture model of chronic white matter injury with maturation arrest of oligodendrocyte progenitors. Mol Neurodegener 2011; 6: 46.

[49] Ngalula KP, Cramer N, Schell MJ, Juliano SL: Transplanted neural progenitor cells from distinct sources migrate differentially in an organotypic model of brain injury. Front Neurol 2015; 6: 212.

[50] Schmidt H, Tlustochowska A, Stuertz K, Djukic M, Gerber J, Schutz E, Kuhnt U, Nau R: Organotypic hippocampal cultures. A model of brain tissue damage in Streptococcus pneumoniae meningitis. J Neuroimmunol 2001; 113: 30–39.

[51] Guldimann C, Lejeune B, Hofer S, Leib SL, Frey J, Zurbriggen A, Seuberlich T, Oevermann A: Ruminant organotypic brain-slice cultures as a model for the investigation of CNS listeriosis. Int J Exp Pathol 2012; 93: 259–268.

[52] Martinez R, Eraso D, Geffin R, McCarthy M: A two-culture method for exposure of human brain organotypic slice cultures to replicating human immunodeficiency virus type 1. J Neurosci Methods 2011; 200: 74–79.

[53] Pandamooz S, Nabiuni M, Miyan J, Ahmadiani A, Dargahi L: Organotypic spinal cord culture: a proper platform for the functional screening. Mol Neurobiol 2015. DOI 10.1007/s12035-015-9403-z

[54] Vanicky I, Urdzikova L, Saganova K, Cizkova D, Galik J: A simple and reproducible model of spinal cord injury induced by epidural balloon inflation in the rat. J Neurotrauma 2001; 18: 1399–1407.

[55] Nagyova M, Slovinska L, Blasko J, Grulova I, Kuricova M, Cigankova V, Harvanova D, Cizkova D: A comparative study of PKH67, DiI, and BrdU labeling techniques for tracing rat mesenchymal stem cells. In Vitro Cell Dev Biol Anim 2014; 50: 656–663.

[56] Jones LL, Tuszynski MH: Spinal cord injury elicits expression of keratan sulfate proteoglycans by macrophages, reactive microglia, and oligodendrocyte progenitors. J Neurosci 2002; 22: 4611–4624.

[57] Bai L, Lennon DP, Caplan AI, DeChant A, Hecker J, Kranso J, Zaremba A, Miller R: Hepatocyte growth factor mediates MSCs stimulated functional recovery in animal models of MS. Nat Neurosci 2012; 15: 862–870.

[58] de Groot MW, van Kleef RG, de Groot A, Westerink RH: In vitro developmental neurotoxicity following chronic exposure to 50 Hz extremely low-frequency electromagnetic fields in primary rat cortical cultures. Toxicol Sci 2016; 149: 433–440.

[59] Daviaud N, Garbayo E, Schiller PC, Perez-Pinzon M, Montero-Menei CN: Organotypic cultures as tools for optimizing central nervous system cell therapies. Exp Neurol 2013; 248: 429–440.

Section 2

Modulating Cellular and Molecular Responses to Spinal Cord Injury

Chapter 3

Protective Role of the Immune System in Spinal Cord Injury: Immunomodulation with Altered Peptide Ligands

Paola Suárez-Meade and Antonio Ibarra

Additional information is available at the end of the chapter

http://dx.doi.org/10.5772/63221

Abstract

Spinal cord injury (SCI) is a phenomenon characterized by damage to the spinal cord and nerve roots, resulting in loss of physiological activity below the lesion. Injury to the spinal cord activates a cascade of cellular and molecular reactions in which the immune system plays an essential role, as there is an uncontrolled immune response that endows further damage to neural tissue. However, the activity of immune system at the site of injury can be modified in order to obtain a neuroprotective environment and promote SCI recovery. This strategy has been designed under the light of the innovative concept "protective autoimmunity" (PA) and can be stimulated with the use of altered peptide ligands (APL). Adequate immunomodulation with APL can be obtained with the peptide A91, which is a safe synthetic peptide derived from the myelin basic protein (MBP) that has proven to be effective in preclinical research. Immunization with A91 is carried out with the objective of preventing further damage and promoting neuroprotection. This peptide has direct influence over SCI secondary mechanisms such as inflammation, lipid peroxidation, and apoptosis. Preclinical results suggest that immunization with A91 could be an effective treatment in the clinical field, providing a better quality of life to SCI patients.

Keywords: spinal cord injury, protective autoimmunity, A91, altered peptide ligand, immunization

1. Introduction

Spinal cord injury (SCI) is perhaps one of the most devastating conditions as it results in a disruption of motor, sensory, and autonomic functions, leading to permanent neurological disability. According to the National Spinal Cord Injury Statistical Center (NSCISC), in 2014 over 276,000 people were suffering from SCI [1]. The incidence ranges over 12,500 new cases each year, with a prevalence of approximately 40 cases per million in the United States [2]. Epidemiological studies indicate that SCI has a higher incidence among male population, and people between 30 and 50 years old [3, 3]. Clinically, the most disabling outcomes of traumatic SCI are motor deficit and sensory loss. Nonetheless, due to autonomic dysfunction and depending on the level and severity of injury, SCI may also alter normal homeostasis and the respiratory, reproductive, urinary, and gastrointestinal systems [4–6]. Besides surgical intervention, the standard of care for SCI in several countries focuses on preventing shock and further damage with the use of methylprednisolone (MP), a synthetic glucocorticoid with anti-inflammatory properties. The National Acute Spinal Cord Injury Study (NASCIS) trials suggest that high-dose MP is effective for the management of acute SCI [5, 8]. However, further studies about NASCIS results indicate that the clinical benefits of the use of MP as a treatment for SCI are questionable [6, 10]. Acute MP therapy reduces cellular damage and secondary injury mechanisms but leads to risks of high-dose steroids [7]. For this reason, MP administration after SCI is still a controversial treatment, and it continues to be debated [8].

Another molecule that has been widely studied for the clinical treatment of SCI is Ganglioside, which is highly expressed in the cell membranes of the central nervous system (CNS). The synthetic form of this glycosphingolipid—monosialotetrahexosylganglioside (GM1)—was known for having anti-apoptotic, anti-excitotoxic, and neuroprotective properties [9, 14]. Therefore, several clinical trials were designed in order to test this drug on SCI [10]. In the most recent study, patients received NASCIS II doses of MP, and different doses of GM1 after the effect of MP was over. Although, GM1 treated patients presented a significant recovery, the beneficial effects related to the drug were inconsistent between different types of injuries and were lost during chronic SCI stages [11, 17]. These results suggest that GM1 has a limited effect and to the date, it is not an approved treatment for SCI [12].

Undoubtedly, the lack of an available treatment for SCI in the clinical field highlights the need to design new and safe therapies for injured patients. Nowadays, research is focused on targeting secondary SCI mechanisms with the objective of minimizing further damage, promoting regeneration and thus, improving functional recovery [13, 19]. One of the most important secondary injury mechanisms is the post-traumatic inflammatory response, which is roughly characterized by the presence of injury-dependent pro-inflammatory cytokines and infiltration of peripheral immune cells to the damaged area [14–22]. It was previously thought that the presence of this uncontrolled immune response in the CNS was harmful and pathological. However, other findings state a controversial theory: immune cells could play an essential role in neuroprotection and regeneration of the spinal cord after injury [15]. A better understanding of how inflammation mediates secondary injury suggests that suppressing all immune responses with the use of glucocorticoids is no longer a rational treatment approach. This information has led scientists to further investigate the beneficial effects of the immune system in several neurological conditions, including SCI [16]. Focusing on the beneficial mechanisms of the immune system after trauma has opened the doors for the design of a new therapeutic strategy. Nevertheless, some questions should first be answered. For instance, how can the immune system be modulated to attain a protective microenvironment? What are the immune-related elements capable of providing the required immune-modulation? And how are they able to provide recovery after SCI?

2. Spinal cord injury pathophysiology

Damage to the spinal cord (SC) causes anatomical and functional deficits to the CNS, that result in the appearance of several long-term medical comorbidities. SCI is characterized by two different pathophysiological phases: primary and secondary injury [17]. Initial trauma to the SC—known as primary injury—is caused by a compressive or contusive mechanism that results in gross anatomical tissue disruption, and immediate hemostatic self-defense events that produce further damage to CNS structures. Direct impact to the SC leads to vascular disturbances such as hemorrhage, ischemia, edema, and hypoperfusion, resulting in tissue necrosis [18]. Hemorrhage and edema formation can raise the risk of developing increased parenchymal pressure and produce more tissue damage [19]. Also, reactive gliosis, demyelination, and axonal loss are often caused by immediate trauma and sustained compression to neural tissue [20]. Depending upon primary injury characteristics, there could be greater tissue damage and worse functional outcomes. Therefore, during this phase, treatment should focus on hemorrhage control to avoid necrosis and early decompression to stabilize intrathecal pressure.

As a consequence of primary injury, there is a cascade of biological reactions that occur minutes after injury and last for several weeks known as secondary injury [21]. This phase is quite complex, as it consists of the development of mechanisms like loss of ATP-dependent cellular functions, ion homeostasis imbalance, excitotoxicity, oxidative stress, lipid peroxidation, inflammation, and apoptosis [22]. There are several secondary mechanisms that are strongly related to the ischemic event observed in SCI. Ischemia produces a depletion of the intracellular amount of ATP, leading to a reduction in the energy-dependent cell function that preserve ion homeostasis [23]. Therefore, the sodium-potassium pump cannot execute its physiological activity, resulting in an elevated potassium (K^+) efflux, and a high influx of sodium (Na^+), calcium (Ca^{2+}), and chloride (Cl^-) into the cell. This homeostasis imbalance alters normal ion concentrations within the intracellular and extracellular spaces, producing a sustained membrane depolarization and a release of excitatory amino acid (EAA) neurotransmitters [24]. The pathological effect related to an increased concentration of EAA neurotransmitters, such as glutamate and aspartate, is known as excitotoxicity. This secondary injury mechanism is characterized by an overstimulation of the NMDA, kainate and AMPA glutamate receptors, which causes massive intracellular Ca^{2+} concentrations, resulting in a pathological neuronal excitation and cell death [25, 32]. Glial cells—especially oligodendrocytes—are very sensitive to excitotoxic damage because of their high expression of ionotropic glutamate receptors [26]. That is why an excessive glutamate accumulation related to SCI can produce oligodendrocyte death, and consequent white matter demyelination [27]. Also, because of glutamate excitotoxicity, there is an increased production of free radicals by reactive microglia, which contribute to lipid peroxidation (LP), and mitochondrial dysfunction [28, 36]. Therefore, this sustained toxic microenvironment is postulated to be one of the most detrimental secondary injury mechanisms related to SCI.

Oxidative stress accompanies secondary injury damage, and is mainly characterized by an increased mitochondrial production of reactive oxygen species (ROS) and reactive nitrogen species (RNS) [29, 38]. The elevation in ROS and RNS concentration is closely related to the aforementioned high Ca^{2+} influx to the cells, as it stimulates free radical production [30]. Free radicals such as superoxide anion (O_2^-), nitric oxide (NO), and peroxynitrite ($ONOO^-$) create a toxic microenvironment by oxidizing nearby molecules producing neural energy failure, blood-brain barrier dysfunction, vascular reactivity, and potentiating inflammation [31, 41]. At high concentrations, these molecules can become cytotoxic and worsen secondary injury mechanisms [32]. Oxidative stress also influences excitotoxicity by exacerbating Ca^{2+} deregulation and thus, glutamate concentrations. The pathological production of ROS that arises after trauma causes oxidative damage, especially on lipids, originating LP. LP is characterized by producing a disruption in the normal structure of the polyunsaturated fatty acids in the cell membrane, such as arachidonic acid, and linoleic acid. In LP, the high concentration of free radicals, results in functional compromise and cell death [33, 43]. Also, structural damage to the cell membrane produces a reduction in the generation and transmission of the electrical potentials leading to synapse dysfunction [34]. Altogether these mechanisms potentiate apoptosis, which is a form of programmed cell death characterized by cell shrinkage, nuclear pyknosis, and chromatin aggregation in a stressful environment [35]. This deleterious event, (apoptosis) occurs after SCI by stimulation of the apoptosis-inducing factor (AIF) to the nucleus, or by direct mitochondrial disruption leading to a subsequent activation of caspase-3 signaling pathways [36, 47]. Evidence supports that secondary injury mechanisms contribute to delayed tissue damage, exacerbating damage, and limiting recovery after traumatic SCI.

2.1. Pathophysiological involvement of the immune system

The immune system has a pivotal and somehow controversial role within the pathophysiology of traumatic SCI. Immediately after trauma there is an activation of the inflammatory response that consists in the proliferation of resident microglia and astrocytes, a high concentration of pro-inflammatory molecules, and infiltration of peripheral immune cells to the site of injury (**Figure 1**). SCI induces the activation of a series of inflammatory stimuli leading to an increased concentration of cytokines and inflammatory cells that will determine the extent of secondary damage [37]. Evidence suggests that in the presence of an excitotoxic and inflammatory microenvironment, microglial cells differentiate into a M1 pro-inflammatory phenotype [38]. Under these conditions, activated microglia is capable of secreting interleukin 1β (IL-1β), IL-6, tumor necrosis factor-alpha (TNFα), and macrophage colony-stimulating factor (MCSF) which are pro-inflammatory in nature [39].

A high free radical and cytotoxic substances secretion is more evident when there is microglial activation starting at day one, and increasing at 7 days post-injury [40]. That is why the immune response is closely related to LP, as these cells are capable of boosting ROS and NO concentrations, favoring oxidative stress, cell membrane dysfunction and thus, apoptosis [41, 50]. At the same time, TNFα stimulates astrocyte proliferation and growth, leading to the formation of the glial scar within the chronic stages of SCI impeding axonal regeneration through the site of injury [42, 53]. Glial cells act immediately after trauma; they secrete pro-inflammatory molecules and promote inflammation, favoring the appearance of secondary injury mechanisms. In spite of the above mentioned deleterious effects, microglial—especially when differentiated into an M2 phenotype (IL-10 and TGF-beta)—and astrocyte activation could produce a beneficial effect through a high production of growth factors like brain derived neurotrophic factor (BDNF), and neurotrophin-3 (NT-3), essential for tissue repair [43]. Also, these cells are capable of expressing glutamate transporters that help reducing harmful

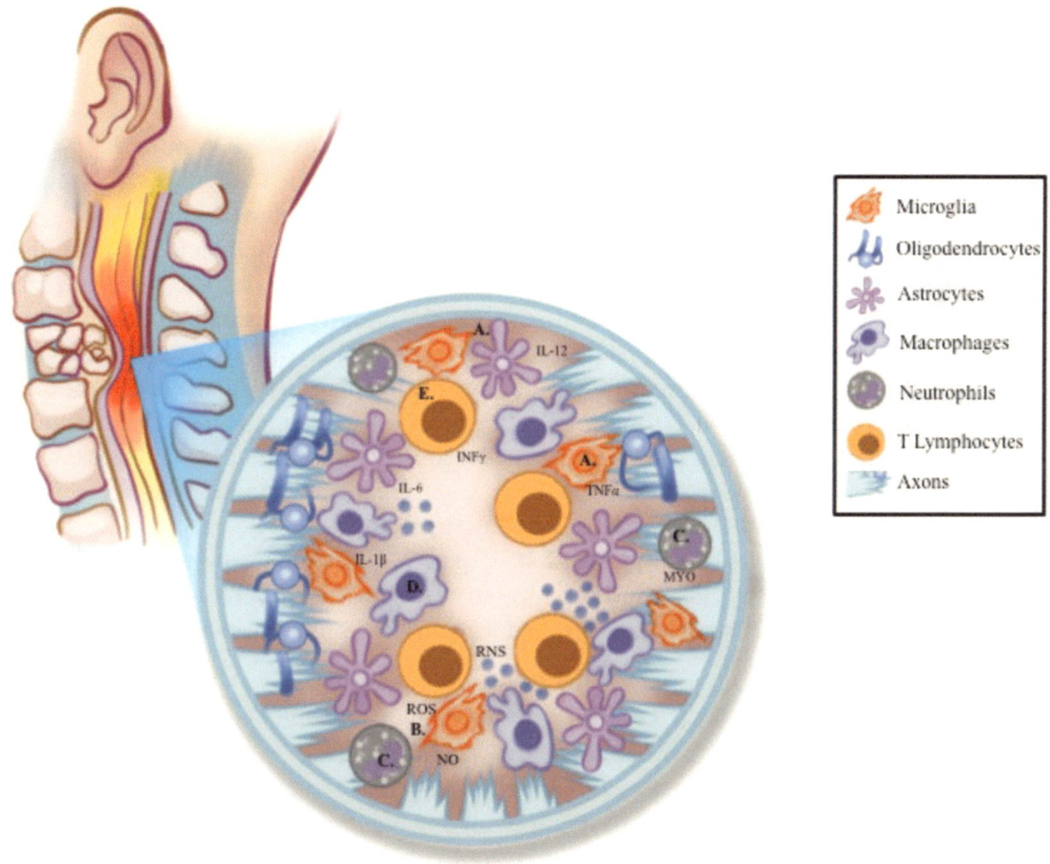

Figure 1. Cellular immune response in SCI. **A.** M1 microglial differentiation, astrocyte activation, and IL-1β, IL-6, and TNFα secretion. **B.** Increase in the concentration of ROS, NO, and RNS. **C.** Peripheral infiltration of neutrophils and myeloperoxidase secretion. **D.** Macrophages arise from peripheral tissue and activate the adaptive immune response. **E.** Infiltration of T-lymphocytes to the site of injury and INFγ secretion. Abbreviations: IL, interleukin; RNS, reactive nitrogen species; ROS, reactive oxygen species; NO, nitric oxide; TNFα, tumor necrosis factor-alpha; INFγ, interferon-gamma; MYO, myeloperoxidase.

concentrations, leading to a reduction in excitotoxicity [44]. Evidence suggests that even though the immune system is considered to be completely pathological in nature, it can also provide beneficial effects for SCI repair.

In normal conditions, inflammatory reaction leads the response to a pathological outcome, promoting damage and spinal cord degeneration. The severity of SCI determines the intensity of the inflammatory response and the glial reaction to SCI. Glial cells are well distributed within the CNS, and have the ability to proliferate and migrate to the site of injury. In response to injury there is a high glial secretion of cytokines and chemokines—such as IL-1, IL-6, and TNFα—that allows migration of peripheral immune cells [45]. TNFα stimulates the expression of adhesion molecules like endothelial intracellular adhesion molecule -1 (ICAM-1) and vascular cell adhesion molecule-1 (VCAM-1) altering the blood-brain barrier permeability and inducing a peripheral infiltration of immune cells to the CNS (**Figure 1**). Cell infiltration to the CNS is considered the principal factor for tissue disruption and sustained neural damage. The first peripheral cells to arrive at the site of injury are neutrophils [46]. These cells have the ability to phagocyte and clear debris, but they also secrete ROS and RNS, as well as other pathological proteolytic and oxidative enzymes like myeloperoxidase, producing greater tissue damage [47, 58]. At the same time, macrophages arise from resident microglia or from peripheral monocytes with the objective of removing cell debris and stimulating angiogenesis [48]. These cells play an essential role in the immune response, as they help in the activation and reclusion of the adaptive immune system cells. Microglia, astrocytes and dendritic cells may act as antigen-presenting cells (APC), leading to T lymphocyte activation, proliferation, and infiltration to the site of injury [49]. Lymphocytes recognize the signal and proliferate creating large numbers of clones, specific to the antigen being presented by the APC. At 3 days post-injury, there is an evident infiltration of T-cells to the CNS, these cells determine the intensity and continue on modulating the immune response to trauma [50]. In SCI, the presence of T-lymphocytes is considered detrimental as they secrete a Th1 cytokine profile including interferon gamma (IFNγ) [51, 63]. IFNγ is a pro-inflammatory cytokine capable of inducing free radical production, increasing IL-6, IL-12, IL-1β, and TNFα concentrations, and activating apoptotic-signaling pathways [52–65]. These events represent the immune activity within the acute phases of SCI and if it is not well controlled it could turn into a chronic and degenerative immune response.

When inflammation is modulated, i.e., we control the intensity of inflammatory response, the type, the action, and the arrival of immune cells, we could expect a change in the final outcome. With this regard, there is a strong evidence suggesting that lymphocytes could also have favorable activity, as they are capable of synthesizing several growth factors, like BDNF, NT3, and nerve growth factor (NGF) [53–68]. These molecules are known for being capable of promoting a protective and regenerative environment for CNS disorders [54].

To the date, it is clear that the immune response appearing after SCI could be pathological if it is not well controlled at the onset of SCI [55]. In a short period of time, this uncontrolled response leads to the extensive recognition of CNS peptides, proteins, lipids, or nucleic acids by the immune system [56]. This interaction between immune cells and CNS constituents—like the MBP—promotes the activation of lymphocytes and thereby, the possible development of an autoimmune response [57, 72, 73]. As a result, higher levels of demyelination are noted, leading to loss of sensitive and motor synapses. Also, several studies have identified that B cells secrete self-reactive antibodies and pro-inflammatory cytokines, promoting autoimmune activity [58, 75]. Therefore, the immune response elicited after SCI is considered to be one of the most important secondary injury mechanisms, as it plays an essential role in stimulating the appearance of a neurotoxic microenvironment after injury. However, further studies about the immune system and its relationship with CNS damage suggest that it is not completely pathological, as it has protective and regenerative properties [59–78].

3. Protective autoimmunity

The reactive immune response against self-constituents appearing after injury has been widely studied, as it can be an excellent target in the design of new therapies for SCI treatment. It was previously thought that the presence of immune activity was detrimental and it had to be suppressed [60–81]. However, more recent findings suggest that such response and the infiltration of peripheral immune cells to the site of injury is a phenomenon destined to protect and restore the CNS after trauma. The phenomenon capable of inducing this beneficial actions has been termed protective autoimmunity (PA) and is a mechanism in which the adaptive immune cells—especially lymphocytes that recognize self-constituents and potentiate an autoreactive response—help maintain tissue integrity in SCI. Researchers have demonstrated that PA is genetically encoded, and it is a physiological phenomenon linked to the inflammatory activity in the CNS, capable of providing protection in several neurodegenerative disorders [61, 83]. The immune system plays an essential role in tissue restoration, angiogenesis, and is capable of increasing functional recovery in CNS trauma [62]. However, in normal conditions the intense inflammatory response appearing after injury overshadows the beneficial effects of PA. For that reason, it was thought that boosting PA after injury could promote the beneficial instead of deleterious effects of the immune response to injury. In an attempt to test this hypothesis, researchers performed a passive transfer of T-cells specific to MBP, and demonstrated that it reduced tissue damage and improved motor recovery in rats with SCI [63, 86]. These studies suggested that the delayed adaptive immune response to injury and the low concentration of autoreactive T-cells are the reasons why PA is not evident, but a higher and earlier presence of these cells could potentiate the beneficial effects of PA over SCI.

Shortly after researchers envisioned that active immunization could elicit a higher proliferation and migration of autoreactive (antigen specific) T-cells to the CNS increasing the action of PA. Therefore, immunization with natural CNS components could help activate this response [64]. In line with this motion, several studies were performed indicating that, immunization with MBP can modulate the immune response, potentiate PA, and provide neuroprotection to the injured tissue [65, 88, 89]. In spite of the encouraging results, immune modulation with neural constituents increases the risk of developing an autoimmune disease such as experimental autoimmune encephalomyelitis (in rodents; EAE) or multiple sclerosis (in humans; MS) [66, 91]. For that reason, neural constituents were studied with the objective of creating a peptide capable of stimulating PA and reducing the risk of developing an autoimmune disease [67, 93]. These experiments led to the creation of altered peptide ligands (APL), which are synthetic peptides with changes in specific amino acid residues, critical for T-cell receptor (TCR) binding [68]. In the normal immune response, the MBP has agonist properties as it interacts with the TCR, leading to lymphocyte differentiation toward a Th1 phenotype [69, 96, 97]. With the objective of altering TCR recognition, a specific amino acid substitution makes APL become partial agonists or antagonists capable of deviating the immune response [70, 98]. That is why APL are able to cause lymphocyte anergy or their differentiation to an anti-inflammatory Th2 phenotype. This way, APL can alter the natural response of the immune system after SCI, by being able to change the whole Th1 (pro-inflammatory) cytokine profile toward a Th2 (anti-inflammatory) profile. Therefore, by altering the immune response, APL represent a good therapeutic approach for the treatment of SCI and other neurodegenerative diseases [71, 99].

3.1. Modulation of protective autoimmunity with the use of altered peptide ligands

A safe and effective way of increasing PA is through immunization with APL [72]. This strategy allows a change in the interaction with the TCR from an agonist to a partial agonist switching the response toward a Th2 cytokine pattern [73]. To create APL, identification of the essential residues of MBP for an acquired immune response to self-determinants was investigated. Evidence indicates that the amino acid sequence including the 87 to 99 residues is the most encephalitogenic portion of the MBP and that it is essential for TCR recognition [74, 102]. This amino acid sequence was fundamental for the creation of several APL and the evaluation of their effect over the immune response [75]. Altering the amino acid sequence by substituting each residue of the encephalitogenic region of the MBP with alanine, led to the discovery of this group of APL [76, 104]. While trying to identify an ideal peptide to promote PA, several APL derived from MBP encephalitogenic epitopes like G91, A96, or A97, along with A91 were tested as therapeutic strategies for CNS trauma. These peptides were capable of controlling the MBP peptide induced autoimmune reaction by altering the MBP specific T-cell responses [77]. Also, these APL demonstrated to be able of providing significant protection by reducing neuronal loss [78]. More importantly, they were limited the extent of the immune secondary injury mechanisms by inducing changes in the cytokine secretion profile of T-cells and enhanced the recovery of motor activity [79, 99, 103]. Studied APL showed different levels of neuroprotection, however, the conclusion of these conducted studies was that the APL A91 provided the best therapeutic effects without the risk of an autoimmune response [80].

Evidence has demonstrated that lysine at the position 91 is an essential residue of the MBP p87–99 for the development of a Th1 immune response. With this respect, it has been shown that when the amino acid 91 (lysine) is replaced with glycine (G91), the peptide which is non-encephalitogenic, regulates the proliferative response and modifies the cytokine secretion profile (toward a Th2 profile) of encephalitogenic MBP 87–99 reactive T-cells [81, 99, 103, 104]. The substitution of lysine at the position 91 for the amino acid alanine led to the creation of the APL: A91. This APL counteracts the production of pro-inflammatory cytokines, generating a microenvironment with anti-inflammatory features [82, 103, 104]. A91 (amino acid sequence:

VHFFANIVTPRTP) is a safe synthetic non-encephalitogenic peptide, capable of inhibiting the development of autoimmune disease while maintaining neuroprotection [83, 104]. This APL (A91) has proven to be an effective TCR partial agonist capable of modulating the immune response after CNS injury, and increasing the beneficial effects of PA. Immunization with A91peptide down regulates Th1 activity and increases the levels of a Th2 cytokine pattern (IL-4 and IL-10) creating an anti-inflammatory microenvironment [84, 105, 106].

3.2. The altered peptide ligand A91 as a potential treatment for spinal cord injury

To increase neuroprotection, A91 was designed to boost PA and to act directly over secondary mechanisms in SCI. Immunization with A91 has been tested as a subcutaneous injection, which has resulted to be an effective and minimally invasive route of administration. The use of this strategy in preclinical studies indicates that active immunization with A91 with a single dose of 150–200 μg improves neurological recovery. It is important to note that in order to avoid the risk of an autoimmune disease while maintaining neuroprotection, immunization with myelin-associated antigens should be fully controlled. A study evaluating the dose and therapeutic window of A91 indicates that beneficial effect of this peptide lies between 10 minutes up to 72 hours after SCI [85]. Further studies also indicate that A91 could be considered as a prophylactic therapeutic vaccine since its administration before SCI could provide high levels of neuroprotection and motor recovery [86]. These results could be of relevant benefit as an approach to provide with prophylactic measures to patients sustaining invasive spinal surgery procedures.

On the other hand, with the objective of evaluating the effect of A91 immunization in the presence of the gold standard treatment for SCI (MP) another study was carried out. The results of this investigation indicated that when these two treatments were administered at the same time, the beneficial properties of A91 were abolished [87]. However, the extensive therapeutic time window of A91 enables immediate MP administration and immunization with A91 up to 48 hours later [88, 109]. This approach has given the possibility of rescuing the beneficial effects elicited by A91, as animals subjected to this combined strategy, present neuroprotection and a higher motor recovery. These results also allow envisioning the possible clinical application of this therapy with no risk of avoiding the therapeutic effects theoretically provided by MP. In the search of increasing the neuroprotective effect of A91, double immunization has also been evaluated [89]. However, unexpectedly a higher concentration of this peptide eliminates the beneficial aftermath of the therapy [90]. Studies in our laboratory have also demonstrated that A91 can be applied at different SCI stages and still be effective. Our investigation suggests that adequate immunization must be performed immediately after injury or during the acute phase [91, 109]. Moreover, studies including vaccination of A91 in chronic SCI are now being conducted, and results have demonstrated to be profitable (Unpublished data).

APL were designed to specifically target the immune-related secondary injury mechanisms in order to attain neuroprotection, promote regeneration, and thus improving motor and sensory recovery in SCI. In line with this, previous studies have shown that immunization with A91 peptide produces an adequate T-cell proliferation characterized by a Th2 phenotype, where the production of IL-4 and IL-10 is increased [92, 110]. Additionally, A91 specific T-cells are capable of producing BDNF, which could be linked directly with the functional recovery appearing after immunization [93]. This anti-inflammatory and permissive microenvironment controls the inflammatory response elicited by SCI, reducing some of the main harmful phenomena developed by inflammation. For instance, it has been demonstrated that A91-immunization is capable of inhibiting LP, which is closely related to the action of immune system and it is one of the most aggressive phenomena related to SCI [94]. LP is present immediately after injury reaching its maximum peak at 4–5 h and has a second increase between 24 hours and 5 days [95]. With this regard, a study conducted to evaluate the impact of A91-immunization on LP showed that A91 is able to reduce the concentration of ROS at the site of injury having a strong impact over the second peak of this phenomenon [96]. A further study indicated that A91-immunization counteracts the production of nitric oxide (NO) and down regulates the expression of the gene encoding for nitric oxide synthase (iNOS) [97]. These are some of the beneficial mechanisms that explain, at least in part, the effect of this strategy on LP.

Apoptotic cell death is another of the main destructive phenomena triggered after SCI. This phenomenon is activated by inflammatory cytokines, free radicals, excitotoxic agents, and increased levels of intracellular calcium [98]. After SCI, neurological recovery depends mainly on the extent of neuronal loss and the functionality of the residual neural tissue. Numerous studies have shown that many neurons die as a consequence of apoptosis. Therefore, regulating apoptotic cell death might play an important role in the neurological recovery following SCI [99, 116]. Recent investigations on the field found that immunizing with A91 decreases caspase-3 activity and TNFα concentrations, reducing the number of apoptotic cells, which is directly correlated with functional improvement after injury [100].

Altogether, the aforementioned observations provide clear evidence on the mechanisms by which A91-immunization exerts its beneficial effects. Besides reducing secondary injury mechanisms, A91 peptide has also proven to prevent tissue damage, as immunized animals presented a higher number of myelinated axons and survival of rubrospinal neurons compared to controls [101, 109, 110]. These results were consistent throughout several SCI preclinical studies. Also it was noted that motor recovery had a direct correlation with neuronal survival, myelin preservation, and apoptosis reduction in treated groups [102, 107, 109, 110, 114, 117, 118]. As a consequence of these encouraging results, we have envisioned the possibility of combining this strategy with others that have also shown beneficial effects [103, 117, unpublished data]. For that reason, A91-immunization was administered along with glutathione monoethyl ester (GSHE), which is an anti-oxidant capable of accelerating the immune response and providing neuroprotection [104, 117]. The results of this study showed that after a contusive or a compressive SCI, this combination induced better motor recovery, higher number of myelinated axons, and better rubrospinal neuron survival than immunization alone. These results open an interesting scenery for clinical studies.

Finally, in order to consider A91-immunization for being used at clinical settings, it is of relevance to contemplate vaccine safety. With this regard, immunizing with A91 shows no signs of autoimmune disease development, possibly due to its low affinity to major histocompatibility complex (MHC) molecules [105]. Furthermore to evaluate vaccine safety, the clinical appearance of treated animals was assessed, and no weight variation or other clinical data of EAE in immunized animals was detected [106]. A91 has proven to be effective in several studies conducted at different time points showing the stability of the vaccine in promoting recovery. Preclinical results of studies evaluating vaccine efficacy indicate that this therapy could be possibly applied to SCI patients and improve their recovery and quality of life.

4. Concluding statement

Injury to the spinal cord stimulates the appearance of innate and adaptive immune responses, which could participate in either the pathogenesis or healing responses to trauma. The immune system should not be suppressed; instead, it must be modulated to attain its beneficial effect. That is why the use of immunosuppressant drugs like MP in the clinical field no longer seems a rational treatment. As a physiological hemostatic self-defense mechanism, PA is an essential mechanism to be considered for the pathophysiology and treatment of SCI. Boosting PA with the use of APL is needed in order to increase the functional recovery in the immune related neurodegenerative diseases. In SCI, immunization with the APL A91 has proven to reduce part of the immune-related secondary injury mechanisms without the risk of developing an autoimmune response. Preclinical results suggest that this therapy could be an effective treatment for SCI recovery, as it is closely related to a higher motor improvement, which is the most evident deficit in SCI patients. However, further studies related to the use of APL in SCI are needed to translate this therapy to the clinical field. For instance, we have to ensure that immunization with this peptide does not cause any side effect (i.e. hypersensitivity or autoimmunity). Additionally, further experiments should be performed in order to find out the best adjuvant to be used in humans, even the investigation should be directed to elucidate if the use of adjuvants is really necessary. Finally, the dosing of the peptide as well as the schedule of administration at clinical settings should also be investigated.

Author details

Paola Suárez-Meade[1] and Antonio Ibarra[1,2*]

*Address all correspondence to: iantonio65@yahoo.com; jose.ibarra@anahuac.mx

1 Faculty of Health Sciences, Anáhuac University, Universidad Anáhuac Av. Huixquilucan Edo. Mexico, Mexico

2 CAMINA Research Project A.C. Mexico City, Mexico

References

[1] National Spinal Cord Injury Statistical Center, University of Alabama at Birmingham. 2015. Annual Statistical Report. Spinal cord injury facts and figures at glance. https://www.nscisc.uab.edu

[2] DeVivo MJ. Epidemiology of traumatic spinal cord injury: trends and future implications. Spinal Cord. 2012; 50: 365–372.

[3] Chiu WT, Lin HC, Lam C, Chu SF, Chiang YH, et al. Epidemiology of traumatic spinal cord injury: comparisons between developed and developing countries. Asia Pac J Public Health. 2015; 22 (1): 9–18.

[4] Karlsson AK. Autonomic dysfunction in spinal cord injury: clinical presentation of symptoms and signs. Prog Brain Res. 2006; 152: 1–8.

[5] Ibarra A, Rios-Hoyo A, Suarez-Meade P, Malagon E, Colin-Rodriguez A. Influence of the level, severity and phase of spinal cord injury on hematological and biochemical parameters. J Trauma Treat. 2014; 3 (4): 1–5.

[6] Hagen EM. Acute complications of spinal cord injuries. World J Orthop. 2015; 6 (1): 17–23.

[7] Bracken MB, Shepard MJ, Collins WF, Holford T, Young W, et al. A randomized, controlled trial of methylprednisolone or naloxone in the treatment of acute spinal-cord injury. Results of the Second National Acute Spinal Cord Injury Study. N Engl J Med. 1990; 332 (20): 1405–1411.

[8] Bracken M, Shepard MJ, Holford T, Leo-Summers L, Aldrich F, et al. Methylprednisolone or tirilazad mesylate administration after acute spinal cord injury: 1-year follow up. Results of the Third National Acute Spinal Cord Injury Randomized controlled Trial. J Neurosurg. 1998; 89 (5): 699–706.

[9] Hulbert J. Methylprednisolone for the treatment of acute spinal cord injury: point. Clin Neurosurg. 2014; 61 (1): 32–35.

[10] Hulbert J. Methylprednisolone for acute spinal cord injury: an inappropriate standard of care. J Neurosurg. 2000; (Spine 1) 93: 1–7.

[11] Rhen T, Cidlowski JA. Anti-inflammatory action of glucocorticoids—new mechanisms for old drugs. N Engl J Med. 2005; 353: 1711–1723.

[12] Ferrari G, Greene LA. Prevention of neuronal apoptotic death by neurotrophic agents and Ganglioside GM1: insights and speculations regarding a common mechanism. Perspect Dev Neurobiol. 1996; 3 (2): 93–100.

[13] Skaper SD, Leon A. Monosialogangliosides, neuroprotection, and neuronal repair processes. J Neurotrauma. 1992; 9 (Suppl 2): S507–516.

[14] Geisler FH, Dorsey FC, Coleman WP. Past and current clinical studies with GM-1 ganglioside in acute spinal cord injury. Ann Emerg Med. 1993; 22 (6): 104–1047.

[15] Geisler FH, Coleman WP, Grieco G, Poonian D, Sygen Study Group. Recruitment and early treatment in a multicenter study of acute spinal cord injury. Spine. 2001; 26 (Suppl 1): S58–67.

[16] Geisler FH, Coleman WP, Griego G, et al. Measurement and recovery patterns in a multicenter study of acute spinal cord injury. Spine. 2001; 26 (Suppl 1): S68–86.

[17] Geisler FH, Coleman WP, Griego G. The Sygen® Multicenter acute spinal cord injury study. Spine. 2001; 26 (Suppl 1): S87–98.

[18] Meurer WJ, Baran WG. Spinal cord injury neuroprotection and the promise of flexible adaptive clinical trials. World Neurosurg. 2014; 82: 3–4.

[19] Kabu S, Gao Y, Kwon BK, Labhasetwar V. Drug delivery, cell-based therapies, and tissue engineering approaches for spinal cord injury. J Control Release. 2015; 219: 141–154.

[20] Stammers AT, Liu J, Kwon BK. Expression of inflammatory cytokines following acute spinal cord injury in a rodent model. J Neurosci Res. 2012; 90: 782–790.

[21] Fleming JC, Norenberg MD, Ramsay DA, Dekaban GA, Marcillo AE, et al. The cellular inflammatory response in human spinal cords after injury. Brain. 2006; 129: 3249–3269.

[22] Karinathan N, Vanathi MB, Subrahmanyam VM, Rao JV. A review on response of immune system in spinal cord injury and therapeutic agents useful in treatment. Curr Pharm Biotechnol. 2015; 16 (1): 26–34.

[23] Schwartz M, Raposo C. Protective autoimmunity: a unifying model for the immune network involved in CNS Repair. Neuroscientist. 2014; 20 (4): 343–358.

[24] Mestre H, Ibarra A. Immunization with neural-derived peptides as a potential therapy in neurodegenerative diseases. Neurodegen Dis Proc Prev Prot Monit. 2011;519–540. ISBN: 978-953-307-485-6.

[25] Fehlings MG, Sekhon LHS. Cellular, ionic and biomolecular mechanisms of the injury process. In: Tator CH, Benzel EC, eds. Contemporary management of spinal cord injury: From Impact to rehabilitation. New York: American Association of Neurological Surgeons. 2000; 33–50.

[26] Mautes A, Weinzierl M, Donovan F, Noble L. Vascular events after spinal cord injury: contribution to secondary pathogenesis. Phys Ther. 2000; 80: 673–687.

[27] Leonard AV, Thornon E, Robert V. The relative contribution of edema and hemorrhage to raised intrathecal pressure after traumatic spinal cord injury. J Neurotrauma. 2015; 32 (6): 397–402.

[28] Rowland J, Hawryluk G, Kwon B, Fehlings M. Current status of acute spinal cord injury pathophysiology and emerging therapies: promise on the horizon. Neurosurg Focus. 2008; 25 (5): E2.

[29] Aidemise Oyinbo C. Secondary injury mechanisms in traumatic spinal cord injury: a nugget of this multiply cascade. Acta Neurobiol Exp. 2011; 71: 281–299.

[30] Xing C, Arai K, Lo EH, Hommel M. Pathophysiologic cascades in ischemic stroke. Int J Stroke. 2012; 7: 378–385.

[31] Mehta A, Prabhakar M, Kumar P, Deshmukh R, Sharma PL. Excitotoxicity: bridge to various triggers in neurodegenerative disorders. Eur J Pharmacol. 2013; 698: 6–18.

[32] Sattler R, Tymianski M. Molecular mechanisms of glutamate receptor-mediated excitotoxic neuronal cell death. Mol Neurobiol. 2001; 24: 107–129.

[33] Matute C, Domercq M, Sanchez-Gomez MV. Glutamate-mediated glial injury: mechanisms and clinical importance. Glia. 2006; 53: 212–224.

[34] Park E, Velumian A, Fehlings MG. The role of excitotoxicity in secondary mechanisms of spinal cord injury: a review with an emphasis on the implications for white matter degeneration. J. Neurotrauma. 2004; 21(6): 754–774.

[35] David S, Kroner A. Repertoire of microglial and macrophage responses after spinal cord injury. Nat Rev Neurosci. 2011; 12: 388–399.

[36] Azbill RD, Mu X, Bruce-Keller A, Mattson MP, Springer JE. Impaired mitochondrial function, oxidative stress and altered antioxidant enzime activities following traumatic spinal cord injury. Brain Res. 1997; 765: 283–290.

[37] Cornelius C, Crupo R, Calabrese V, Graziano A, Milone P, et al. Traumatic brain injury: oxidative stress and neuroprotection. Antioxid Redox Signal. 2013; 19 (8): 836–853.

[38] Visavadiya PN, Patel SP, Venrooyen JL, Sullivan P, Rabchevsky A. Cellular and subcellular oxidative stress parameters following severe spinal cord injury. Redox Biol. 2016; 8: 59–67.

[39] Nathan C, Cunningham-Brussel A. Beyong oxidative stress: an immunologist's guide to reactive oxygen species. Net Rev Immunol. 2013; 13 (5): 349–361.

[40] Hall ED, Wang JA, Bosken JM, Singh IN. Lipid peroxidation in brain or spinal cord mitochondria after injury. J Bioenerg Biomembr. 2015. 48 (2): 169–174.

[41] Gilgun-Sherki Y, Rosenbaum Z, Melamed E, Offen D. Antioxidant therapy in acute central nervous system injury: current state. Pharmacol Rev. 2002; 54: 271–284.

[42] O'Connel KM, Littleton-Kearney MT. The role of free radicals in traumatic brain injury. Biol Res Nurs. 2012; 15 (3): 253–263.

[43] Farmer E, Mueller M. ROS-mediated lipid peroxidation and RES-activated signaling. Ann Rev Plant Biol. 2013; 64: 429–450.

[44] Ibarra A, Diaz-Ruiz A. Inhibition of lipid peroxidation by cyclosporin after spinal cord injury in rats. Humana Press. 2003: 283–298.

[45] Ekshyyan O, Aw TY. Apoptosis in acute and chronic neurological disorders. Front Biosci. 2004; 9: 1567–1576.

[46] Chun-Shu P, Loane DJ, Stoica BA, Shihong L, Hanscom M. Combined inhibition of cell death induced by apoptosis inducing factor and caspases provides additive neuroprotection in experimental traumatic brain injury. Neurobiol Dis. 2012; 46: 745–758.

[47] Springer JE, Azbill R, Knapp P. Activation of the caspase-3 apoptotic cascade in traumatic spinal cord injury. Nat Med. 1999; 5: 943–946.

[48] Stammers AT, Liu J, Kwon BK. Expression of inflammatory cytokines following acute spinal cord injury in a rodent model. J Neurosci Res. 2012; 90 (4): 782–790.

[49] Domercq M, Vázquez-Villoldo N, Matute C. Neurotransmitter signaling in the pathophysiology of microglia. Front Cell Neurosci. 2013; 49: 122–138.

[50] Hao C, Parney I, Roa W, Turner J, Petruk K, et al. Cytokine and cytokine receptor mRNA expression in human glioblastomas: evidence of Th1, Th2 and Th3 cytokine dysregulation. Acta Neuropathol. 2002; 103: 171–178.

[51] Hausmann ON. Post-traumatic inflammation following spinal cord injury. Spinal Cord. 2003; 41: 369–378.

[52] Dougherty KD, Dreyfus C, Black IB. Brain-derived neurotrophic factor in astrocytes, oligodendrocytes, and microglia/macrophages after spinal cord injury. Neurobiol Dis. 2000; 7 (6): 574–585.

[53] Camand E, Morel MP, Faissner A, Sotelo C, Dusart I. Long-term changes in the molecular composition of the glial scar and progressive increase of serotoninergic fibre sprouting after hemisection of the mouse spinal cord. Eur J Neurosci. 2004; 20 (5): 1161–1176.

[54] McPhail LT, Plunet WT, Partha D, Ramer M. The astrocytic barrier to axonal regeneration at the dorsal root entry zone is induced by rhizotomy. Eur J Neurosci. 2005; 21 (1): 267–270.

[55] Van Landeghem F, Stover JF, Bechmann I, Bruck W, Unterberg A, et al. Early expression of glutamate transporter proteins in ramified microglia after controlled cortical impact injury in the rat. Glia. 2201; 35 (3): 167–179.

[56] Esposito E, Cuzzocrea S. Anti-TNF therapy in the injured spinal cord. Trends Pharmacol Sci. 2011; 32 (2): 107–115.

[57] Neirinckx V, Coste C, Franzen R, Gothet A, Rogister B, et al. Neutrophil contribution to spinal cord injury and repair. J Neuroinflammation. 2014; 11: 150.

[58] Taoka Y, Okajima K, Uchiba M, Murakami K, Kushimoto S, Johno M. Role of neutrophils in spinal cord injury in the rat. Neuroscience. 1997; 79 (4): 1177–1182.

[59] Greenhalgh A, David S. Differences in the phagocytic response of microglia and pripheral macrophages after spinal cord injury and its effects on cell death. J Neurosci. 2014; 34 (18): 6316–6322.

[60] Popovich PG, Jones TB. Manipulating neuroinflammatory reactions in the injured spinal cord: back to basics. Trends Pharmacol Sci. 2003; 24 (1): 13–17.

[61] Triveldi A, Olivas A, Noble-Haeusslein L. Inflammation and spinal cord injury: infiltrating leukocytes as determinants of injury and repair processes. Clin Neurosci Res. 2006; 6: 283–292.

[62] Hu JG, Shi LL, Chen YJ, Xie XM, Zhang N, et al. Differential effects of myelin basic protein-activated Th1 and Th2 cells on the local immune microenvironment of injured spinal cord. Exp Neurol. 2016; 277: 190–201.

[63] Shaked I, Tchiresh D, Gersner R, Meiri G, Mordechai S, et al. Protective autoimmunity: interferon-γ enables microglia to remove glutamate without evoking inflammatory mediators. J Neurochem. 2005; 92: 997–1009.

[64] Mir M, Tolosa L, Asensio V, Llado J, Olmos G. Complementary roles of tumor necrosis factor alpha and interferón gamma in inducible microglial nitric oxide generation. J Neuroimmunol. 2008; 204 (1–4): 101–109.

[65] Esposito E, Cuzzocrea S. TNF-alpha as a therapeutic target in inflammatory diseases, ichemia-reperfusion injury and trauma. Curr Med Chem. 2009; 16 (24): 3152–3167.

[66] Stadelmann C, Kerschensteriner M, Misgeld T, Bruck W, Hohlfeld R, et al. BDNF and gp145trkB in multiple sclerosis brain lesions: neuroprotective interactions between immune and neuronal cells. Brain. 2002; 125: 75–85.

[67] Chen Q, Smith G, Shine D. Immune activation is required for NT-3-induced azonal plasticity in chronic spinal cord injury. Exp Neurol. 1008; 209 (2): 497–509.

[68] Stantambrogio L, Benedetti M, Chao M, Muzaffar R, Kulig K, et al. Nerve growth factor production by lymphocytes. J Immunol. 1994; 153: 4488–4495.

[69] Suarez-Meade P, Carvajal HG, Yasuhara T, Taijiri N, Date I, et al. Regenerative medicine for central nervous system disorders: role of therapeutic molecules in stem cell therapy. Brain Circul. 2015; 1 (2): 125–132.

[70] Saltzman JW, Battaglino RA, Stott HL, Morse LR. Neurotoxic or neuroprotective? Current controversies in SCI-induced autoimmunity. Curr Phys Med Rehabil Rep. 2013; 1: 174–177.

[71] Ankeny DP, Popovich PG. Mechanisms and implications of adaptive immune responses after traumatic spinal cord injury. Neuroscience. 2009; 158: 1112–1121.

[72] Schwab JM, Zhang Y, Kopp M, Brommer B, Popovich PG. The paradox of chronic neuroinflammation, systemic immune suppression, autoimmunity after traumatic chronic spinal cord injury. Exp Neurol. 2014; 258: 121–129.

[73] Zajarías-Fainsod D, Carrillo-Ruiz J, Mestre H, Grijalva I, Madrazo I, et al. Autoreactivity against myelin basic protein in patients with chronic paraplegia. Eur Spine J. 2012; 21: 964–970.

[74] Archelos JJ, Storch MK, Hartung HP. The role of B cells and autoantibodies in multiple sclerosis. Ann Neurol. 2000; 47 (6): 694–702.

[75] Fillatreau S, Sweenie CH, McGeachy MJ, Gray D, Anderton SM. B cells regulate autoimmunity by provision of IL-10. Nat Immunol. 2002; 3 (10): 944–950.

[76] Schwartz M, Kipnis J. Protective autoimmunity and neuroprotection in inflammatory and non-inflammatory neurodegenerative diseases. J Neurol Sci. 2005; 233 (1–2): 163–166.

[77] Schwartz M, Kipnis J. Protective autoimmunity: regulation and prospects for vaccination after brain and spinal cord injuries. Trends Mol Med. 2001; 7 (6): 252–258.

[78] Yoles E, Hauben E, Palqi O, Agranov E, Gothilf A, et al. Protective autoimmunity is a physiological response to CNS trauma. J Neurosci. 2001; 21 (11): 3740–3748.

[79] Hall E, Braughler M. Glucocorticoid mechanisms in acute spinal cord injury: a review and therapeutic rationales. Surg Neurol. 1982; 18 (5): 320–327.

[80] Schwartz M, Cohen I. Autoimmunity can benefit self-maintenance. Immunol Today. 2000; 21 (6): 265–268.

[81] Yoles E, Hauben E, Palgi O, Agranof E, Gothilf A, et al. Protective autoimmunity is a physiological response to CNS trauma. J Neurosci. 2001; 21 (11): 3740–3748.

[82] Kipnis J, Yoles E, Schori H, Hauben E, Shaked I, et al. Neuronal survival after CNS insult is determined by a genetically encoded autoimmune response. J Neurosci. 2001; 21: 4564–4571.

[83] Angelov DN, Waibel S, Guntinas-Lichius O, Lenzen M, Neiss WF, et al. Therapeutic vaccine for acute and chronic motor neuron diseases: implications for amyotrophic lateral sclerosis. PNAS. 2003; 100: 4790–4795.

[84] Schwartz M, Moalem G, Leibowitz-Amit R, Cohen I. Innate and adaptive immune responses can be beneficial for CNS repair. Trends Neurosci. 1999; 22: 295–299.

[85] Hauben E, Butovsky O, Nevo U, Yoles E, Moalem G, et al. Passive or active immunization with myelin basic protein promotes recovery from spinal cord contusion. J Neurosci. 2000; 10: 6421–6430.

[86] Kipnis J, Mizrahi T, Hauben E, Shaked I, Shevach E. Neuroprotective autoimmunity: naturally occurring CD4+CD25+ regulatory T cells suppress the ability to withstand injury to the central nervous system. PNAS. 2002; 99 (24): 15620–15625.

[87] Schwartz M, Raposo C. Protective autoimmunity: a unifying model for the immune network involved in CNS repair. Neuroscientist. 2014; 20 (4): 343–358.

[88] Barouch R, Schwartz M. Autoreactive T cells induce neurotrophin production by immune and neural cells in injured rat optic nerve: implications for protective autoimmunity. FASEB J. 2002; 16: 1304–1306.

[89] Aharoni R, Arnon R, Eilam R. Neurogenesis and neuroprotection induced by peripheral immunomodulatory treatment of experimental autoimmune encephalomyelitis. J Neurosci. 2005; 25: 8217–8228.

[90] Sakai K, Sinha A, Mitchel D, Zamvil S, Rothbard J, et al. Involvement of distinct murine T-cell receptors in the autoimmune encephalitogenic response to nested epitopes of myelin basic protein. Proc Natl Acad Sci. 1988; 85: 8608–8612.

[91] Sakai K, Zamvil S, Mitchel DJ, Lim M, Rothbard J, et al. Characterization of a major encephalitogenic T cell epitope in SJL/J mice with synthetic oligopeptides of myelin basic protein. J Neuroimmunol. 1988; 19: 21–32.

[92] Nicholson L, Greer J, Sobel R, Lees M, Kuchroo V. An altered peptide ligand mediates immune deviation and prevents autoimmune encephalomyelitis. Immunity. 1995; 3: 397–405.

[93] Hauben E, Agranov E, Gothlif A, Nevo U, Cohen A, et al. Posttraumatic therapeutic vaccination with modified myelin self-antigen prevents complete paralysis while avoiding autoimmune disease. J Clin Invest. 2001; 108: 591–599.

[94] Winghagen A, Scholz C, Hollsberg P, Fukaura H, Sette A, et al. Modulation of cytokine patters of human autoreactive T cell cones by a single amino acid substitution of their peptide ligand. Immunity. 1995; 2: 373–380.

[95] Jameson S, Bevan M. T cell receptor antagonists and partial agonists. Immunity. 1995; 2 (1): 1–11.

[96] Nel A. T-cell activation through the antigen receptor. Part 1: signaling components, signaling pathways, and signal integration at the T-cell antigen receptor synapse. J Allergy Clin Immunol. 2002; 109 (5): 758–770.

[97] Evavold BD, Allen PM. Sparation of IL-4 production from Th cell proliferation by an altered T cell receptor ligand. Science. 1991; 252: 1308–1310.

[98] Hauben E, Ibarra A, Mizrahi T, Barouch R, Agranov E, et al. Vaccination with a Nogo-A-derived peptide after incomplete spinal cord injury promotes recovery via a T-cell mediated neuroprotective response: comparison with other myelin antigens. PNAS. 2001; 98 (26): 15173–15178.

[99] Nel AE, Slaughter N. T-Cell activaction through the antigen receptor. Part 2: role of signaling cascades in T-cell differentiation, anergy, immune senescence, and development of immunotherapy. J Allergy Clin Immunol. 2002; 109 (6): 901–915.

[100] Yu M, Johnson J, Tuohy V. A predictable sequential determinant spreading cascade invariably accompanies progression of experimental autoimmune encephalomyelitis: a basis for peptide-specific therapy after onset of clinical disease. J Exp Med. 1996; 183: 1777–1788.

[101] Tuohy V, Yu M, Yin L, Kawczak J, Johnson J, et al. The epitope spreading cascade during progression of experimental autoimmune encephalomyelitis and multiple sclerosis. Immunol Rev. 1998; 164 (1): 93–100.

[102] Karin N, Mitchell D, Brocke S, Ling N, Steinman L. Reversal of experimental autoimmune encephalomyelitis by a soluble peptide variant of a myelin basic protein epitope: T cell receptor antagonism and reduction of interferon γ and tumor necrosis factor α production. J Exp Med. 1994; 180: 2227–2237.

[103] Gaur A, Boehme S, Chalmers D, Crowe P, Pahuja A. Amelioration of relapsing experimental autoimmune encephalomyelitis with altered myelin basic protein peptides involves different cellular mechanism. J Neuroimmunol. 1997; 74: 149–158.

[104] Willenbong D, Staykova M. Cytokines in the pathogenesis and therapy of autoimmune encephalomyelitis and multiple sclerosis. Adv Exp Med Biol. 2003; 520: 96–119.

[105] Martiñón S, García E, Gutierrez-Ospina G, Mestre H, Ibarra A. Development of protective autoimmunity by immunization with a neural derived peptide is ineffective in severe spinal cord injury. PLoS ONE. 2012; 7 (2): 1–7.

[106] Del rayo Garrido M, Silva-García R, García E, Martiñón S, Morales M, et al. Therapeutic window for combination therapy of A91 peptide and glutathione allows delayed treatment after spinal cord injury. Basic Clin Pharmacol Toxicol. 2013; 112: 314–318.

[107] Ibarra A, Sosa M, García E, Flores A, Cruz Y, et al. Prophylactic neuroprotection with A91 improves the outcome of spinal cord injured rats. Neurosci Lett. 2013; 554: 59–63.

[108] Ibarra A, Hauben E, Butovsky O, Schwartz M. The therapeutic window after spinal cord injury can accommodate T cell-based vaccination and methylprednisolone in rats. Eur J Neurosci. 2004; 19: 2985–2990.

[109] Martiñón S, García E, Flores N, González I, Ortega T. Vaccination with a neural-derived peptide plus administration of glutathione improves the performance of paraplegic rats. Eur J Neurosci. 2007; 26: 403–412.

[110] Ibarra A, García E, Flores N, Martiñón S, Reyes R. Immunization with neural-derived antigens inhibits lipid peroxidation after spinal cord injury. Neurosci Lett. 2010; 476: 62–65.

[111] Christie SD, Corneau B, Myers T, Sadi D, Purdy M, et al. Duration of lipid peroxidation after acute spinal cord injury in rats and the effect of methylprednisolone. J Neurosurg. 2008; 25 (5): E5.

[112] García E, Silva-García R, Mestre H, Flores N, Martiñón S. Immunization with A91 peptide or Copolymer-1 reduces the production of nitric oxide and inducible nitric oxide synthase gene expression after spinal cord injury. J Neurosci Res. 2012; 90: 656–663.

[113] Lou J, Lenke LG, Ludwig FJ, O'Brien MF. Apoptosis as a mechanism of neuronal cell death following acute experimental spinal cord injury. Spinal Cord. 1998; 36 (10): 683–690.

[114] Lee YJ, Choi SY, Oh TH, Yune TY. Estradiol inhibits apoptotic cell death of oligodendrocytes by inhibiting RhoA-JNK3 activation after spinal cord injury. Endocrinology. 2012; 153 (8): 3815–3827.

[115] Zhang N, Xu SJ, Chen WS, Yin Y, Wu YP. Inflammation and apoptosis in spinal cord injury. Indian J Med Res. 2012; 135 (3): 287–296.

[116] Rodríguez-Barrera R, Fernández-Presas A, García E, Flores-Romero A, Martiñón S, et al. Immunization with a neural-derived peptide protects the spinal cord from apoptosis after traumatic injury. Bio Med Res. 2013: 2013: 1–8.

[117] Hauben E, Ibarra A, Mizrahi T, Barouch R, Agranov E, et al. Vaccination with a Nogo-A-derived peptide after incomplete spinal-cord injury promotes recovery via a T-cell mediated neuroprotective response: comparison with other myelin antigens. PNAS. 2001; 98 (26): 15173–15178.

Chapter 4

Role of the Neuroinflammation in the Degree of Spinal Cord Injury: New Therapeutic Strategies

Irene Paterniti, Emanuela Esposito and
Salvatore Cuzzocrea

Additional information is available at the end of the chapter

http://dx.doi.org/10.5772/63222

Abstract

A case of spinal cord injury (SCI) is defined as the occurrence of an acute traumatic lesion of neural elements in the spinal canal (spinal cord and cauda equina), resulting in temporary or permanent sensory and/or motor deficit. Most studies on traumatic SCI show a bimodal age distribution, with a first peak in young adulthood and a second peak in older adults. Spinal cord trauma activates a cascade of events that exacerbates the damage such as activation of inflammatory process that determinates cytokine and chemokine production and that generates reduction in functional recovery resulting in necrosis or apoptosis of neurons. However, the precise mechanism of SCI-induced inflammatory response remains not fully understood at present. Current strategy to treat damage to the spinal cord is limited, only the treatment with methylprednisolone (MP), if administered in excessive dose during the acute phase of the damage, could ameliorate patients with severe SCI. However, associated to the beneficial effects, there are growing evidence that high-dose of MP is correlated to increased risk of infections, pneumonia and gastrointestinal bleeding. Therefore, there is a necessity to develop new therapies to treat SCI; one of these is to selectively reduce inflammation that possess unique role in the processes of injury and recovery.

Keywords: Immune response, oxidative stress, spinal cord injury, inflammation, neuroprotection

1. Inflammation response after spinal cord injury

Spinal cord injury (SCI) is damage caused to the spinal cord that compromise the major functions of the spinal cord and remains actually the most important cause of mortality in the society. In addition to its cost to the individual, physically as well as the health care system and society financially, SCI has profound psychosocial effects that are devastating for patients, families and friends. SCI usually begins with a sudden, traumatic blow to the spine that fractures or dislocates vertebrae; long-term mechanical compression of the spinal cord gradually causes various pathologic changes in neural tissue. The pathophysiology of SCI comprises both primary and secondary mechanisms of injury; the "primary injury" refers to the forces that impart the primary mechanical insult to the spinal cord, which in its mildest form causes a cord concussion with brief transient neurologic deficits and in its most severe form causes complete and permanent paralysis. The primary damage to tissue is followed by a second phase of tissue degeneration that might occur over weeks or even months and further generate progressive destruction of the tissue surrounding the necrotic core that expands from the injury "epicenter" and is known as secondary injury, that is a persistence of some crucial events of the acute phase such as edema and apoptotic cell death as well as generation of oxidative stress, activation of immune system response and inflammation process. In particular we focus our attention on some mechanisms that occur after spinal cord injury such as on the involvement of the inflammation process and immune system response.

Inflammation is a physiological process that removes damaged stimuli and initiates the healing process; however, if it persists and if it is over-activated, then the inflammation becomes devastating; inflammation is a key element in the pathophysiology of some disorders such as chronic pain, neurodegenerative pathology, trauma and spinal cord injury [1–5]. Principal pro-inflammatory markers that are both cellular components, such as neutrophils, macrophages and T cells, and non-cellular components, such as cytokines, prostaglandins and complement, have been found in spinal cord tissue that received a mechanical insult. Following spinal cord trauma, the site of injury is penetrated by neutrophils, that determinate release of cytokines that may progressive damage local tissue and recruit other inflammatory cells [6]; moreover, monocytes/macrophages are released and locally activated in microglia, that subsequently invade the injured tissue [7]. The pro-inflammatory cytokines that are produced at the site of injury, such as tumor necrosis factor (TNF-α), interleukins and interferons, mediate the inflammatory response and can generate further tissue damage [8,9]. Furthermore, cytokines can induce the expression of cyclo-oxygenase (COX) 2 and thus promote the breakdown of arachidonic acid into pro-inflammatory prostanoids (prostaglandins, prostacyclin and thromboxanes) that mediate vascular permeability/resistance and platelet aggregation/adherance [10,11]. The involvement of the cyclo-oxygenases in the generation of these inflammatory mediators represents a potential target for intervention, because inhibitors of these enzymes are in widespread clinical use. Additionally, TNF-α contributes to the tissue injury induced by neutrophils by directly activating them [12,13] as well as by increasing the expression of such molecules as ICAM-1 and E-selectin, which cause the activated neutrophils to adhere to the surface of the endothelial cells; it has also been shown that the inhibition of neutrophil adhesion to the endothelial cell surface markedly reduces the severity of the SCI induced by compressive trauma [14]. These observations indicate that the interaction of activated neutrophils with the surface of the endothelial cells is another important mediator in the secondary tissue damage of the spinal cord.

1.1. Cytokine responses to inflammation

Cytokines are small and non-structural proteins with no amino acid sequence motif, their biological activities allow us in turn to group them into different classes: exit 18 cytokines called interleukin (IL), some of these promote inflammation and are named pro-inflammatory cytokines such as IL1β and IL1α, IL6, IL8 and TNF-α, whereas other cytokines suppress the activity of pro-inflammatory cytokines and are called anti-inflammatory cytokines such as IL-4, IL-10, TGFβ. The hypothesis that some cytokine functions primarily induce inflammation while others suppress inflammation is essential to cytokine biology and also to clinical medicine.

Cytokines are secreted by a variety of immune cells such as T-lymphocytes and macrophages, as well as b non-immune cells such as fibroblasts; the physiological effects mediated by cytokines comprise the stimulation or inhibition of cell growth, cytotoxicity/apoptosis, antiviral activity and inflammatory responses. The main function of cytokines is the regulation of T-cell differentiation from undifferentiated cells to T-helper 1 and 2, regulatory T cells, and T-helper 17 cells [15]. These regulatory proteins include ILs, interferons (IFNs) and TNFs. Many of these cytokines have already been shown to be produced by neurons or glia in central nervous system (CNS) disorders in which they are notably increased.

The cytokine class of inflammatory mediators is secreted by microglia and astrocytes and their production is increased in inflammatory states; moreover they act by modulating the intensity and duration of the immune response. Pro-inflammatory cytokines and chemokines up-regulate microbicidal activity of neutrophils, and they can be considered as additional immunomodulatory agents to treat serious or refractory infections in humans.

Through cytokines IL-1 the immune response is initiated, having a crucial role in the onset and expansion of a complex hormonal and cellular inflammatory cascade; the IL-1 family of cytokines includes IL-1α and IL-1β, which generate cell activation upon binding with specific membrane receptors and has been documented that IL-1 plays a role in neuronal degeneration. In astrocytes, IL-1 induces IL-6 production, stimulates iNOS activity [16], enhances neuronal acetylcholinesterase activity, microglial activation and additional IL-1 production, and astrocyte activation.

Another important pro-inflammatory cytokine is the IL-6, a multifunctional cytokine that plays an important role in host defence [17] and possesses main effects during the inflammatory response [18]. IL-6 is associated to the family of neuropoietin cytokine and it possesses direct and indirect neurotrophic effects on neurons [19]; moreover, IL-6 promotes astrogliosis [20], activates microglia [21], and stimulates the release of acute phase molecules.

1.2. Inflammatory mediator: crucial role of TNF-α

Through all the cytokines involved in the secondary damage, TNF-α plays a crucial role; in fact it releases shortly after injury, it can accumulate rapidly at the site of injury, and it is produced by a number of different cell populations, such as neutrophils, macrophages and microglia, astrocytes and T cells [22]. Several cell types are able to produce TNF-α, including macrophages after its activation, dendritic cells, monocytes, NK cells, CD4+ T cells, CD8+ T cells, microglia and astrocytes. Macrophages/monocytes are able to produce TNF-α in the acute phase of inflammation and this cytokines drives several range of signalling events within cells, leading to necrosis or apoptosis.

Several biological functions are ascribed to the TNF-α and for this reason the mechanism of action is somewhat complex; although it inhibits the growth of tumor cells and it has an enhancing effect on the proliferation of normal cells [23]. TNF-α takes part in septic shock, autoimmunity, and inflammatory disorders. The major role of TNF-α is explicated as mediator in resistance against infections; moreover, it was postulated that TNF plays a pathological role in a number of autoimmune pathology such as graft vs host rejection or rheumatoid arthritis. Moreover, TNF-α possesses potent pro-inflammatory effects that are associated to its capacity to generate endothelial cell adhesion molecules and subsequently support neutrophil adherence to vascular endothelium. Neutrophils are exquisite targets of TNF-α that is under certain conditions it strengthens their expression of adhesion molecules induces their degranulation and successive release of lysosomal enzymes, causing the production of highly reactive oxygen species. TNF-α induces the migration of neutrophils mediating the production of chemotactic factors, including IL-8; this testifies cytokine networking involvement in inflammatory cell recruitment and an active role in inflammation.

TNF-α works by binding and clustering high-affinity receptors that are present in a great numbers on most cell membranes [24], the ligand/receptor complex is easily internalised via clathrin-coated pits and ends up in secondary lysozymes where it is degraded. Interestingly, the binding of TNF-α to the 75 kDa TNFR-2 is not sufficient to reach cytotoxicity, but rather binding to the 55 kDa TNFR-1 is sufficient to reach TNF-α mediated cell killing. TNF-α exerts its effects by activating several secondary proteins that provoke a variety of responses within the cell such as activation of gene transcription and/or production of reactive oxygen or nitrogen radicals (e.g., NO). Activated proteins include Gprotein, transcription factors such as NF-κB and AP-1 and serine and cysteine proteases, known as caspases. Many members of the TNF receptor superfamily have intracellular "death domains" which represent protein interaction domains each consisting of 65–80 amino acids; these proteins participate in TNF-α mediated apoptosis process; many evidence demonstrated that TNF–TNFR interactions are implicated in the pathogenesis of CNS disorders such as EAE and MS. These interactions are able to monitor the disease outcome by modifying immune response and the interactions between CNS-resident cells and effector immune cells in the CNS.

However, recent studies showed a dual nature for TNF-α that it can be not only neurotoxic but also neuroprotective; a study conducted with transgenic mice for TNF-α receptors demonstrated that the mice lacking TNF-α showed more tissue loss and functional deficits compared to wild-type mice, implying that TNF-α mediated a neuroprotective effect [25]. The beneficial or deleterious effects of TNF-α dependent when it is being released and on cellular population that is acting on, the conflicting actions of TNF-α described above reflects a growing view of inflammation as a "dual-edged sword" having neurotoxic and neuroprotective properties [26].

Thus, comprehension of their profile, kinetics of expression and interactions between TNF-α ligands and their TNFRs on different CNS residents and infiltrating immune cells would aid to better design strategies to control neuroinflammation and CNS autoimmunity. Blockers of TNF-α have been acknowledged for human use in treating TNF-linked autoimmune and inflammatory disorders. Pathways downstream of receptor ligation supply critical points for interjection for planning new therapeutic strategies.

1.3. Microglia activation

Moreover, other important mediators of inflammation that respond rapidly to disturbances within the microenvironment by change in morphology are the microglia, the expression "activated microglia" is used to define cells that change their immunophenotype and their morphology after a specific stimuli; the principal role of microglia at the lesion site is a rapid phagocytosis of fragments and induction of apoptosis [27]. The different response of microglia *in vitro* suggests that these cells may elicit unique functional properties and consequently control the inflammatory response at the injury site. Microglial activation has been well-known in the spinal cord tissue that has received a trauma and has shown to occur from caudal to lumbar enlargement, based on that there are papers supporting the role of microglia in pain after injury and showing activation of microglia post-SCI.

Thus, we postulated that activated spinal microglia have a role in chronic pain after SCI.

Microglia activate the innate immune system and are key regulators of inflammatory processes in CNS pathologies such as trauma and neurodegenerative diseases participation in both acute and chronic phase of the inflammatory responses. Activated microglia secrete cytotoxic substances including various cytokines such as TNF-α, IL-1, reactive free radicals, and nitric oxide. However, the principal effects of microglia at the levels of the lesion core are probably rapid phagocytosis of debris rather than induction of apoptosis. Microglia when activated can cause neuronal and glial toxicity through the release of cytokines, free radicals, eicosanoids, activated neutrophils, and macrophages [28]. On the other hand, microglia activation leads to beneficial effects producing growth factors that are fundamental for neuronal and tissue restoration. Moreover, it has been demonstrated that transplantation of peripherally activated macrophages has beneficial effects on spinal cord regeneration.

1.4. Apoptosis

In the last decade the generation of apoptotic process after spinal cord trauma was also confirmed, apoptosis can be triggered by a variety of insults including cytokines, inflammatory injury, free radical damage, and excitotoxicity.

The apoptotic process after spinal cord trauma is activated in neurons, oligodendrocytes, microglia, and perhaps, astrocytes; apoptosis in microglia contributes to inflammatory secondary injury.

Two main pathways of apoptosis—extrinsic or receptor-dependent and intrinsic or receptor-independent—have been well characterized, and both appear to be active in SCI; the extrinsic or receptor-dependent pathway is mediated by Fas ligand and Fas receptor [29] and/or inducible nitric oxide synthase production by macrophages [30], while intrinsic or receptor-independent pathway is mediated via direct caspase-3 pro-enzyme activation [31] and/or mitochondrial damage, release of cytochrome c and activation of the inducer caspase-9, pathways of caspase-mediated apoptotic death [32].

Receptor-dependent apoptosis is evoked by extracellular signals, the most significant of which is TNF, so it is termed as "extrinsic" pathway; TNF is known to rapidly accumulate in the injured spinal cord, and activation of the Fas receptor of neurons, microglia, and oligodendrocytes induces a programmed sequence of caspase activation. Moreover, additional control of cell death/survival is provided by the balance between major pro-apoptotic proteins such as Bax, Bad, and Bid and anti-apoptotic proteins such as Bcl-XL and Bcl-2.

Apoptotic cells were reached in the grey matter after injury, starting from 1h with a proliferation during the other 8 h [33]. The number of apoptotic cells is increased at the site of injury and are related with axons degeneration [34].

Apoptotic process that is activated in the secondary injury in SCI has recently come under close study, and the precise contribution and potential therapeutic implications of apoptosis in SCI could be helpful to generate new therapeutic approach to treat the secondary events associated to spinal cord injury.

2. Inflammatory/immunologic response

The inflammatory and immunological response to injury within the CNS is different than that which is occurring in other tissues [35]. The inflammatory and immunologic responses to injury involve activation of innate immune cells that provide immediate defence against inflammatory stimuli and in turn help to recruit cells of the adaptive immune system (i.e., T- and B-lymphocytes). The activation of immune system is driven by interactions involving presentation of antigen and release of various inflammatory mediators [36]. Also, cells present at the injury site may sequester debris and carry CNS antigens to secondary lymphoid organs [37], where trigger lymphocyte activation. Recent studies done on mice showed that the number of activated T and B cells increases in the spleen and bone marrow within 24 hours of trauma [38].

2.1. Lymphocytes infiltration

T-lymphocytes are distributed in the intact spinal cord and gradually grow in number after trauma in parallel with the stimulation of microglia and influx of peripheral macrophages. Lymphocytes infiltrate the spinal cord tissue starting from 24 hours until 7 days after injury and return gradually back to normal levels in 4 to 5 weeks [14].

Under normal conditions, activated T cells can cross the Add Blood–brain barrier (BBB) and enter the CNS parenchyma. In contrast with other inflammatory cells enrolled after a trauma, the number of lymphocytes remains low [39]; however, T-lymphocytes play an important role in the CNS immune system, since on activation, T-lymphocytes may kill target cells and produce cytokines [40].

Once lymphocytes enter the lesion site, they persist indeterminately [38,41], whereas T and B cells increase at the lesion site at least 9 weeks post-injury [42,43], suggesting that cytokine/chemokine gradients exist chronically and regulate integrin expression on endothelia and cells [44,45]. These chemokine gradients and adhesion molecules represent molecular targets for manipulating the effects of intraspinal lymphocytes after SCI [46–48]; the progressive increase in lymphocyte numbers may also be justified by lymphocyte activation and proliferation within the injured centre of spinal cord.

Moreover, induction of immune response could be generated as impaired nerve transmission; increasing the production of pro-inflammatory cytokines in chronic phase of SCI could worsen the damage increasing the axonal injury and demyelination. Furthermore, there are evidences that autoreactive lymphocytes promote neuronal survival *in vivo* through activation not only of autoreactive T cell but also through activation of other non-CNS reactive T cells or B cells such as resident microglia and infiltrating macrophages.

Thus, because lymphocytes remain for long term at the site of the lesion; new strategy of treatment could orientate on these cells that possess a fundamental role in regulating degenerative and regenerative processes after injury.

3. Pharmacologic interventions for acute spinal cord injury

The temporal profile of the secondary injury cascade provides a window within which it is theoretically possible to reduce the pathophysiological processes; many of the current pharmacological and surgical strategies for the treatment of SCI are based on minimising secondary injury and preserving neurological function following trauma to the brain and spinal cord. Over the past couple of decades, a myriad of agents have been nominated as putative neuroprotective therapies, several of these have been tested in the pre-clinical and clinical studies.

The following section briefly highlights some of the most promising neuroprotective approaches that are being pursued.

3.1. Corticosteroids

In the last decade one of the most used approaches to treat patients with a severe SCI is the use of corticosteroids that possess a well-recognized anti-inflammatory properties reducing spinal cord edema. However, the exact mechanisms by which corticosteroids mediated neuroprotection are not yet completely understood but seems that they induce a reduction of inflammatory cytokines production, modulation of the inflammatory/immune cells, inhibition of lipid peroxidation and reduction of oxidative stress. In this regard, methylprednisolone (MP) appears to be particularly efficacious compared with other glucocorticoids. According to the National Acute Spinal Cord Injury Study 2 (NASCIS 2) protocol, MP is usually administered within 8 h after trauma in a high concentration of 30 mg/kg, followed by an infusion of 5.4 mg/kg/h for 23 hours [49,50]. MP is the only well-known pharmacological treatment of SCI injury patients; however, its administration has been shown to be controversial. Some toxic effects such as infection rates, pulmonary embolism, severe pneumonia and sepsis and even death secondary to respiratory complications appeared to be higher with steroid use.

The anti-inflammatory properties of MP are mediated by different mechanisms that are known as transrepression, this mechanism involves interference with pro-inflammatory transcription factor signalling (such as NF-κB) which is upstream of several inflammatory mediators including COX2, chemokines and cytokines.

Together with the minor functional improvement in humans and risk of adverse side effects, these studies highlighted the compelling need to develop better neuroprotective agents with more convincing efficacy.

3.2. Estrogen as a neuroprotective agent

At present, several effects have been associated to estrogen that acts with different mechanism of action [51]. Recently, the neuroprotective and anti-inflammatory effect of estrogen are of great interest; leukocyte adhesion and microglia activation are also sensitive to estrogen and show significantly decreased superoxide dismutase production and phagocytic activity when treated with estrogen *in vitro* [52].

Moreover, cell death is associated to decreases blood flow in spinal cord and estrogen are involved in increasing post-traumatic blood flow induced by ischemia [53] and TBI [54]. Thus, estrogen treatment has been related with increased expression of pro-apoptotic Bcl-2 in the spinal cord injured tissue, this anti-apoptotic increase in Bcl-2 may be mediated by Akt activation with downstream phosphorylation of cAMP response element binding protein (CREB) [55].

However, estrogen may also act on Add N-methyl-D-aspartate receptor (NMDA) receptors, indicating a potential to limit secondary cell death due to excitotoxicity [56].

3.3. Nuclear hormone receptors family: PPARs receptor

Other members of the nuclear hormone receptors family (NHRs) are now explored for their anti-inflammatory properties in experimental models, including SCI.

Peroxisome proliferator-activated receptors (PPARs) are part of the nuclear hormone receptor superfamily, upon ligand activation regulate gene expression and have been shown to be anti-inflammatory in different model of inflammatory pathology, including SCI. PPAR exists as three isoforms (α, β/δ and γ) that control many cellular functions including lipid metabolism, glucose absorption, cell growth and differentiation, and inflammation.

One mechanism involves direct interaction of PPAR with pro-inflammatory transcription factors, most importantly NFκB and AP-1, and the subsequent reduction of gene transcription. Pioglitazone and rosiglitazone are PPARγ agonists that are in common clinical use for type II diabetes. Beyond their metabolic effects, interest in PPAR γ ligand has grown due to their anti-inflammatory, neuroprotective, and even anti-neoplastic properties, suggesting its potential use after spinal cord trauma [57]. As such, PPAR agonists have already been clinically tested in other disorders with inflammatory pathology, such as Alzheimer's disease (AD), rheumatoid arthritis (RA), and ischemia reperfusion injury, but not in SCI yet. Moreover, in the last few years a great interest has been focused on other PPAR receptors agonist such as for PPARα and β/δ receptors. One of the first reports indicating that PPARα is involved in attenuating inflammation demonstrated that the eicosanoid LTB4 binds and activates PPARα [58]. Several studies on inflammatory cytokine produced in aged mice demonstrated an active interaction of PPARα with NFκB; in fact the oxidative stress in different tissue leads to active NFκB. Treatment with PPARα agonists were found to restore the alteration of oxidative mediators, to inhibit the activation of NFκB and to remove IL-6 and IL-12 produced [59,60].

These features were accompanied by enhanced functional motor recovery and reduced hyperalgesia.

Since PPAR agonists are currently used in medical treatment of diabetes, clinical studies for stroke and different CNS pathologies are to be expected. The knowledge about anti-inflammatory properties of PPAR ligands obtained from cell cultures and animal model of SCI demonstrate that PPARs signalling may be therapeutic targets after spinal cord injury.

4. Conclusion

Thus, recent researches are moving to develop new pharmacological approaches that may offer an effective neuroprotection after spinal cord injury. After spinal cord injury, inflammatory reactions account for a large proportion of the secondary damage to neurons and oligodendrocytes.

Promising research is being carried out to better understand the aspects of inflammation, lipid peroxidation and apoptotic cell death that may be the target of pharmacologic intervention.

Few agents have been studied demonstrating efficacy in animal models of spinal cord injury and may become appropriate for testing in the human setting in the near future.

Clearly, much effort has to be done to bring experimental strategies to clinical fruition, but they do represent promising potential interventions.

Thus, the current medical and surgical interventions for the acutely cord-injured patient attempt to minimize the inflammatory process that possess a crucial role in generating and maintaining secondary damage associated to injury and defend the neural cells that initially survived the mechanical injury.

Author details

Irene Paterniti, Emanuela Esposito* and Salvatore Cuzzocrea

*Address all correspondence to: eesposito@unime.it

Department of Chemical, Biological, Pharmaceutical and Environmental Sciences, University of Messina, Messina, Italy

References

[1] Giovannini MG, Scali C, Prosperi C, Bellucci A, Vannucchi MG, Rosi S, et al. Beta-amyloid-induced inflammation and cholinergic hypofunction in the rat brain in vivo: involvement of the p38MAPK pathway. Neurobiology of disease. 2002; 11(2): 257–74.

[2] Dauer W, Przedborski S. Parkinson's disease: mechanisms and models. Neuron. 2003; 39(6): 889–909.

[3] Tenorio G, Kulkarni A, Kerr BJ. Resident glial cell activation in response to perispinal inflammation leads to acute changes in nociceptive sensitivity: implications for the generation of neuropathic pain. Pain. 2013; 154(1): 71–81. doi:10.1016/j.pain.2012.09.008.

[4] Najjar S, Pearlman DM, Alper K, Najjar A, Devinsky O. Neuroinflammation and psychiatric illness. Journal of neuroinflammation. 2013; 10: 43. doi: 10.1186/1742-2094-10-43.

[5] Iadecola C, Anrather J. The immunology of stroke: from mechanisms to translation. Nature medicine. 2011; 17(7): 796–808. doi:10.1038/nm.2399.

[6] Popovich PG, Wei P, Stokes BT. Cellular inflammatory response after spinal cord injury in Sprague–Dawley and Lewis rats. The journal of comparative neurology. 1997; 377(3): 443–64.

[7] Dusart I, Schwab ME. Secondary cell death and the inflammatory reaction after dorsal hemisection of the rat spinal cord. The European journal of neuroscience. 1994; 6(5): 712–24.

[8] Bartholdi D, Schwab ME. Expression of pro-inflammatory cytokine and chemokine mRNA upon experimental spinal cord injury in mouse: an in situ hybridization study. The European journal of neuroscience. 1997; 9(7): 1422–38.

[9] Klusman I, Schwab ME. Effects of pro-inflammatory cytokines in experimental spinal cord injury. Brain research. 1997; 762(1–2): 173–84.

[10] Tonai T, Taketani Y, Ueda N, Nishisho T, Ohmoto Y, Sakata Y, et al. Possible involvement of interleukin-1 in cyclooxygenase-2 induction after spinal cord injury in rats. Journal of neurochemistry. 1999; 72(1): 302–9.

[11] Dubois RN, Abramson SB, Crofford L, Gupta RA, Simon LS, Van De Putte LB, et al. Cyclooxygenase in biology and disease. FASEB journal : official publication of the Federation of American Societies for Experimental Biology. 1998; 12(12): 1063–73.

[12] Genovese T, Mazzon E, Di Paola R, Cannavo G, Muia C, Bramanti P, et al. Role of endogenous ligands for the peroxisome proliferators activated receptors alpha in the secondary damage in experimental spinal cord trauma. Experimental neurology. 2005; 194(1): 267–78. doi:10.1016/j.expneurol.2005.03.003.

[13] Paterniti I, Genovese T, Crisafulli C, Mazzon E, Di Paola R, Galuppo M, et al. Treatment with green tea extract attenuates secondary inflammatory response in an experimental model of spinal cord trauma. Naunyn-Schmiedeberg's archives of pharmacology. 2009; 380(2): 179–92. doi:10.1007/s00210-009-0414-z.

[14] Taoka Y, Okajima K. Role of leukocytes in spinal cord injury in rats. Journal of neurotrauma. 2000; 17(3): 219–29.

[15] Steinman L. A brief history of T(H)17, the first major revision in the T(H)1/T(H)2 hypothesis of T cell-mediated tissue damage. Nature medicine. 2007; 13(2): 139–45. doi: 10.1038/nm1551.

[16] Hausmann ON. Post-traumatic inflammation following spinal cord injury. Spinal cord. 2003; 41(7): 369–78. doi:10.1038/sj.sc.3101483.

[17] Okada S, Nakamura M, Mikami Y, Shimazaki T, Mihara M, Ohsugi Y, et al. Blockade of interleukin-6 receptor suppresses reactive astrogliosis and ameliorates functional recovery in experimental spinal cord injury. Journal of neuroscience research. 2004; 76(2): 265–76. doi:10.1002/jnr.20044.

[18] Roxburgh CS, McMillan DC. Therapeutics targeting innate immune/inflammatory responses through the interleukin-6/JAK/STAT signal transduction pathway in patients with cancer. Translational research: the journal of laboratory and clinical medicine. 2016; 167(1): 61–6. doi:10.1016/j.trsl.2015.08.013.

[19] Teng FY, Tang BL. Axonal regeneration in adult CNS neurons-signaling molecules and pathways. Journal of neurochemistry. 2006; 96(6): 1501–8. doi:10.1111/j.1471-4159.2006.03663.x.

[20] Morales I, Farias G, Maccioni RB. Neuroimmunomodulation in the pathogenesis of Alzheimer's disease. Neuroimmunomodulation. 2010; 17(3): 202–4. doi: 10.1159/000258724.

[21] Inoue K. Microglial activation by purines and pyrimidines. Glia. 2002; 40(2): 156–63. doi:10.1002/glia.10150.

[22] Yan P, Li Q, Kim GM, Xu J, Hsu CY, Xu XM. Cellular localization of tumor necrosis factor-alpha following acute spinal cord injury in adult rats. Journal of neurotrauma. 2001; 18(5): 563–8. doi:10.1089/089771501300227369.

[23] Mandi Y, Endresz V, Krenacs L, Regely K, Degre M, Beladi I. Tumor necrosis factor production by human granulocytes. International archives of allergy and applied immunology. 1991; 96(2): 102–6.

[24] Loetscher H, Gentz R, Zulauf M, Lustig A, Tabuchi H, Schlaeger EJ, et al. Recombinant 55-kDa tumor necrosis factor (TNF) receptor. Stoichiometry of binding to TNF alpha and TNF beta and inhibition of TNF activity. The Journal of biological chemistry. 1991; 266(27): 18324–9.

[25] Kim GM, Xu J, Xu J, Song SK, Yan P, Ku G, et al. Tumor necrosis factor receptor deletion reduces nuclear factor-kappaB activation, cellular inhibitor of apoptosis protein 2 expression, and functional recovery after traumatic spinal cord injury. The journal of neuroscience : the official journal of the society for neuroscience. 2001; 21(17): 6617–25.

[26] Bethea JR. Spinal cord injury-induced inflammation: a dual-edged sword. Progress in brain research. 2000; 128: 33–42. doi:10.1016/S0079-6123(00)28005-9.

[27] Shuman SL, Bresnahan JC, Beattie MS. Apoptosis of microglia and oligodendrocytes after spinal cord contusion in rats. Journal of neuroscience research. 1997; 50(5): 798–808.

[28] Schwartz M. Autoimmune involvement in CNS trauma is beneficial if well controlled. Progress in brain research. 2000; 128: 259–63. doi:10.1016/S0079-6123(00)28023-0.

[29] Leskovar A, Moriarty LJ, Turek JJ, Schoenlein IA, Borgens RB. The macrophage in acute neural injury: changes in cell numbers over time and levels of cytokine production in mammalian central and peripheral nervous systems. The journal of experimental biology. 2000; 203(Pt 12): 1783–95.

[30] Satake K, Matsuyama Y, Kamiya M, Kawakami H, Iwata H, Adachi K, et al. Nitric oxide via macrophage iNOS induces apoptosis following traumatic spinal cord injury. Brain research molecular brain research. 2000; 85(1–2): 114–22.

[31] Citron BA, Arnold PM, Sebastian C, Qin F, Malladi S, Ameenuddin S, et al. Rapid upregulation of caspase-3 in rat spinal cord after injury: mRNA, protein, and cellular localization correlates with apoptotic cell death. Experimental neurology. 2000; 166(2): 213–26. doi:10.1006/exnr.2000.7523.

[32] Hartley CJ, Reddy AK, Madala S, Martin-McNulty B, Vergona R, Sullivan ME, et al. Hemodynamic changes in apolipoprotein E-knockout mice. American journal of physiology-heart and circulatory physiology. 2000; 279(5): H2326–34.

[33] Zurita M, Vaquero J, Zurita I. Presence and significance of CD-95 (Fas/APO1) expression after spinal cord injury. Journal of neurosurgery. 2001; 94(2 Suppl): 257–64.

[34] Casha S, Yu WR, Fehlings MG. Oligodendroglial apoptosis occurs along degenerating axons and is associated with FAS and p75 expression following spinal cord injury in the rat. Neuroscience. 2001; 103(1): 203–18.

[35] Schwartz M, Moalem G, Leibowitz-Amit R, Cohen IR. Innate and adaptive immune responses can be beneficial for CNS repair. Trends in neurosciences. 1999; 22(7): 295–9.

[36] Ling C, Sandor M, Fabry Z. In situ processing and distribution of intracerebrally injected OVA in the CNS. Journal of neuroimmunology. 2003; 141(1–2): 90–8.

[37] Karman J, Ling C, Sandor M, Fabry Z. Initiation of immune responses in brain is promoted by local dendritic cells. Journal of immunology. 2004; 173(4): 2353–61.

[38] Ankeny DP, Lucin KM, Sanders VM, McGaughy VM, Popovich PG. Spinal cord injury triggers systemic autoimmunity: evidence for chronic B lymphocyte activation and lupus-like autoantibody synthesis. Journal of neurochemistry. 2006; 99(4): 1073–87. doi: 10.1111/j.1471-4159.2006.04147.x.

[39] Schnell L, Fearn S, Klassen H, Schwab ME, Perry VH. Acute inflammatory responses to mechanical lesions in the CNS: differences between brain and spinal cord. The European journal of neuroscience. 1999; 11(10): 3648–58.

[40] Kierdorf K, Wang Y, Neumann H. Immune-mediated CNS damage. Results and problems in cell differentiation. 2010; 51: 173–96. doi:10.1007/400_2008_15.

[41] Sroga JM, Jones TB, Kigerl KA, McGaughy VM, Popovich PG. Rats and mice exhibit distinct inflammatory reactions after spinal cord injury. The journal of comparative neurology. 2003; 462(2): 223–40. doi:10.1002/cne.10736.

[42] Bilgen M, Dogan B, Narayana PA. In vivo assessment of blood-spinal cord barrier permeability: serial dynamic contrast enhanced MRI of spinal cord injury. Magnetic resonance imaging. 2002; 20(4): 337–41.

[43] Whetstone WD, Hsu JY, Eisenberg M, Werb Z, Noble-Haeusslein LJ. Blood-spinal cord barrier after spinal cord injury: relation to revascularization and wound healing. Journal of neuroscience research. 2003; 74(2): 227–39. doi:10.1002/jnr.10759.

[44] Lee YL, Shih K, Bao P, Ghirnikar RS, Eng LF. Cytokine chemokine expression in contused rat spinal cord. Neurochemistry international. 2000; 36(4–5): 417–25.

[45] Babcock AA, Kuziel WA, Rivest S, Owens T. Chemokine expression by glial cells directs leukocytes to sites of axonal injury in the CNS. The journal of neuroscience: the official journal of the society for neuroscience. 2003; 23(21): 7922–30.

[46] Bao F, Chen Y, Dekaban GA, Weaver LC. Early anti-inflammatory treatment reduces lipid peroxidation and protein nitration after spinal cord injury in rats. Journal of neurochemistry. 2004; 88(6): 1335–44.

[47] Eng LF, Lee YL. Response of chemokine antagonists to inflammation in injured spinal cord. Neurochemical research. 2003; 28(1): 95–100.

[48] Gonzalez R, Glaser J, Liu MT, Lane TE, Keirstead HS. Reducing inflammation decreases secondary degeneration and functional deficit after spinal cord injury. Experimental neurology. 2003; 184(1): 456–63.

[49] Bracken MB. Methylprednisolone in the management of acute spinal cord injuries. The medical journal of Australia. 1990; 153(6): 368.

[50] Bracken MB, Shepard MJ, Collins WF, Holford TR, Young W, Baskin DS, et al. A randomized, controlled trial of methylprednisolone or naloxone in the treatment of acute spinal cord injury. Results of the Second National Acute Spinal Cord Injury Study.

The New England journal of medicine. 1990; 322(20): 1405–11. doi:10.1056/NEJM199005173222001.

[51] Sribnick EA, Wingrave JM, Matzelle DD, Ray SK, Banik NL. Estrogen as a neuroprotective agent in the treatment of spinal cord injury. Annals of the New York Academy of Sciences. 2003; 993: 125–33; discussion 59–60.

[52] Bruce-Keller AJ, Keeling JL, Keller JN, Huang FF, Camondola S, Mattson MP. Antiinflammatory effects of estrogen on microglial activation. Endocrinology. 2000; 141(10): 3646–56. doi:10.1210/endo.141.10.7693.

[53] He Z, He YJ, Day AL, Simpkins JW. Proestrus levels of estradiol during transient global cerebral ischemia improves the histological outcome of the hippocampal CA1 region: perfusion-dependent and independent mechanisms. Journal of the neurological sciences. 2002; 193(2): 79–87.

[54] Roof RL, Hall ED. Estrogen-related gender difference in survival rate and cortical blood flow after impact-acceleration head injury in rats. Journal of neurotrauma. 2000; 17(12): 1155–69. doi:10.1089/neu.2000.17.1155.

[55] Honda K, Shimohama S, Sawada H, Kihara T, Nakamizo T, Shibasaki H, et al. Nongenomic antiapoptotic signal transduction by estrogen in cultured cortical neurons. Journal of neuroscience research. 2001; 64(5): 466–75.

[56] Nilsen J, Chen S, Brinton RD. Dual action of estrogen on glutamate-induced calcium signaling: mechanisms requiring interaction between estrogen receptors and src/mitogen activated protein kinase pathway. Brain research. 2002; 930(1–2): 216–34.

[57] Cuzzocrea S. Peroxisome proliferator-activated receptors gamma ligands and ischemia and reperfusion injury. Vascular pharmacology. 2004; 41(6): 187–95. doi:10.1016/j.vph.2004.10.004.

[58] Devchand PR, Keller H, Peters JM, Vazquez M, Gonzalez FJ, Wahli W. The PPAR alpha-leukotriene B4 pathway to inflammation control. Nature. 1996; 384(6604): 39–43. doi:10.1038/384039a0.

[59] Esposito E, Cuzzocrea S. Palmitoylethanolamide is a new possible pharmacological treatment for the inflammation associated with trauma. Mini reviews in medicinal chemistry. 2013; 13(2): 237–55.

[60] Esposito E, Cuzzocrea S. Targeting the peroxisome proliferator-activated receptors (PPARs) in spinal cord injury. Expert opinion on therapeutic targets. 2011; 15(8): 943–59. doi:10.1517/14728222.2011.581231.

Chapter 5

Normal Distribution and Plasticity of Serotonin Receptors after Spinal Cord Injury and Their Impacts on Motor Outputs

Mengliang Zhang

Additional information is available at the end of the chapter

http://dx.doi.org/10.5772/63759

Abstract

Following spinal cord injury (SCI) a series of anatomical and functional plastic changes occur in the spinal cord, including reorganization of the spinal neuronal network, alteration of properties of interneurons and motoneurons as well as up- or down-regulation of different neurotransmitter receptors. In mammalian spinal cord, one of the important neurotransmitters, serotonin (5-HT), plays an essential role in modulating sensory, motor and autonomic functions. Following SCI, especially complete spinal cord lesion, the descending supply of 5-HT is lost. As a consequence different 5-HT receptors undergo variant degrees of plastic changes.

In this chapter I have systematically reviewed the distribution of different 5-HT receptors in the spinal cord and their plastic changes following SCI where applicable. In addition, the plastic changes of 5-HT supplying system in reaction to SCI have also been reviewed. These results indicate that 5-HT receptors are important factors not only for modulation of normal motor function, their plastic changes are also critical for motor functional recovery and, quite often, for the development of certain pathological states after SCI. Pharmacological and/or genetic intervention of selected 5-HT receptors and/or intrinsic 5-HT producing system in the spinal cord may pave new ways for the restoration of motor functions after SCI.

Keywords: monoamine, monoamine receptor, spinal cord, motor control, intraspinal 5-HT cell

1. Introduction

Spinal cord injury (SCI) is a devastating condition with an incidence of 10–83 per million people per year worldwide according to statistical data from different countries [1]. It leads to an extensive and usually irreversible loss of sensory functions, voluntary motor control, and autonomic functions below injury level. A variety of primary and secondary complications occur depending on the severity of the injury and time course of its development. These symptoms may involve different systems, manifesting as, e.g., paralysis, spasticity, neuropathic pain, pulmonary and cardiovascular problems, osteoporosis, anemia, pressure ulcers, bladder and bowel problems, and sexual dysfunction [2–8]. Currently, there is no cure for SCI and thus improving quality of life, such as restoration of partial motor and sensory functions, has become a priority for setting up the treatment strategy. The primary cause of these problems is the loss of both descending and ascending projecting pathways in the spinal cord. The descending pathways include direct motor-initiating pathways, such as cortical spinal tracts, and modulatory pathways, such as serotonergic, dopaminergic, and noradrenergic pathways. These monoaminergic systems are so important that in either acute or chronic SCI direct stimulation of the receptors of these monoamines with drugs could regain locomotor activity in animals [9–17]. Thus, restoring the function of monoaminergic systems has become a key strategy to restore motor function and ameliorate secondary symptoms [18–23].

So far a great number of studies have been focusing on the serotonergic system in SCI. In the mammalian spinal cord, serotonin (5-HT) originates mainly in the raphe nuclei of the brainstem and plays an important role in modulating sensory, motor, and autonomic function [24–27]. Following SCI, especially complete spinal cord lesion, the descending supply of 5-HT is lost and as a consequence different 5-HT receptors undergo variant degrees of plastic changes [22, 28–36]. In addition, a potential intraspinal 5-HT-producing system in the spinal cord, i.e., aromatic L-amino acid decarboxylase (AADC) cells, also undergoes plastic changes to increase their potency to produce 5-HT from its precursor [37–40]. Although these plastic changes may induce pathological symptoms such as spasticity and chronic central pain [34, 41, 42], they are essential for spinal function recovery (for review see [43–45]). In this chapter, I will make a systematic review according to up-to-date literature related to the distribution and plastic changes of 5-HT receptors in the spinal cord in normal or SCI states with a note on the intraspinal 5-HT-producing cells.

2. 5-HT in the spinal cord in health

In mammals, including humans, 5-HT axons in the spinal cord almost exclusively originate from the brainstem raphe nuclei [46–49]. Their terminals are distributed in all parts of the gray matter at all levels of the spinal cord [50, 51]. The cell bodies with descending 5-HT projections are located in the caudal part of the raphe nuclei, which include the raphe magnus, raphe obscurus, raphe pallidus, ventral lateral medulla, and the area postrema [52]. In the spinal cord, 5-HT projecting fibers descend in the white matter through two different routes: one with fibers from the raphe magnus in the dorsal part of the lateral funiculus which terminates mainly in the dorsal horn, and the other with fibers from raphe obscurus and raphe pallidus in the ventral funiculus which terminates mainly in the ventral horn and the intermediate zone.

In addition to the descending projecting system, there are indeed 5-HT neurons in the spinal cord although in normal states their contribution of 5-HT can be ignored. So far a small number of intraspinal 5-HT neurons have been reported in macaque monkey (ca. 150 cells per monkey [53]), rat (3–9 cells per rat [54, 55]), and mouse [51]. In the rat spinal cord, 5-HT cells were distributed in different parts of the spinal cord with the exception of cervical segments; in the monkey spinal cord most of the cells were observed in the cervical segments with a small number in other segments; whereas in the mouse spinal cord they were exclusively located in the sacral segments. In the rat spinal cord, the 5-HT cells were found to be located in laminae VII and X in the gray matter, whereas in monkey and mouse spinal cord they were exclusively found in lamina X.

Serotonin in the spinal cord plays an important role in sensory information processing, motor control, and autonomic function. Traditionally, it is hypothesized that 5-HT in the spinal cord exerts its effects by inhibiting sensory systems and facilitating motor systems [56]. However, now it is known that the effects of 5-HT are very complicated both in sensory and motor aspects. In sensory aspect, 5-HT not only has antinociceptive but also pronociceptive effects (e.g., [57, 58]). In motor aspect, except for facilitating motor output, 5-HT also inhibits motor behavior (e.g., [59, 60]). The different functions that 5-HT exert at different circumstances depend on many factors, such as the brainstem origins of the descending projections, the termination localizations of these fibers in the spinal cord, and the activation states of its different receptors.

3. 5-HT receptors in the spinal cord in health

The diverse functions of 5-HT in the spinal cord are achieved through the activation of different 5-HT receptors. As seen in **Table 1**, seven families (or types) and at least 14 subfamilies (or subtypes) of 5-HT receptors have been identified so far [61]. In these seven families, with exception of 5-HT3 receptors that are ligand-gated ion channels, all other families are G protein-coupled receptors [62]. To better understand the diversity of 5-HT functions, it is fundamentally important to have the knowledge of the anatomical localizations of different 5-HT receptors in the spinal cord. A majority, though not all, of 5-HT receptor subfamilies have been found to be expressed in the spinal cord (for reviews see [63, 64]). Here, I will make a systematic review of these receptors in terms of their cellular as well as subcellular localizations in the spinal cord based on available data. One should keep in mind that due to the existence of a great number of splices and editing variants for several 5-HT receptors, a greater degree of operational diversity could be expected, though this issue is not the focus of the present review.

Receptor family (year of molecular gene clone)*	Receptor subfamily (year of molecular gene clone)*	Expression in the spinal cord	Functions at normal states	Expression changes following SCI	Functions at SCI states
5-HT1	1A (1987)	Primary afferent fibers in dorsal horn [66]; neuronal somata in different laminae of gray matter [31,69]; axon initial segments [31,71];	Antinociception [73,76]; pronociception [77]; increases motoneuron excitability [60]; induces central fatigue [81]	Upregulation at least to 30 days after SCI [28,31]	Promotes motor functional recovery [13,14,172]
	1B (1992)	Primary afferent fibers in dorsal horn [83]; neuronal somata at least in intermediate zone [38]	Antinociception [72]; autoreceptor [89]; inhibits activity of AADC cells [38]	--	Inhibits mono- and polysynaptic reflexes [99,174]
	1D (1991)	Primary afferent fibers in dorsal horn [92]; gamma motoneurons in ventral horn [94]	Antinociception, [93]; modulates proprioceptive circuits [94]	--	Inhibits polysynaptic reflex [95]??
	1E (1992)	--	--	--	--
	1F (1993)	Substantia gelatinosa of spinal dorsal horn [98]	Antinociception [101,102]??	--	Inhibits polysynaptic reflex [99]??
5-HT2	2A (1988)	Different laminae of the spinal gray matter but largely in the superficial dorsal horn and lamina IX	Pronociceptive [57,112]; antinociceptive [115]; excites motoneuron [117]; facilitates micturition reflex [119]; facilitates sexual behavior	Upregulation [32,33,35]	Locomotor functional recovery [12,14,43]; 5-HT supersensitivity and muscle spasm [42]

Receptor family (year of molecular gene clone)*	Receptor subfamily (year of molecular gene clone)*	Expression in the spinal cord	Functions at normal states	Expression changes following SCI	Functions at SCI states
		[104,107,108]	[120,121]		
	2B (1992)	Dorsal horn (probably primary afferent fibers) [109]	Pronociception [109,124,126]	Constitutive activation [182]	Motoneuron hyperexcitability and muscle spasm [182]
	2C (1988) (Named 1C before 1993)	Different laminae of the spinal gray matter [36,104,107]	Pronociception [57,112]; antinociception [96,115,133]; induces long-lasting amplification of spinal reflexes [73,134]; inhibits micturition reflex [127,138]	Constitutive activation [34,182]; upregulation [22,36,177]	Motor functional recovery [34,182]; 5-HT supersensitivity, motoneuron hyperexcitability, and muscle spasm [34,42,182]
5-HT3	3A (1991) 3B (1999) 3C (2003) 3D (2003) 3E (2003) [62,139]	Different laminae of the spinal gray matter [107,142]	Antinociception [145,146]; pronociception [149]; mediates tail-flick reflexes [117]; inhibits bladder function [152]	--	Promotes motor function recovery [151]
5-HT4 (1995)		Ventral horn, some sympathetic neurons [153]	Pronociception [154]	--	--
5-HT5	5A (1994)	Dorsal horn, intermediate lateral nucleus, and Onuf's nucleus [110,156]	Antinociception [58,157]; autonomic and micturition control [156]	--	--
	5B (1993)	--	--	--	--
5-HT6 (1993)		Different laminae of the spinal gray matter [159]	Pronociception [160]	--	--
5-HT7 (1993)		Dorsal horn, intermediate zone, and ventral horn	Pronociception [164–166]; promotes locomotion		Promotes locomotor functional

Receptor family (year of molecular gene clone)*	Receptor subfamily (year of molecular gene clone)*	Expression in the spinal cord	Functions at normal states	Expression changes following SCI	Functions at SCI states
		with a dorsoventral density gradient [16,162]	[16,167,169]		recovery [43,172]

* Year of molecular gene clone is based on Wikipedia (https://en.wikipedia.org/wiki/5HT_receptor) except 5-HT3 receptors; --: no data available; ??: data not conclusive.

Table 1. 5-HT receptors in the spinal cord and plastic changes following SCI.

3.1. 5-HT1 receptors

As listed in **Table 1**, 5-HT1 receptors include five subfamilies: 1A, 1B, 1D, 1E, and 1F. Although all of these receptors have been detected in the brain by different techniques [65], there is no report to my knowledge demonstrating the expression of 5-HT1E receptors in the spinal cord. In addition, the evidence of the existence of 5-HT1F in the spinal cord is mainly from physiological experiments. Nonetheless, I will describe 5-HT1A, 1B, 1D, and 1F in the spinal cord according to the available data.

5-HT1A receptors: Data from both autoradiographic (radioligand binding) and immunohistochemical experiments have demonstrated the presence of 5-HT1A receptors in different regions of the spinal gray matter across different spinal segments in rats [31, 66–69]. 5-HT1A receptor binding sites were predominantly seen in the dorsal horn especially laminae I and II [67], where they were partly located in the primary afferent fibers [66]. In autoradiographic images, it is difficult to identify the components located in cell bodies; however, with immunohistochemistry with a 5-HT1A antibody generated from an intracellular epitope, it was clear that 5-HT1A receptors were expressed in cell bodies in the spinal cord [31]. The immunolabeled cell bodies were located in different spinal regions in the gray matter including the dorsal horn, intermediate zone, and ventral horn [31, 69, 70]. In addition, using a different 5-HT1A antibody generated from an extracellular epitope, the receptors were also shown to be present in the axon hillock [31, 71]. There are no studies to investigate 5-HT1A receptor localization at an ultrastructural level and therefore no data available for their subcellular distribution.

It is commonly believed that 5-HT1A receptors exert an inhibitory effect in sensory information transmission including nociception in the spinal dorsal horn (e.g., [72–76]). For example, in mice intrathecal injection of 5-HT1A receptor agonist 8-hydroxy-2-(di-*n*-propylamino) tetralin (8-OH-DPAT) could inhibit the tail-flicks induced by noxious radiant heat [72]. In neonatal rat spinal cord in vitro experiments, Hochman et al. [73] showed that 8-OH-DPAT depressed evoked excitatory postsynaptic potentials (EPSPs) in the deep dorsal horn neurons, whereas 5-HT1A receptor antagonist WAY-100635 (*N*-[2-[4-(2-methoxyphenyl)-1-

piperazinyl]ethyl]-*N*-(2-pyridyl)cyclohexanecarboxamide) facilitated evoked EPSPs. Data from the same group also indicated that the activation of 5-HT1A receptors facilitated long-term depression in the dorsal horn neurons. However, the effects of 5-HT1A receptors in the dorsal horn are not always inhibitory. For example, the activation of 5-HT1A receptors has been reported to facilitate nociceptive [77, 78] and itch transmission [79], and to induce spontaneous tail-flicks [80].

As 5-HT1A receptors have been found to be present both at the neuronal somata and the axon initial segments in spinal ventral horn neurons, including motoneurons [31], it is speculated that 5-HT1A receptors may have heterogeneous functions on motor outputs, i.e., both excitatory and inhibitory [59, 60]. Indeed, using a turtle spinal cord, slice preparation, and intracellular recording technique, Perrier and Cotel [60] demonstrated that the activation of 5-HT1A receptors by 8-OH-DPAT induced an increased excitability in a large fraction (9/11) of sampled motoneurons; whereas in a small fraction of motoneurons (2/11) 8-OH-DPAT gave a hyperpolarizing effect. Subsequent data from the same research group have demonstrated that the inhibitory effect was due to the activation of extrasynaptic 5-HT1A receptors located at the axon initial segments, a mechanism supposed to underlie central fatigue [81, 82].

5-HT1B receptors: To the best of my knowledge, there are no systematic immunohistochemical studies on the distribution of 5-HT1B receptors in the spinal cord. Previous studies using autoradiography have demonstrated that 5-HT1B receptors did not have any dominant expression region in the spinal gray matter although the intermediate zone seemed to dwell slightly higher labeled profiles [67, 68]. Although it is difficult to differentiate labeled cell bodies from nerve fibers with autoradiography, results from studies using other methods including lesion, pharmacology, and reverse transcription polymerase chain reaction (RT-PCT) indicated the existence of this receptor subfamily both at presynaptic (primary afferent fibers) [83] and postsynaptic locations (motoneurons) [84, 85]. Recently by using immunohistochemistry, Wienecke et al. [38] have found that 5-HT1B receptors were indeed expressed in the cell bodies at least in the intermediate zone in the rat spinal cord.

Similar to 5-HT1A receptors, a major role of 5-HT1B receptors is inhibition in sensory transmission, especially nociception [72, 86, 87]. For example, Eide et al. [72] showed that in mice intrathecal injection of 5-HT1B receptor antagonist RU-24969 (5-methoxy-3(1,2,3,6-tetrahydropyridin-4-yl)-1*H*-indole) induced a significant increase of tail-flick latencies. Another role of 5-HT1B receptors is to inhibit the release of 5-HT from its fibers via autoreceptor mechanism. Although both 5-HT1A and 1B receptors have been demonstrated to be autoreceptors in the brain, in the spinal cord it is most likely that 5-HT1B receptors play a more important role than 5-HT1A receptors in controlling the release of 5-HT from 5-HT fiber terminals [88–90]. Thus, Brown et al. [89] using rat spinal cord synaptosomes preparation showed that the 5-HT1B receptor agonists 1-(*m*-trifluoromethylphenyl)piperazine and 1-(*m*-chlorophenyl) piperazine concentration-dependently decreased [3*H*]5-HT release. In addition, 5-HT1B receptors could also inhibit the production of 5-HT from AADC cells in the spinal cord through feed-forward mechanism so that the AADC cells do not produce 5-HT in normal physiological states [38]. Another function of 5-HT1B receptors, as noted in mice, is to delay the maturation of γ-aminobutyric acid (GABA) phenotype in spinal cord during its development [91].

5-HT1D receptors: Data concerning the anatomical localization of 5-HT1D receptors in the spinal cord are relatively poor. The available data indicate that 5-HT1D receptors exist both in the dorsal and the ventral horn. Using immunohistochemistry, 5-HT1D receptors were found to be expressed in the primary afferent fibers in the superficial dorsal horn of the rat spinal cord [92, 93]. At the ultrastructural level, 5-HT1D receptors in the spinal cord dorsal horn were found to be localized exclusively within dense core vesicles of synaptic terminals and not the plasma membrane [92]. Using in situ hybridization and transgenic mouse model, Enjin et al. [94] found that 5-HT1D receptors were specifically expressed in γ motoneurons in the ventral horn as well as in some proprioceptive sensory neurons in different spinal regions which were coexpressed with parvalbumin (used as a proprioceptive neuronal marker in the study).

The available data indicate an effect of 5-HT1D receptors in the suppression of sensory, especially nociceptive, information transmission [58, 93, 95]. However, different results were also present. For example, in a formalin-induced hindpaw pain model, Jeong et al. [96] showed that the 5-HT1D receptor agonist GR-46611 (3-[3-(2-dimethylaminoethyl)-1*H*-indol-5-yl]-*N*-(4-methoxybenzyl)acrylamide) did not suppress the formalin-induced flinching responses and the 5-HT1D receptor antagonist BRL-15572 (3-(4-(4-chlorophenyl)piperazin-1-yl)-1,1-diphenyl-2-propanol) failed to reverse the antinociceptive effects of 5-HT. Other functions of 5-HT1D receptors include, e.g., depressing the spinal monosynaptic reflex induced by endogenously released 5-HT [97], and shaping proprioceptive circuits to receive and relay accurate sensory information in the spinal cord motor network [94]. In addition, since 5-HT1D receptors were expressed in γ, but not α, motoneurons, they could be used as a marker to identify γ motoneurons in the spinal cord [94].

5-HT1F receptors: To my knowledge, there is no systematic investigation concerning the expression of 5-HT1F receptors in the spinal cord of any species. However, there are indeed some pieces of evidence from studies using radioligand or physiological technique indicating that this receptor subfamily is present in the spinal cord dorsal horn. Castro et al. [98] used [3*H*]sumatriptan as a radioligand in the presence of suitable concentrations of 5-carboxamidotryptamine (5-CT) to define 5-HT1F receptors in the human spinal cord, and they found significant levels of binding sites in substantia gelatinosa in the cervical spinal cord. However, because 5-CT is not a specific 5-HT1F agonist, the data cannot be taken as granted. Using an in vitro sacrocaudal spinal cord preparation from spinal transected rats, Murray et al. [99] showed that the EPSPs and associated long polysynaptic reflexes were consistently inhibited by 5-HT1F-specific agonist LY-344864 (*N*-[(3*R*)-3-(dimethylamino)-2,3,4,9-tetrahydro-1*H*-carbazol-6-yl]-4-fluorobenzamide), indicating the existence of 5-HT1F in the spinal cord. However, the exact locations of these receptors are yet to be determined.

Due to the lack of related anatomical data, it is difficult to unveil the functions of 5-HT1F in the spinal cord. Considering that 5-HT1F receptors are expressed in the trigeminal and spinal dorsal root ganglia [100] and their agonists have been used to treat migraine [101, 102], it is most likely that this receptor subfamily exerts an antinociceptive effect in spinal cord.

3.2. 5-HT2 receptors

As listed in **Table 1**, 5-HT2 receptors include three subfamilies, i.e., 5-HT2A, 2B, and 2C. Before 1993, 5-HT2C receptors were named 5-HT1C receptors [103]. By using different experimental techniques including autoradiography, in situ hybridization, Western blot and immunohistochemistry all these three receptor subfamilies have been detected in the spinal cord in different species [104–109] although 5-HT2C subfamily is probably not expressed in cat spinal cord [105]. 5-HT2A and 2C receptors are likely among the most thoroughly investigated 5-HT receptors in the spinal cord due to their important functions in both sensory information processing and motor control.

5-HT2A receptors: Using various techniques, the existence of 5-HT2A receptors has been confirmed at both mRNA and protein level in the spinal cord of different species [104–108, 110]. By using polymerase chain reaction (PCR) together with Southern hybridization technique, Helton et al. [105] showed that spinal cord tissues from rat, cat, monkey, and human contained 5-HT2A receptor mRNAs. By using in situ hybridization, Pompeiano et al. [104] showed that 5-HT2A receptor mRNAs were present at intermediate density in the ventral horn. This distribution pattern has been confirmed with immunohistochemistry [106, 108]. Doly et al. [108] systematically investigated the distribution of 5-HT2A receptor immunoreactivity in rat spinal cord and the results indicated that 5-HT2A receptors were distributed in all the spinal segments with a similar immunolabeling pattern. The most prominent labeling was found in lamina IX, where many, but not all, motoneurons were labeled. At lumbar five to six level, 5-HT2A receptors were densely expressed in Onuf's nucleus that contains the motoneurons innervating pelvic striated muscles controlling sexual behavior and micturition [110]. Another region with dense immunolabeling was lamina II. The remaining laminae of the gray matter displayed a weak to moderate labeling. Doly et al. [108] also examined the subcellular localization of 5-HT2A receptors in laminae II and IX and they demonstrated that most immunolabeled profiles were postsynaptic, i.e., dendrites and cell somata, although a small number of axons and axon terminals were also labeled. The immunoreactive product was localized mainly on the plasma membrane where synaptic specifications were lacking.

The localization of 5-HT2A receptors in the neurons in both the spinal dorsal and ventral horn endows their functions in both sensory information transmission and motor control. For the sensory information modulation, evidence to date largely favors in their pronociceptive role [57, 111–114]. For example, Kjørsvik et al. [112] showed that in formalin-induced pain model, intrathecal injection of DOI ((±)-2,5-dimethoxy-4-iodoamphetamine hydrochloride), a 5-HT2A/2C receptor agonist, augmented nociceptive response in rats. This effect could be completely abolished when ketanserin (a 5-HT-2A receptor antagonist) was coadministrated. Rahman et al. [57] investigated the effects of DOI, ketanserin, and ritanserin (another 5-HT2A/2C antagonist) on the evoked responses of dorsal horn neurons to electrical, mechanical, and thermal stimulation, and found that the activation of 5-HT2A receptors facilitated the spinal nociceptive transmission under normal physiological states. However, there is also evidence indicating that 5-HT2A receptors exert an antinociceptive effect [115, 116]. For example, using a rat spinal cord slice preparation Xie et al. [115] found that bath application of 5-HT increased the frequency of spontaneous inhibitory postsynaptic currents in GABAergic and glycinergic neurons in substantia gelatinosa. TCB-2 (4-bromo-3,6-dimethoxybenzocyclobuten-1-yl)methylamine hydrobromide), a 5-HT2A receptor agonist, could mimic the 5-HT effect, and ketanserin could partially inhibit the effect of 5-HT and completely inhibit the effect of TCB-2.

It is not surprising that 5-HT2A receptors play a significant role in motor control considering their intensive expression in ventral horn motoneurons. Indeed, direct stimulation of 5-HT2 receptors in motoneurons in vivo with selective 5-HT2 receptor agonist DOI or DOM (2,5-dimethoxy-alpha,4-dimethylbenzene ethamine hydrochloride) produced dose-related back muscle contractions and wet dog shakes which could be markedly attenuated by ritanserin, ketanserin, or mianserin, suggesting an effect from 5-HT2A receptors [117]. Their direct facilitating effect on spinal motoneurons was also evidenced by application of DOI in rat spinal cord in vitro experiments [118]. In addition, pharmacological experiments showed that 5-HT2A receptor activation facilitated micturition reflex and activated the external urethral sphincter in female rats [119], whereas in both male and female rats 5-HT2A receptors seemed to involve sexual behavior [120, 121].

5-HT2B receptors: In comparison with 5-HT2A and 5-HT2C, 5-HT2B receptors in the spinal cord have been less investigated and the available data are inconsistent. Using in situ hybridization expression of 5-HT2B receptors was not found in rat spinal cord and even brain [104]. However, using several other techniques, the receptors have been detected in the spinal cord. Thus, using reverse transcription polymerase chain reaction (RT-PCR) 5-HT2B receptor mRNAs have been detected in spinal cord tissue in many different species including rat, cat, monkey, and human [105]. Using microarray global gene expression technique [122] and immunohistochemistry [123], 5-HT2B receptors have been detected in the rat spinal cord motoneurons. In addition, using Western blot it was shown that the receptor proteins were also present in the dorsal part of the spinal cord [109]. Considering that with Western blot and immunohistochemistry 5-HT2B receptors have been demonstrated to be expressed in the dorsal root ganglia [109, 124], their expression in the spinal dorsal horn is likely originating from the primary afferent fibers from the dorsal root ganglia, although it cannot be excluded that they might be also expressed in neuronal somata (e.g., [125]).

It is presumable that 5-HT2B receptors are largely related with sensory information transmission considering their localization in dorsal root ganglia and dorsal horn. Thus, evidence from a few studies related to 5-HT2B receptor functions in the spinal cord favors that the receptors are responsible for facilitating mechanical hyperalgesia, tactile allodynia, and nociception [109, 124, 126]. Studies concerning the receptors' motor function are rare. One study showed that 5-HT2B receptors likely increased urethral smooth muscle tone since the 5-HT2B receptor antagonist RS-127445 (3-(4-(4-chlorophenyl)piperazin-1-yl)-1,1-diphenyl-2-propanol) blocked increase in urethral pressure in female rats [127]. In frog, the activation of 5-HT2B receptors by α-methey-5-HT (a 5-HT2B receptor agonist) facilitates *N*-methyl-D-aspartate (NMDA)-induced depolarization of motoneurons [128]. In addition, 5-HT2B receptors seemed to modulate respiratory activity in rats [123].

5-HT2C receptors: 5-HT2C receptor mRNAs and proteins were widely distributed in different laminae of the spinal gray matter including motoneurons as demonstrated by different experimental methods, such as PCR [105], autoradiography [68, 129], in situ hybridization [104, 107], and immunohistochemistry [36, 130–132]. Using PCR combined with Southern hybridization 5-HT2C receptor mRNAs were detected in spinal cord tissue from rat, monkey, and human, but not in cat spinal cord [105]. By using in situ hybridization, Fonseca et al. [107] showed that 5-HT2C receptor mRNAs were present at high levels in most parts of the spinal gray matter, except lamina II. Using immunohistochemistry, Ren et al. [36] have investigated 5-HT2C receptor expression in both normal and spinalized rats and the results showed that 5-HT2C receptors were widely distributed in different regions of the spinal gray matter (except lamina II) and were predominantly located in the neuronal somata and their dendrites although they also seemed to be present in axonal fibers in the superficial dorsal horn. Thus, the data from in situ hybridization and immunohistochemistry fit very well for this receptor subfamily.

The wide distribution of 5-HT2C receptors in different laminae of the spinal cord endows the receptors' role both in sensory information transmission and motor control. For the sensory information transmission available data point to that 5-HT2C receptors play roles both in pronociception [57, 112] and antinociception [96, 115, 133]. For their role on pronociception, refer to the part concerning 5-HT2A receptors since most studies used DOI (a common agonist for 5-HT2A and 2C receptors) to stimulate and ketanserin to inhibit the receptors in response to different nociceptive stimulations. However, because ketanserin is mainly a 5-HT2A receptor antagonist some researchers argued that the pronociception effect should preferably attribute to 2-HT2A than 2C receptors. Their effects on antinociception seem to be adequately evidenced. For instance, in one study Jeong et al. [96] showed that in formalin-induced pain model 5-HT2C receptor specific antagonist D-MC (*N*-ormethylclozapine/8-chloro-11-(1-piperazinyl)-5*H*-dibenzo[*b*,*e*][1,4]diazepine) could block the suppression effect of 5-HT, whereas 5-HT2C receptor specific agonist MK-212 (6-chloro-2-(1-piperazinyl)pyrazine hydrochloride) could suppress the formalin response. In another study, Xie et al. [115] showed that a 5-HT2C receptor agonist WAY-161503 (8,9-dichloro-2,3,4,4a-tetrahydro-1*H*-pyrazino[1,2-*a*]quinoxalin-5(6*H*)) mimicked the 5-HT antinociceptive effect in dorsal horn neurons and this effect could be blocked by a 5-HT2C receptor antagonist, *N*-desmethylclozapine.

In motor control, one of the functions of 5-HT2C receptors is the induction of a long-lasting amplification of spinal reflex [73, 134–136]. Machacek et al. [134] showed that, in an in vitro neonatal rat spinal cord preparation, superfusion of 5-HT depressed reflex responses recorded in the ventral roots which was induced by electrical stimulation of primary afferents. However, following 5-HT washout, a long-lasting reflex facilitation was observed. Further pharmacological analysis indicated that it was the activation of 5-HT2C but not 5-HT2A receptors that was required for this long-lasting reflex. Although 5-HT2C receptors play a major role in long-term motor reflexes, they also play an inhibitory role in some physiological states. For example, in mice, when activated by DOI, 5-HT2C receptors inhibited the locomotor activity which opposed the effects of 5-HT2A receptors [137]. In addition, 5-HT2C receptors were also demonstrated to inhibit the micturition reflex [119, 127, 138]. Thus, Conlon et al. [138] showed that, in guinea pigs, Ro-600175 ((*α**S*)-6-chloro-5-fluoro-*α*-methyl-1*H*-

indole-1-ethanamine fumarate), a 5-HT2C receptor agonist, increased peak urethral pressure in a dose-dependent manner. This effect was reversed by a selective 5-HT2C receptor antagonist SB-242084 (6-chloro-2,3-dihydro-5-methyl-*N*-[6-[(2-methyl-3-pyridinyl)oxy]-3-pyridinyl]-1*H*-indole-1-carboxyamide) but not a 5-HT2A or 2B receptor antagonist. Similar results were also observed in rats [119, 127]. Clinically, duloxetine, a serotonin-norepinephrine reuptake inhibitor, has been used to treat stress urinary incontinence. One possible mechanism for this effect may be the activation of 5-HT2C receptors in motoneurons in Onuf's nucleus, which leads to an increased activity of pudendal motor neurons and a subsequent increase in the strength of urethral sphincter contractions.

3.3. 5-HT3 receptors

Although genes encoding the molecular structures of five different 5-HT3 receptor subfamilies (A–E) have been cloned, it is demonstrated so far that only the 5-HT3A subfamily is functional in homomeric form, and all other subfamilies require coassembling with 5-HT3A as functional heteromers [62, 139]. Therefore, here 5-HT3 receptors will be described together as one receptor unity. In the spinal cord, 5-HT3 receptors in the beginning were detected mainly in the dorsal horn with autoradiography and immunohistochemistry in rats and humans [140, 141]. Later by using in situ hybridization and immunohistochemistry, they were found to be expressed in different laminae across the spinal gray matter [107, 142]. By using immunohistochemistry, Morales et al. [142] observed labeled cell bodies in the dorsal horn among the densely labeled fiber terminals. In the ventral horn, large neurons, likely motoneurons, were densely labeled. By using in situ hybridization, Fonseca et al. [107] found that 5-HT3 receptor mRNAs were expressed in different laminae in the rat spinal cord with very low levels in the dorsal horn, slightly higher levels in laminae VI through X and the highest level in lamina IX. Maxwell et al. [143] have studied the ultrastructure of 5-HT3 immunolabeled profiles in the dorsal horn of the rat spinal cord. They found that 5-HT3-immunopositive terminals invariably formed asymmetric synaptic junctions with dendritic profiles and often contained a mixture of granular and agranular vesicles. Immunoreactive cells were found to contain intense patches of reaction product within their cytoplasm. Although there are no data available regarding the subcellular morphology of 5-HT3 receptors in the ventral horn neurons, from the light microscopic data, it can be concluded that the receptor immunoreactive product was located at least in the cytoplasm [142].

It has long been known that 5-HT3 receptors modulate spinal nociceptive reflexes [144]. A large part of literature demonstrated a role of 5-HT3 receptors in antinociception in the spinal cord (e.g., [145, 146]). This is likely due to, for instance, that the receptors interact with inhibitory interneurons such as GABA interneurons in the dorsal horn [147]. However, there are also data indicated that 5-HT3 receptors have a pronociceptive effect. For example, Guo et al. [148] showed that when the spinal 5-HT3 receptors were activated by intrathecal injection of a selective 5-HT3 receptor agonist SR-57227 (1-(6-chloropyridin-2-yl)piperidin-4-amine) spinal glial hyperactivity, neuronal hyperexcitability, and pain hypersensitivity were induced in rats. These diverse effects could be explained by, e.g., the expression of 5-HT3 receptors in different neuronal components and/or the different effects of assemblies formed from different receptor subfamilies [149, 150].

Although 5-HT3 receptors are expressed in the ventral horn neurons data concerning their motor functions are scarce. A study by Guertin and Steuer [151] showed that in hindlimb paralyzed mice 5-HT3 receptor agonist SR-57227 could produce hindlimb movements although with a low score. This result indicates that 5-HT3 receptors might also modulate spinal motoneuron activity in normal states. In addition, the activation of 5-HT3 receptors by 2-methyl-5-HT, another 5-HT3 receptor agonist, could induce sideward tail-flick reflex in rats [117], which might likely involve both sensory and motor components in the spinal cord. Further, 5-HT3 receptors have been reported to inhibit micturition in cats in both normal and spinalized situation [152].

3.4. 5-HT4 receptors

Data concerning 5-HT4 receptors in the spinal cord are scarce. As far as I know, so far only one article reported the expression of 5-HT4 receptors in the spinal cord [153]. Using immunohistochemistry, Suwa et al. [153] investigated 5-HT4 receptor cell distribution in the brain and spinal cord in juvenile rats and found a high density of immunostained neurons in the ventral horn of the spinal cord. In addition, several sympathetic neurons were also seen to be immunopositive.

Similarly, studies about the functions of 5-HT4 receptors in the spinal cord are also rare. Using pharmacological method, Godínez-Chaparro et al. [154] showed that 5-HT in the spinal cord promotes the development and maintenance of secondary allodynia and hyperalgesia caused by formalin stimulation via the activation of 5-HT4/6/7 receptors. Considering the anatomical distribution of 5-HT4 receptors in the spinal cord, they should also play a role in some motor functions. Whether this is the case needs to be investigated further.

3.5. 5-HT5 receptors

The 5-HT5 receptor family comprises two members: 5-HT5A and 5-HT5B. Although 5-HT5B receptors have been found in some structures in rat and mouse brain, they are not expressed in humans [155]. Therefore, I will only describe the 5-HT5A receptors in this chapter.

5-HT5A receptors were first identified in the rat spinal cord by Doly et al. [156]. They showed that in the rat spinal cord, 5-HT5A receptors were expressed with high density in the superficial dorsal horn (laminae I and II) especially in lamina II. In addition, they were also expressed in other regions including the intermediolateral nucleus in the thoracolumbar region and Onuf's nucleus in lumbosacral region. Ventral horn motoneurons in different regions were weakly labeled. Subcellularly, the receptors were found both in the cytoplasm and on the cell membrane of neuronal somata and dendrites. In the cytoplasm, they were associated with Golgi apparatus, rough endoplasmic reticulum, and vesicles. On the membrane, they were exclusively located on the postsynaptic density that was in clear contrast with the subcellular localization of 5-HT2A receptors [108, 110].

According to their locations in the spinal cord, it is speculated that 5-HT5A receptors are related to spinal modulation of pain, autonomic function, and control of micturition. Indeed, data from recent pharmacological studies have demonstrated that 5-HT-induced antinociceptive effect was mediated by spinal 5-HT5A receptors in several pain models, such as that induced by formalin, capsaicin, or acetic acid [58, 157]. For example, injection of 5-HT or 5-CT (an agonist of 5-HT5A receptors) could dose-dependently prevent nociception induced by formalin [157]. However, the speculated effects of the receptors on autonomic function and control of micturition yet need to be demonstrated.

3.6. 5-HT6 receptors

Using RT-PCR, Gérard et al. [158] discovered the existence of 5-HT6 receptor mRNAs at a moderate level in the rat spinal cord. Later, using immunoautoradiogram, data from the same group showed that 5-HT6 receptor immunoreactive product seemed to be present across all laminae of the spinal gray matter with a denser labeling in the superficial dorsal horn and lamina IX [159]. No data are available about the subcellular distribution of 5-HT6 receptors in the spinal cord. However, according to the electron microscopic data from other brain regions such as the striatum and the hippocampus, 5-HT6 receptors were mainly associated with postsynaptic dendrites and no immunopositive axon terminals were found [159].

The exclusive roles of 5-HT6 receptors in the spinal cord yet remain to be elaborated. Using a formalin pain model in rats, Castañeda-Corral et al. [160] suggested that 5-HT6 receptors play a pronociceptive role in the spinal cord since intrathecal injection of EMD-386088 (5-chloro-2-methyl-3-(1,2,3,6-tetrahydro-4-pyridinyl)-1*H*-indole), a selective 5-HT6 receptor agonist, enhanced formalin-induced nociception. It is unknown whether 5-HT6 receptors play any role in motor control.

3.7. 5-HT7 receptors

As there were no specific radioligands for 5-HT7 receptors available, data concerning their distribution in the spinal cord acquired using autoradiography had been inconclusive [161] until 2005 when Doly et al. [162] used immunohistochemistry to study their distribution in the rat spinal cord. Doly et al. [162] showed that in the rat lumbar spinal cord 5-HT7 receptors were mainly located in two superficial laminae of the dorsal horn. Except in the Onuf's nucleus where the labeling was relatively denser, immunolabeling in the ventral horn motoneuron region was generally weak. At subcellular level, the receptors were found in the postsynaptic locations in neuronal cell bodies and dendrites as well as presynaptic locations in unmyelinated and thin myelinated axonal fibers. In addition, immunolabeling was also found in astrocytes. In cats, Noga et al. [16] found that in thoracolumbar spinal cord 5-HT7-immunolabeled cells spread across different laminae in the gray matter with a dorsoventral density gradient.

Available data showed that 5-HT7 receptors exert multiple roles in modulating both sensory and motor behavior. In sensory aspect 5-HT7 receptors have been demonstrated to exert dual but diverse actions in nociception depending on the different situations. In healthy rats, 5-HT7 receptor agonists exerted a pronociceptive action but in neuropathic animals they exerted an antinociceptive action [163]. Yesilyurt et al. [164] showed that intrathecal application of SB-269970 ((2*R*)-1-[(3-hydroxyphenyl)sulfonyl]-2 -(2-(4-methyl-1-piperidinyl)ethyl)pyrrolidine), a 5-HT7 receptor antagonist, blocked both opioid and nonopioid type stress-induced analgesia, and this effect was mediated by descending serotonergic pathways and the spinal 5-HT7 receptors. Several pieces of evidence have indicated that the nonopioid analgesic drug Nefopam also took its effects via activation of 5-HT7 receptors [165, 166].

5-HT7 receptors have been demonstrated to be critical for 5-HT-induced locomotor-like activity [16, 167–169]. Liu and Jordan [167] showed that in rats 5-HT7 receptor antagonists blocked locomotor-like activity induced by stimulating mid-medulla region and also decreased step cycle duration. These results have been verified in 5-HT7 knockout mice [169]. Considering that 5-HT7 receptor antagonists blocked locomotor-like activity when applied only above the L3 segments [167], it is possible that they activated the central pattern generator neurons above this level that expressed 5-HT7 receptors and responded to 5-HT stimulation. Indeed, in decerebrated cats in which locomotion was induced by electrical stimulation of the mesencephalic locomotor region abundant c-Fos immunoreactive cells were observed in laminae VII and VIII throughout the thoracolumbar segments [16].

4. Expression changes of different 5-HT receptors and their significance in motor outputs following SCI

Following SCI the descending 5-HT projections are interrupted and as a consequence, a number of 5-HT receptors undergo different degrees of plastic changes below the lesion depending on the severity of injury, which on one hand will facilitate the re-establishment of neuronal circuits in the spinal cord below the lesion and thus promote functional recovery, and on the other hand will result in pathological symptoms. These changes can occur at both anatomical and functional levels. However, due to the fact that more functional than anatomical data are available, for some receptors only functional changes have been reported. So far 5-HT receptors that have been confirmed to undergo anatomical changes include, but are not limited to, 5-HT1 and 5-HT2 receptor families. In some other receptors, functional (activity) changes are indeed detected although there are no data revealing their anatomical changes. This group of receptors includes 5-HT3 and 5-HT7 receptors. So far there are no reports as to the anatomical or functional changes for 5-HT4, 5-HT5, and 5-HT6 receptors following SCI. Below I will mainly describe the 5-HT receptors that have been clearly demonstrated to undergo anatomical and/or functional changes in relation to their impact on motor outputs.

4.1. 5-HT1 receptors

Among the different 5-HT1 subfamilies, 5-HT1A receptors were mostly investigated in terms of their anatomical and functional changes probably due to their direct involvement in functional recovery following SCI. For other subfamilies, such as 5-HT1B, 1D, and 1F, related studies were less abundant and results relating to their roles in motor functional outputs were also less conclusive.

5-HT1A receptors: Using autoradiography, the expression of 5-HT1A receptors have been shown to increase in the rat spinal cord 3 weeks following destruction of descending serotonergic fibers with 5,7-dihydroxytryptamine [83]. In cats, using the same technique, it was found that after spinal cord transection at T13 level binding density was significantly increased in laminae II, III, and X of lumbar segments at 15 and 30 days, but at 60 days the binding density recovered to the control level [28]. It should be addressed that using binding technique it is difficult to differentiate whether the labeled profiles were from neuronal cell bodies, their dendrites or axon fiber terminals. Using immunohistochemistry with two different 5-HT1A antibodies, one labeling neuronal somata and the other labeling the axon initial segments, Otoshi et al. [31] reported that 8 weeks following complete spinal transection at T7-T8 level the expression of 5-HT1A receptors in axon hillock was increased in laminae III, IV, VII, and IX, whereas the expression in neuronal somata and dendrites were increased in laminae VII and IX. This upregulation, both in the axon hillock and neuronal somata and dendrites, was dependent on the sensory input since the receptors were not upregulated when the spinal cord was isolated. Using in situ hybridization, Cornide-Petronio et al. [170] saw a similar upregulation time course for 5-HT1A receptors in lampreys as in cats. They reported an acute upregulation of 5-HT1A receptors in the spinal cord after SCI both in the rostral and caudal part of the lesion site, and the upregulation recovered to normal levels at 3 weeks. This quick recovery of 5-HT1A receptor expression may be due to that in lamprey serotonergic descending projecting neurons in the rhombencephalon could regenerate their axons across the lesion site after complete spinal cord transection [171]. Thus, the variation of results from these studies may partly reflect the different receptor responses to SCI in different species.

There is ample evidence that the activation of 5-HT1A receptors could induce motor functional recovery after SCI [13, 84, 172]. Antri et al. [13] found that, in thoracic spinal cord transected rats, after daily systemic application of 5-HT1A receptor agonist 8-OH-DPAT, locomotor function was significantly improved when compared with control spinalized animals. The agonist had both short- and long-term effects for motor functional improvement. A similar result was also demonstrated by Jackson and White [84] that in acute C1 spinal cord transected rats, after intravenous administration of 8-OH-DPAT, the excitability of spinal motoneurons was markedly enhanced. However, local application of 8-OH-DPAT directly into the ventral horn by microiontophoresis inhibited the glutamate-evoked firing of motoneurons. These results indicate that when 8-OH-DPAT was directly applied into the vicinity of the motoneurons it may activate 5-HT1A receptors in the axon hillock which inhibits the motoneuron firing [81]. However, the marked increase in firing of motoneurons induced by systemic administration of 8-OH-DPAT suggests that 5-HT1A receptors in other locations, likely at sites presynaptic to the motoneurons, have also been activated. In addition to the functions described above, 5-HT1A receptors have been reported to increase bladder capacity under saline or acid infused conditions in SCI cats [173].

5-HT1B receptors: In comparison with 5-HT1A receptors, studies concerning plastic changes of 5-HT1B receptors following SCI are sparse. Using autoradiography, Laporte et al. [83]

reported that when descending serotonergic projections were destroyed by 5,7-dihydroxy-tryptamine the labeling of 5-HT1B receptors was decreased (−12%) in the dorsal horn at the cervical but not at the lumbar level in rats. Interestingly, when noradrenergic systems had been lesioned by DSP-4 (*N*-(2-chloroethyl)-*N*-ethyl-2-bromobenzylamine) there was an increase of labeling of 5-HT1B receptors both at the cervical level (+31%) and the lumbar level (+17%). In a C2 hemisection rat model, using quantitative RT-PCR, Mantilla et al. [86] did not detect expression changes of 5-HT1B receptors in phrenic motoneurons 2 or 3 weeks following the injury.

Similar to their functions in normal physiological states, in SCI states 5-HT1B receptors also play an inhibitory role for motor outputs possibly through inhibitions on both mono- and polysynaptic reflexes. In acute C1 spinalized rats, Honda et al. [174] showed that serotonergic depression of monosynaptic reflex transmission induced by application of 5-HTP was mediated by 5-HT1B receptors. In S2 spinal cord transection model (also called tail spasticity model), Murray et al. [99] showed that polysynaptic EPSPs that trigger muscle spasms after SCI were inhibited by 5-HT1B receptors.

5-HT1D and 1F receptors: To my knowledge, no studies have investigated the expression changes of these two receptors following SCI. Functionally, the activation of 5-HT1D receptors seemed to reduce sensory transmission in both monosynaptic and polysynaptic reflexes in humans [95], and to inhibit bladder activity in cats after SCI [175]. The activation of 5-HT1F seemed to inhibit long polysynaptic reflexes in rats after SCI [99]. However because the agonists used in these studies were not specific enough for selected receptors the results were not conclusive.

4.2. 5-HT2 receptors

5-HT2, especially 5-HT2A and 2C, receptors are the most intensely studied receptors among all 5-HT receptor families mostly due to their considerable effects on the motor functional recovery and perhaps also on the pathological symptoms developed following SCI such as spasticity. Due to the close relationship and similar functions of these three receptor subfamilies, their influences on the motor outputs after SCI will be described together.

5-HT2A receptors: Using different SCI animal models such as contusion, hemisection, and complete spinal transection, it is confirmed that 5-HT2A receptors underwent different degrees of plastic changes following SCI. In thoracic contusive rats using immunohistochemistry, Lee et al. [30] found a moderate yet significantly increased 5-HT2A receptor expression (~1.2-fold of control) in the motoneurons at L5-L6 level after 4 weeks of injury. With the same method in a C2 hemisection rat model Fuller et al. [29] demonstrated a significant upregulation (~1.7-fold of control) of 5-HT2A receptors in the ipsilateral phrenic motoneurons after 2 weeks of injury. In a S2 spinal transection model, Kong et al. [32, 33] reported a dramatic increase of 5-HT2A receptor immunoreactivity (~5.6-fold of control) in the motoneurons below the lesion. The upregulation began as early as 1 day after injury, reached a maximal level by 28 days and lasted at least until 60 days, the longest time interval investigated. Similarly an upregulation of 5-HT2A receptors were also observed in chronic (6 weeks) thoracic spinal transected rats. Navarrett et al. [35] reported a ~1.3-fold increase of 5-HT2A receptor mRNAs in the spinal tissue (including both white and gray matter) below the lesion with RT-PCR. Upregulation of 5-HT2A receptor mRNAs was also reported in mice subjected to an acute thoracic spinal transection. Thus, Ung et al. [176] found that 3 h after the lesion 5-HT2A receptor mRNA expression levels were increased 2.5-fold in the lateral intermediate zone in L1-L2 segments and they remained to be elevated for at least 2 weeks. However, no significant change was found in the ventral horn motoneuron regions, which was strikingly different from that in the rat.

5-HT2B receptors: No expression changes have been reported for this receptor subfamily in the spinal cord following SCI. With microarray global gene analysis technique, Wienecke et al. [122] did not detect significant changes of 5-HT2B receptor mRNAs in S2 spinal transected rats.

5-HT2C receptors: Similar to 5-HT2A receptors, 5-HT2C receptor expression changes have been investigated in different SCI animal models with different techniques. However, discrepancies exist as to whether 5-HT2C receptors are upregulated or not following SCI. In chronic SCI rats (~15 weeks) severe contusion or transection at thoracic level (T9) could induce a significant increase of 5-HT2C receptor immunoreactivity in lumbar spinal cord [22]. The increase could reach 4–7-fold in the ventral horn and ~17-fold in the dorsal horn over control level. In thoracic (T8-T9) spinal transected neonatal rats, following 4 weeks injury 5-HT2C receptor immunoreactivity was seen to increase 4–5-fold both in the spinal dorsal and ventral horn [177]. In a S2 spinal transection rat model, data from our group [36] indicated that 5-HT2C receptor immunoreactivity increased in all parts of the spinal gray matter below the lesion from 2 weeks but did not reach a significant level until 3 weeks (~1.4-fold over control animals). The increase sustained thereafter and a maximal level was reached at 45 days (~1.7-fold) and maintained at 60 days, the longest investigated interval. It is somehow perplexing that although upregulation was observed at protein level no significant increase at mRNA level was detected in different SCI animal models [34, 35, 122, 178]. However, although no significant changes of the total amount of 5-HT2C receptor mRNAs were detected, Murray et al. [34] did detect certain constitutive isoforms, such as INI isoform, that were significantly increased in the motoneurons 6 weeks after S2 spinal transection.

Functional significance for motor outputs of 5-HT2 receptors: The activation of 5-HT2 receptors has different effects on motor outputs after SCI, which include promoting motor functional recovery and causing maladaptive pathological motor symptoms such as spasticity. Due to uncertainty of the expression of 5-HT2B receptors in the spinal cord most studies have been focused on 5-HT2A and 2C receptors. There is ample evidence for the roles of 5-HT2A and 2C receptors in motor functional recovery following SCI from different studies (e.g., [9, 12, 14, 34, 43, 84, 134, 176, 179, 180], for reviews see [44, 45]). For example, in thoracic spinalized cats, when a 5-HT2A/C receptor agonist (e.g., quipazine or DOI) was administrated α-motoneuron excitability was increased and hindlimb motor activity was enhanced [9]. Similar results were also demonstrated in SCI rats [12, 14] and mice [176]. Although 5-HT2A and 2C receptors both play a common role for motor functional recovery each subfamily may also exert different functions in different aspects of the motor outputs. Using different agonists and antagonists specific for each of these two receptor subfamilies it is found that 5-HT2A receptors might contribute to locomotor network activation and locomotor-like movement generation

[15, 43, 176]. Direct stimulation of 5-HT2C receptors with its agonist meta-chlorophenylpiperazine improved weight-supported locomotion in adult rats spinalized as neonates [177, 181]. 5-HT2C, probably also 2B, but not 2A, receptors could become constitutively active which could contribute to motor functional recovery following SCI [34, 182].

One maladaptive consequence for 5-HT2 receptor plastic changes is the induction of muscle spasm due to increased motoneuron excitability. The rapid and robust upregulation of 5-HT2A receptors in spinal motoneurons might be responsible for 5-HT supersensitivity after SCI [32, 33]. Activation of 5-HT2C receptors could induce long-lasting reflexes of motoneurons in the in vitro spinal cord preparations [134, 135]. These long-lasting reflexes could be enhanced when 5-HT2C receptors became constitutively active following SCI [34, 182]. One of the cellular mechanisms for the increased motoneuron excitability is that the activation of 5-HT2 receptors could enhance calcium and/or sodium persistent inward currents [42, 183].

In addition to promoting locomotion, 5-HT2 (especially 2A) receptors also play a significant role for respiratory functional recovery after cervical spinal hemisection [179] and in enhancing bladder function in thoracic spinal transected rats [184].

It should be addressed that the upregulation of 5-HT2 receptors does not by all means lead the motoneurons toward a hyperexcitatory state. Recently one interesting finding is presented by Bos et al. [185] who showed that the activation of 5-HT2A receptors could increase K(+)-Cl(−) cotransporter (KCC2) expression on cell membrane in the spinal cord motoneurons after SCI. The upregulation of KCC2 receptors in turn increased the activity of GABA A and glycine receptors which would restore endogenous inhibition and reduce spasticity after SCI in rats [186]. These results indicate that the upregulation of 5-HT2A receptors would not simply produce an excitatory effect. Rather, their activation will trigger an inhibitory factor which attempts to balance the excitatory effect. This effect seems to be paradoxical to the 5-HT2A receptors' direct excitatory effect on motoneurons. However, this might be one of the common functional mechanisms of a spinal network—different factors interact and compensate each other, and the final motor output is determined by a summed vector of these push-pull forces acted on the motoneurons. In fact, any motor action cannot be arisen solely from the activation of a single factor; instead it needs a concert activity of multiple factors including both excitatory and inhibitory. For instance, Hayashi et al. [22] have showed that in contusive SCI rats, application of 5-HT1A or 5-HT2C receptor agonists alone or in combination could not improve hindlimb motor function; rather, motor functional improvement could be achieved only when the 5-HT precursor 5-HTP was administrated, indicating that simultaneously multiple 5-HT receptor activations are needed for motor functional recovery. This concept is reinforced by the results from Noga et al. [16] who showed that in paralyzed, decerebrated cats, when locomotion was induced by electrical stimulation of the mesencephalic locomotor region, most locomotor-activated cells, labeled with c-Fos, colocalized with 5-HT1A, 5-HT2A, and 5-HT7 receptors in laminae VII and VIII in the thoracolumbar spinal region.

4.3. 5-HT3 receptors

There are no data demonstrating the expression changes of 5-HT3 following SCI. Laporte et al. [83] did not detect 5-HT3 receptor expression changes with binding technique in rat spinal cords whose descending serotonergic projections had been destroyed by 5,7-dihydroxytryptamine. However, lesions in peripheral nerves could reduce 5-HT3 receptor expression in the spinal motoneurons in rats [187].

Most studies concerning 5-HT3 receptor functions have been focused on sensory aspects, especially nociception. Studies relating to their functions in motor outputs after SCI are scarce. So far there is only one study having investigated the influence of the activation of 5-HT3 receptors on motor outputs in SCI mice. In this study, Guertin and Steuer [152] showed that in hindlimb paralyzed mice 5-HT3 receptor agonist SR-57227 could produce hindlimb movements although with a low score. This result, anyhow, provided the first evidence that 5-HT3 receptors could modulate spinal motoneuron activity after SCI.

4.4. 5-HT7 receptors

So far there are no data available with respect to the expression changes of 5-HT7 receptors following SCI. However, the activation of 5-HT7 receptor has been shown to be related to locomotor functional recovery in SCI states [23, 43, 172]. Landry et al. [172] showed that in thoracic spinal transected mice systemic application of 8-OH-DPAT, an agonist for both 5-HT1A and 5-HT7 receptors, acutely induced hindlimb movements with characteristics similar to normal locomotion. When the animals were pretreated with SB-269970, a selective 5-HT7 receptor antagonist, 8-OH-DPAT-induced movements were reduced. Sławińska et al. [23] showed that, in thoracic spinal transected rats, grafting of neurons from the B1, B2, and B3 descending 5-HT system from the brainstem into the spinal cord below the lesion effectively restored coordinated plantar stepping, and the application of SB-269970 disrupted the inter- and intralimb coordination. Further evidence from the same group indicated that 8-OH-DPAT facilitated plantar stepping in chronic spinalized rats [43]. Since 5-HT7 receptor agonists mainly improved coordination movement the authors assumed that 5-HT7 receptors mainly facilitated the activity of the central pattern generator interneurons. This assumption is supported by anatomical data that 5-HT7 receptors were mainly expressed in the neurons in the dorsal horn and the intermediate zone of the spinal gray matter [16]. In addition to the effects on locomotion, it has been reported that the activation of 5-HT7 receptors by their agonist LP44 (4-[2-(methylthio)phenyl]-*N*-(1,2,3,4-tetrahydronaphthalen-1-yl)-1-piperazinehexanamide) increased bladder voiding efficiency in chronic thoracic spinal transected rats [188].

5. Plasticity of 5-HT innervations after SCI

It is evidenced that a small number of 5-HT receptors, or more precisely receptor isoforms, could become active following SCI without ligand activation—so-called constitutive activation. However, for most of the 5-HT receptors that do not have constitutive isoforms the presence of their ligand—5HT is a necessity for their activation. Then, where could 5-HT originate following SCI? After contusion spinal cord injury or partial spinal cord transections there are still spared supraspinal serotonergic projections and these serotonergic fibers could undergo plastic changes to eventually supplement lost 5-HT supply in the injured spinal cord. For example, in contusion injury the density of spared 5-HT fibers below the lesion varies depending on the locations along the dorsoventral axis and the severity of the injury [22, 189, 190], and 5-HT innervation could be partially restored with time which is responsible at least partly for motor functional recovery [190]. In thoracic hemisection injury, the density of 5-HT fibers in the ipsilateral ventral horn varied from 8% to 30% of the control value according to studies with a postinjury interval 4–7 days [39, 191–194]. The data are inconsistent as to whether 5-HT fibers increase with time following hemisection. Some researchers reported a gradual increase of 5-HT fibers on the ipsilateral side below the lesion (e.g., [193, 195]), whereas some others did not see apparent changes (e.g., [39, 194]). For example, Saruhashi et al. [193] observed that 5-HT-immunoreactive fibers recovered from 20% to about 75% of the normal value in the ventral horn during first 4 weeks. Camand et al. [195] also reported a similar finding in the intermediate zone. However, Filli et al. [194] reported a decrease to about 10% by 4 weeks from about 30% at day 4 in ventral horn motoneuron region. Azam et al. [39] reported that by 60 days the density of 5-HT-immunoreacitve fibers in the intermediate zone was reduced to 11% from 23% at 5 days, whereas in the ventral horn it was not reduced (23% vs. 22%). Following complete spinal transection, some 2–15% of the normal content of 5-HT remained in the spinal cord below the lesion ([196]; for review see [25]).

The next question would be then where the residual 5-HT originates following complete spinal transection. One origin might be the intraspinal serotonergic neurons. However, intraspinal serotonergic neurons are very few in number and sparsely distributed (see Section 1). Then, what are the other possible sources? Recent findings from our [38] and Bennett's group [37] indicated that AADC cells in the spinal cord might be another origin. AADC is an essential enzyme for the synthesis of 5-HT, dopamine, and certain trace amines from their respective precursors. AADC cells are widely distributed in different regions of the spinal cord [38], not limiting to the area around the central canal as reported previously [197]. Following SCI the ability of AADC cells in the spinal cord to synthesize 5-HT/dopamine from 5-HTP/L-dopa was dramatically increased and 5-HT/dopamine produced in the AADC was responsible for the increased motoneuron ability recorded both in vivo and in vitro [37, 38, 40, 198]. Nonetheless, we have to admit that without 5-HTP application 5-HT could not be detected in the spinal AADC cells. This might be due to that the detecting techniques used in related studies were not sensitive enough to disclose a small amount of 5-HT, or the turnover rate of 5-HT produced in the AADC cells was so high that once produced it was immediately metabolized. One piece of evidence to support the speculation that monoamine transmitters could be produced from AADC cells in the spinal cord after SCI comes from Hou et al. [199], who showed that the number of dopamine-producing cells, which contained both AADC and tyrosine hydroxylase, was increased in lumbosacral spinal cord in thoracic spinal transected rats; and with enzyme-linked immunosorbent assay (ELISA) dopamine with a content of about 10% of its normal value could be detected in this part of the spinal cord even without L-dopa application. At the same time they also showed that dopamine produced from the spinal cord below the lesion was implicated for micturition functional recovery following SCI.

6. Conclusions

The serotonin system in the spinal cord is an important modulator for sensory, motor as well as autonomic function. This system normally exercises its function via the interaction between ligand 5-HT and a number of 5-HT receptors expressed in different structures in the spinal cord. Among the 14 5-HT receptor subfamilies at least 12 have been detected in the spinal cord, in which 5-HT1A, 2A, 2C, and 7 receptors have been demonstrated to be more important for motor control. In normal physiological states, these receptors coordinate with each other and also with other monoamine systems to enable smooth and controllable motor outputs for our physical activity [200]. Following SCI extensive plastic changes occur for a number of 5-HT receptor subfamilies, mostly with increased receptor numbers and/or constitutive activity. In addition, plasticity also occurs for descending serotonergic fibers (in the case of incomplete SCI) and intraspinal serotonin-producing cells. The coeffects of these plastic changes, together with the plastic changes of other monoamine systems, ultimately lead to increased motoneuron excitability in the chronic phase [17, 21, 108]. These plastic changes have both beneficial and detrimental effects for spinal motor outputs after SCI. Although the plastic changes can result in an adaptive compensation of the lost transmitters and thus assist in motor functional recovery, they can also result in a plethora of maladaptive problems, such as spasticity. In clinical practice, a strategy needs to be set so as to maximally take advantage of the positive side of the plasticity to promote motor functional recovery and meanwhile to reduce negative effects to a minimal extent. To reach this endpoint, pharmacological and/or genetic interferences need to be utilized so that the activity of different 5-HT receptors and 5-HT supply in the spinal cord reach a new balance and consequently an appropriate motor behavior is generated. Such a strategy would certainly have great implications for future treatment of SCI patients.

Acknowledgements

This work was supported by the Lundbeck Foundation and the Danish Medical Research Council.

Abbreviations

5-CT: 5-carboxamidotryptamine

5-HT: 5-hydroxytryptomine, serotonin

8-OH-DPAT: 8-hydroxy-2-(di-*n*-propylamino) tetralin

AADC: aromatic L-amino acid decarboxylase

http://dx.doi.org/10.5772/63759

BRL-15572: 3-(4-(4-chlorophenyl)piperazin-1-yl)-1,1-diphenyl-2-propanol

C, T, L, and S: cervical, thoracic, lumbar, and sacral spinal cord, respectively

D-MC: *N*-ormethylclozapine/8-chloro-11-(1-piperazinyl)-5*H*-dibenzo[*b,e*][1,4]diazepine

DOI: (±)-2,5-dimethoxy-4-iodoamphetamine hydrochloride

DOM: 2,5-dimethoxy-alpha,4-dimethyl-benzene ethamine hydrochloride

DSP-4: *N*-(2-chloroethyl)-*N*-ethyl-2-bromobenzylamine

ELISA: enzyme-linked immunosorbent assay

EMD-386088: 5-chloro-2-methyl-3-(1,2,3,6-tetrahydro-4-pyridinyl)-1*H*-indole

EPSP: excitatory postsynaptic potential

GABA: γ-aminobutyric acid

GR-46611: 3-[3-(2-dimethylaminoethyl)-1*H*-indol-5-yl]-*N*-(4-methoxybenzyl)acrylamide

KCC2: K(+)-Cl(–) cotransporter

L-dopa: L-3,4-dihydroxyphenylalanine

LP44: 4-[2-(methylthio)phenyl]-*N*-(1,2,3,4-tetrahydronaphthalen-1-yl)-1-piperazinehexanamide

LY-344864: *N*-[(3*R*)-3-(dimethylamino)-2,3,4,9-tetrahydro-1*H*-carbazol-6-yl]-4-fluorobenzamide

MK-212: 6-chloro-2-(1-piperazinyl)pyrazine hydrochloride

mRNA: messenger ribonucleic acid

NMDA: *N*-methyl-D-aspartate

PCR: polymerase chain reaction

Ro-600175: (α*S*)-6-chloro-5-fluoro-α-methyl-1*H*-indole-1-ethanamine fumarate

RS-127445: (3-(4-(4-chlorophenyl)piperazin-1-yl)-1,1-diphenyl-2-propanol)

RT-PCT: reverse transcription polymerase chain reaction

RU-24969: 5-methoxy-3(1,2,3,6-tetrahydropyridin-4-yl)-1*H*-indole

SB-242084: 6-chloro-2,3-dihydro-5-methyl-*N*-[6-[(2-methyl-3-pyridinyl)oxy]-3-pyridinyl]-1*H*-indole-1-carboxyamide

SB-269970: (2*R*)-1-[(3-hydroxyphenyl)sulfonyl]-2 -(2-(4-methyl-1-piperidinyl)ethyl)pyrrolidine

SCI: spinal cord injury

SR-57227: 1-(6-chloropyridin-2-yl)piperidin-4-amine

TCB-2: 4-bromo-3,6-dimethoxybenzocyclobuten-1-yl)methylamine hydrobromide

WAY-100635: *N*-[2-[4-(2-methoxyphenyl)-1-piperazinyl]ethyl]-*N*-(2-pyridyl)cyclohexanecarboxamide

WAY-161503: 8,9-dichloro-2,3,4,4a-tetrahydro-1*H*-pyrazino[1,2-*a*]quinoxalin-5(6*H*)

Author details

Mengliang Zhang[1,2]

Address all correspondence to: mzhang@sund.ku.dk

1 Department of Neuroscience and Pharmacology, University of Copenhagen, Copenhagen, Denmark

2 Neuronano Research Center, Department of Experimental Medical Science, Lund University, Lund, Sweden

References

[1] Witiw CD, Fehlings MG. Acute spinal cord injury. J Spinal Disord Tech. 2015;28:202–210. DOI: 10.1097/BSD.0000000000000287.

[2] Jensen MP, Kuehn CM, Amtmann D, Cardenas DD. Symptom burden in persons with spinal cord injury. Arch Phys Med Rehabil. 2007;88:638–645. DOI: 10.1016/j.apmr.2007.02.002.

[3] Nielsen JB, Crone C, Hultborn H. The spinal pathophysiology of spasticity-from a basic science point of view. Acta Physiol (Oxf). 2007;189:171–180. DOI: 10.1111/j.1748-1716.2006.01652.x.

[4] Sheean G, McGuire JR. Spastic hypertonia and movement disorders: pathophysiology, clinical presentation, and quantification. PM R. 2009;1:827–833. DOI: 10.1016/j.pmrj.2009.08.002.

[5] Gunduz H, Binak DF. Autonomic dysreflexia: an important cardiovascular complication in spinal cord injury patients. Cardiol J. 2012;19:215–219. DOI: 10.5603/CJ.2012.0040.

[6] Felix ER. Chronic neuropathic pain in SCI: evaluation and treatment. Phys Med Rehabil Clin N Am. 2014;25:545–571. DOI: 10.1016/0006-8993(88)91548-X.

[7] Nas K, Yazmalar L, Şah V, Aydın A, Öneş K. Rehabilitation of spinal cord injuries. World J Orthop. 2015;6:8–16. DOI: 10.5312/wjo.v6.i1.8.

[8] Guertin PA. New pharmacological approaches against chronic bowel and bladder problems in paralytics. World J Crit Care Med. 2016;5:1–6. DOI: 10.5492/wjccm.v5.i1.1.

[9] Barbeau H, Rossignol S. The effects of serotonergic drugs on the locomotor pattern and on cutaneous reflexes of the adult chronic spinal cat. Brain Res. 1990;514:55–67. DOI: 10.1016/0006-8993(90)90435-E.

[10] Kiehn O, Kjaerulff O. Spatiotemporal characteristics of 5-HT and dopamine-induced rhythmic hindlimb activity in the in vitro neonatal rat. J Neurophysiol. 1996;75:1472–1482.

[11] McEwen ML, Van Hartesveldt C, Stehouwer DJ. L-DOPA and quipazine elicit air-stepping in neonatal rats with spinal cord transections. Behav Neurosci. 1997;111:825–833. DOI: 10.1037/0735-7044.111.4.825.

[12] Antri M, Orsal D, Barthe JY. Locomotor recovery in the chronic spinal rat: effects of long-term treatment with a 5-HT2 agonist. Eur J Neurosci. 2002;16:467–476. DOI: 10.1046/j.1460-9568.2002.02088.x.

[13] Antri M, Mouffle C, Orsal D, Barthe JY. 5-HT1A receptors are involved in short- and long-term processes responsible for 5-HT-induced locomotor function recovery in chronic spinal rat. Eur J Neurosci. 2003;18:1963–1972. DOI: 10.1046/j.1460-9568.2003.02916.x.

[14] Antri M, Barthe JY, Mouffle C, Orsal D. Long-lasting recovery of locomotor function in chronic spinal rat following chronic combined pharmacological stimulation of serotonergic receptors with 8-OHDPAT and quipazine. Neurosci Lett. 2005;384:162–267. DOI: 10.1016/j.neulet.2005.04.062.

[15] Landry ES, Guertin PA. Differential effects of 5-HT1 and 5-HT2 receptor agonists on hindlimb movements in paraplegic mice. Prog Neuropsychopharmacol Biol Psychiatry. 2004;28:1053–1060. DOI: 10.1016/j.pnpbp.2004.05.001.

[16] Noga BR, Johnson DM, Riesgo MI, Pinzon A. Locomotor-activated neurons of the cat. I. Serotonergic innervation and co-localization of 5-HT7, 5-HT2A, and 5-HT1A receptors in the thoraco-lumbar spinal cord. J Neurophysiol. 2009;102:1560–1576. DOI: 10.1152/jn.91179.2008.

[17] Musienko P, van den Brand R, Märzendorfer O, Roy RR, Gerasimenko Y, Edgerton VR, Courtine G. Controlling specific locomotor behaviors through multidimensional monoaminergic modulation of spinal circuitries. J Neurosci. 2011;31:9264–9278. DOI: 10.1523/JNEUROSCI.5796-10.2011.

[18] Feraboli-Lohnherr D, Orsal D, Yakovleff A, Giménez y Ribotta M, Privat A. Recovery of locomotor activity in the adult chronic spinal rat after sublesional transplantation of embryonic nervous cells: specific role of serotonergic neurons. Exp Brain Res. 1997;113:443–454. DOI: 10.1007/PL00005597.

[19] Orsal D, Barthe JY, Antri M, Feraboli-Lohnherr D, Yakovleff A, Giménez y Ribotta M, Privat A, Provencher J, Rossignol S. Locomotor recovery in chronic spinal rat: long-

term pharmacological treatment or transplantation of embryonic neurons? Prog Brain Res. 2002;137:213–230.

[20] Kubasak MD, Jindrich DL, Zhong H, Takeoka A, McFarland KC, Muñoz-Quiles C, Roy RR, Edgerton VR, Ramón-Cueto A, Phelps PE. OEG implantation and step training enhance hindlimb-stepping ability in adult spinal transected rats. Brain. 2008;131:264–276. DOI: 10.1093/brain/awm267.

[21] Courtine G, Gerasimenko Y, van den Brand R, Yew A, Musienko P, Zhong H, Song B, Ao Y, Ichiyama RM, Lavrov I, Roy RR, Sofroniew MV, Edgerton VR. Transformation of nonfunctional spinal circuits into functional states after the loss of brain input. Nat Neurosci. 2009;12:1333–1342. DOI: 10.1038/nn.2401.

[22] Hayashi Y, Jacob-Vadakot S, Dugan EA, McBride S, Olexa R, Simansky K, Murray M, Shumsky JS. 5-HT precursor loading, but not 5-HT receptor agonists, increases motor function after spinal cord contusion in adult rats. Exp Neurol. 2010;221:68–78. DOI: 10.1016/j.expneurol.2009.10.003.

[23] Sławińska U, Miazga K, Cabaj AM, Leszczyńska AN, Majczyński H, Nagy JI, Jordan LM. Grafting of fetal brainstem 5-HT neurons into the sublesional spinal cord of paraplegic rats restores coordinated hindlimb locomotion. Exp Neurol. 2013;247:572–581. DOI: 10.1016/j.expneurol.2013.02.008.

[24] Jacobs BL, Fornal CA. Serotonin and motor activity. Curr Opin Neurobiol. 1997;7:820–825. DOI: 10.1016/S0959-4388(97)80141-9.

[25] Schmidt BJ, Jordan LM. The role of serotonin in reflex modulation and locomotor rhythm production in the mammalian spinal cord. Brain Res Bull. 2000;53:689–710. DOI: 10.1016/S0361-9230(00)00402-0.

[26] Millan MJ. Descending control of pain. Prog Neurobiol. 2002;66:355–474. DOI: 10.1016/S0301-0082(02)00009-6.

[27] Pearlstein E, Ben Mabrouk F, Pflieger JF, Vinay L. Serotonin refines the locomotor-related alternations in the in vitro neonatal rat spinal cord. Eur J Neurosci. 2005;21:1338–1346. DOI: 10.1111/j.1460-9568.2005.03971.x.

[28] Giroux N, Rossignol S, Reader TA. Autoradiographic study of alpha1- and alpha2-noradrenergic and serotonin1A receptors in the spinal cord of normal and chronically transected cats. J Comp Neurol. 1999;406:402–414. DOI: 10.1002/(SICI)1096-9861(19990412)406:3<402::AID-CNE8>3.0.CO;2-F.

[29] Fuller DD, Baker-Herman TL, Golder FJ, Doperalski NJ, Watters JJ, Mitchell GS. Cervical spinal cord injury upregulates ventral spinal 5-HT2A receptors. J Neurotrauma. 2005;22:203–213. DOI: 10.1089/neu.2005.22.203.

[30] Lee JK, Johnson CS, Wrathall JR. Up-regulation of 5-HT2 receptors is involved in the increased H-reflex amplitude after contusive spinal cord injury. Exp Neurol. 2007;203:502–511. DOI: 10.1016/j.expneurol.2006.09.003.

[31] Otoshi CK, Walwyn WM, Tillakaratne NJ, Zhong H, Roy RR, Edgerton VR. Distribution and localization of 5-HT(1A) receptors in the rat lumbar spinal cord after transection and deafferentation. J Neurotrauma. 2009;26:575–584. DOI: 10.1089/neu.2008.0640.

[32] Kong X-Y, Wienecke J, Hultborn H, Zhang M. Robust upregulation of serotonin 2A receptors after chronic spinal transection of rats: an immunohistochemical study. Brain Res. 2010;1320:60–68. DOI: 10.1016/j.brainres.2010.01.030.

[33] Kong XY, Wienecke J, Chen M, Hultborn H, Zhang M. The time course of serotonin 2A receptor expression after spinal transection of rats: an immunohistochemical study. Neuroscience. 2011;177:114–126. DOI: 10.1016/j.neuroscience.2010.12.062.

[34] Murray KC, Nakae A, Stephens MJ, Rank M, D'Amico J, Harvey PJ, Li X, Harris RL, Ballou EW, Anelli R, Heckman CJ, Mashimo T, Vavrek R, Sanelli L, Gorassini MA, Bennett DJ, Fouad K. Recovery of motoneuron and locomotor function after spinal cord injury depends on constitutive activity in 5-HT2C receptors. Nat Med. 2010;16:694–700. DOI: 10.1038/nm.2160.

[35] Navarrett S, Collier L, Cardozo C, Dracheva S. Alterations of serotonin 2C and 2A receptors in response to T10 spinal cord transection in rats. Neurosci Lett. 2012;506:74–78. DOI: 10.1016/j.neulet.2011.10.052.

[36] Ren LQ, Wienecke J, Chen M, Møller M, Hultborn H, Zhang M. The time course of serotonin 2C receptor expression after spinal transection of rats: an immunohistochemical study. Neuroscience. 2013;236:31–46. DOI: 10.1016/j.neuroscience.2012.12.063.

[37] Li Y, Li L, Stephens MJ, Zenner D, Murray KC, Winship IR, Vavrek R, Baker GB, Fouad K, Bennett DJ. Synthesis, transport, and metabolism of serotonin formed from exogenously applied 5-HTP after spinal cord injury in rats. J Neurophysiol. 2014;111:145–163. DOI: 10.1152/jn.00508.2013.

[38] Wienecke J, Ren LQ, Hultborn H, Chen M, Møller M, Zhang Y, Zhang M. Spinal cord injury enables aromatic L-amino acid decarboxylase cells to synthesize monoamines. J Neurosci. 2014;34:11984–12000. DOI: 10.1523/JNEUROSCI.3838-13.2014.

[39] Azam B, Wienecke J, Jensen DB, Azam A, Zhang M. Spinal cord hemisection facilitates aromatic L-amino acid decarboxylase cells to produce serotonin in the subchronic but not the chronic phase. Neural Plast. 2015;2015:549671. DOI: 10.1155/2015/549671.

[40] Zhang M. Aromatic L-amino acid decarboxylase cells in the spinal cord: a potential origin of monoamines. Neural Regen Res. 2015;10:715–717. DOI: 10.4103/1673-5374.156960.

[41] Hains BC, Everhart AW, Fullwood SD, and Hulsebosch CE. Changes in serotonin, serotonin transporter expression and serotonin denervation supersensitivity: involvement in chronic central pain after spinal hemisection in the rat. Exp Neurol. 2002;175:347–362. DOI: 10.1006/exnr.2002.7892.

[42] Harvey PJ, Li X, Li Y, Bennett DJ. 5-HT2 receptor activation facilitates a persistent sodium current and repetitive firing in spinal motoneurons of rats with and without

chronic spinal cord injury. J Neurophysiol. 2006;96:1158–1170. DOI: 10.1152/jn.01088.2005.

[43] Sławińska U, Miazga K, Jordan LM. 5-HT2 and 5-HT7 receptor agonists facilitate plantar stepping in chronic spinal rats through actions on different populations of spinal neurons. Front Neural Circuits. 2014;8:95. DOI: 10.3389/fncir.2014.00095.

[44] Ghosh M, Pearse DD. The role of the serotonergic system in locomotor recovery after spinal cord injury. Front Neural Circuits. 2015;8:151. DOI: 10.3389/fncir.2014.00151.

[45] Nardone R, Höller Y, Thomschewski A, Höller P, Lochner P, Golaszewski S, Brigo F, Trinka E. Serotonergic transmission after spinal cord injury. J Neural Transm (Vienna). 2015;122:279–295. DOI: 10.1007/s00702-014-1241-z.

[46] Dahlstroem A, Fuxe K. Evidence for the existence of monoamine containing neurons in the central nervous system. I. Demonstration of monamines in the cell bodies of brain stem neurons. Acta Physiol Scand Suppl. 1964;62:1–55.

[47] Takeuchi Y, Kimura H, Sano Y. Immunohistochemical demonstration of serotonin neurons in the brainstem of the rat and cat. Cell Tissue Res. 1982;224:247–267. DOI: 10.1007/BF00216872.

[48] Skagerberg G, Björklund A. Topographic principles in the spinal projections of serotonergic and non-serotonergic brainstem neurons in the rat. Neuroscience. 1985;15:445–480. DOI: 10.1016/0306-4522(85)90225-8.

[49] Hornung JP. The human raphe nuclei and the serotonergic system. J Chem Neuroanat. 2003;26:331–343. DOI: 10.1016/j.jchemneu.2003.10.002.

[50] Azmitia EC, Gannon PJ. The primate serotonergic system: a review of human and animal studies and a report on macaca fasicularis. Adv Neurol. 1986;43:407–468.

[51] Ballion B, Branchereau P, Chapron J, Viala D. Ontogeny of descending serotonergic innervation and evidence for intraspinal 5-HT neurons in the mouse spinal cord. Brain Res Dev Brain Res. 2002;137:81–88. DOI: 10.1016/S0165-3806(02)00414–5.

[52] Jacobs BL, Azmitia EC. Structure and function of the brain serotonin system. Physiol Rev. 1992;72:165–229.

[53] Lamotte CC, Johns DR, de Lanerolle NC. Immunohistochemical evidence of indolamine neurons in monkey spinal cord. J Comp Neurol.1982; 206:359–570. DOI: 10.1002/cne.902060404.

[54] Newton BW, Maley BE, Hamill RW. Immunohistochemical demonstration of serotonin neurons in autonomic regions of the rat spinal cord. Brain Res. 1986;376:155–163. DOI: 10.1016/0006-8993(86)90910-8.

[55] Newton BW, Hamill RW. The morphology and distribution of rat serotoninergic intraspinal neurons: an immunohistochemical study. Brain Res Bull. 1988;20:349–360. DOI: 10.1016/0361-9230(88)90064-0.

[56] Jacobs BL, Fornal CA. 5-HT and motor control: a hypothesis. Trends Neurosci. 1993;16:346–352. DOI: 10.1016/0166-2236(93)90090-9.

[57] Rahman W, Bannister K, Bee LA, Dickenson AH. A pronociceptive role for the 5-HT2 receptor on spinal nociceptive transmission: an in vivo electrophysiological study in the rat. Brain Res. 2011;1382:29–36. DOI: 10.1016/j.brainres.2011.01.057.

[58] Cervantes-Durán C, Rocha-González HI, Granados-Soto V. Peripheral and spinal 5-HT receptors participate in the pronociceptive and antinociceptive effects of fluoxetine in rats. Neuroscience. 2013;252:396–409. DOI: 10.1016/j.neuroscience.2013.08.022.

[59] Beato M, Nistri A. Serotonin-induced inhibition of locomotor rhythm of the rat isolated spinal cord is mediated by the 5-HT1 receptor class. Proc Biol Sci. 1998;265:2073–2080. DOI: 10.1098/rspb.1998.0542.

[60] Perrier JF, Cotel F. Serotonin differentially modulates the intrinsic properties of spinal motoneurons from the adult turtle. J Physiol. 2008;586:1233–1238. DOI: 10.1113/jphysiol.2007.145706.

[61] Nichols DE, Nichols CD. Serotonin receptors. Chem Rev. 2008;108:1614–1641. DOI: 10.1021/cr078224o.

[62] Hannon J, Hoyer D. Molecular biology of 5-HT receptors. Behav Brain Res. 2008;195:198–213. DOI: 10.1016/j.bbr.2008.03.020.

[63] Werry TD, Loiacono R, Sexton PM, Christopoulos A. RNA editing of the serotonin 5HT2C receptor and its effects on cell signalling, pharmacology and brain function. Pharmacol Ther. 2008;119:7–23. DOI: 10.1016/j.pharmthera.2008.03.012.

[64] Perrier JF, Rasmussen HB, Christensen RK, Petersen AV. Modulation of the intrinsic properties of motoneurons by serotonin. Curr Pharm Des. 2013;19:4371–4384. DOI: 10.2174/13816128113199990341.

[65] Lanfumey L, Hamon M. 5-HT1 receptors. Curr Drug Targets CNS Neurol Disord. 2004;3:1–10. DOI: 10.2174/1568007043482570.

[66] Daval G, Vergé D, Basbaum AI, Bourgoin S, Hamon M. Autoradiographic evidence of serotonin1 binding sites on primary afferent fibres in the dorsal horn of the rat spinal cord. Neurosci Lett. 1987;83:71–76. DOI: 10.1016/0304-3940(87)90218-7.

[67] Marlier L, Teilhac JR, Cerruti C, Privat A. Autoradiographic mapping of 5-HT1, 5-HT1A, 5-HT1B and 5-HT2 receptors in the rat spinal cord. Brain Res. 1991;550:15–23. DOI: 10.1016/0006-8993(91)90400-P.

[68] Thor KB, Nickolaus S, Helke CJ. Autoradiographic localization of 5-hydroxytryptamine1A, 5-hydroxytryptamine1B and 5-hydroxytryptamine1C/2 binding sites in the rat spinal cord. Neuroscience. 1993;55:235–252. DOI: 10.1016/0306-4522(93)90469-V.

[69] Kia HK, Miquel MC, Brisorgueil MJ, Daval G, Riad M, El Mestikawy S, Hamon M, Vergé D. Immunocytochemical localization of serotonin1A receptors in the rat central

nervous system. J Comp Neurol. 1996;365:289–305. DOI: 10.1002/(SICI)1096-9861(19960205)365:2<289::AID-CNE7>3.0.CO;2-1.

[70] Talley EM, Bayliss DA. Postnatal development of 5-HT(1A) receptor expression in rat somatic motoneurons. Brain Res Dev Brain Res. 2000;122:1–10. DOI: 10.1016/S0165-3806(00)00036-5.

[71] Kheck NM, Gannon PJ, Azmitia EC. 5-HT1A receptor localization on the axon hillock of cervical spinal motoneurons in primates. J Comp Neurol. 1995;355:211–220. DOI: 10.1002/cne.903550205.

[72] Eide PK, Joly NM, Hole K. The role of spinal cord 5-HT1A and 5-HT1B receptors in the modulation of a spinal nociceptive reflex. Brain Res. 1990;536:195–200. DOI: 10.1016/0006-8993(90)90025-7.

[73] Hochman S, Garraway SM, Machacek DW, Shay BL. 5-HT receptors and the neuromodulatory control of spinal cord function. In: Cope TC, editor. Motor Neurobiology of the Spinal Cord. CRC Press: Boca Raton; 2001. p. 47–87.

[74] Nadeson R, Goodchild CS. Antinociceptive role of 5-HT1A receptors in rat spinal cord. Br J Anaesth. 2002;88:679–684. DOI: 10.1093/bja/88.5.679.

[75] Buritova J, Larrue S, Aliaga M, Besson JM, Colpaert F. Effects of the high-efficacy 5-HT1A receptor agonist, F 13640 in the formalin pain model: a c-Fos study. Eur J Pharmacol. 2005;514:121–130. DOI:10.1016/j.ejphar.2005.03.016.

[76] Kim JM, Jeong SW, Yang J, Lee SH, Kim WM, Jeong S, Bae HB, Yoon MH, Choi JI. Spinal 5-HT1A, not the 5-HT1B or 5-HT3 receptors, mediates descending serotonergic inhibition for late-phase mechanical allodynia of carrageenan-induced peripheral inflammation. Neurosci Lett. 2015;600:91–97. DOI: 10.1016/j.neulet.2015.05.058.

[77] Alhaider AA, Wilcox GL. Differential roles of 5-hydroxytryptamine1A and 5-hydroxytryptamine1B receptor subtypes in modulating spinal nociceptive transmission in mice. J Pharmacol Exp Ther. 1993;265:378–385.

[78] Ali Z, Wu G, Kozlov A, Barasi S. The actions of 5-HT1 agonists and antagonists on nociceptive processing in the rat spinal cord: results from behavioural and electrophysiological studies. Brain Res. 1994;661:83–90. DOI:10.1016/0006-8993(94)91184-3.

[79] Zhao ZQ, Liu XY, Jeffry J, Karunarathne WK, Li JL, Munanairi A, Zhou XY, Li H, Sun YG, Wan L, Wu ZY, Kim S, Huo FQ, Mo P, Barry DM, Zhang CK, Kim JY, Gautam N, Renner KJ, Li YQ, Chen ZF. Descending control of itch transmission by the serotonergic system via 5-HT1A-facilitated GRP–GRPR signaling. Neuron. 2014;84:821–834. DOI: 10.1016/j.neuron.2014.10.003.

[80] Bervoets K, Rivet JM, Millan MJ. 5-HT1A receptors and the tail-flick response. IV. Spinally localized 5-HT1A receptors postsynaptic to serotoninergic neurones mediate spontaneous tail-flicks in the rat. J Pharmacol Exp Ther. 1993;264:95–104.

[81] Cotel F, Exley R, Cragg SJ, Perrier JF. Serotonin spillover onto the axon initial segment of motoneurons induces central fatigue by inhibiting action potential initiation. Proc Natl Acad Sci USA. 2013;110:4774–4779. DOI: 10.1073/pnas.1216150110.

[82] Perrier JF, Cotel F. Serotonergic modulation of spinal motor control. Curr Opin Neurobiol. 2015;33:1–7. DOI: 10.1016/j.conb.2014.12.008.

[83] Laporte AM, Fattaccini CM, Lombard MC, Chauveau J, Hamon M. Effects of dorsal rhizotomy and selective lesion of serotonergic and noradrenergic systems on 5-HT1A, 5-HT1B, and 5-HT3 receptors in the rat spinal cord. J Neural Transm Gen Sect. 1995;100:207–223. DOI: 10.1007/BF01276459.

[84] Jackson DA, White SR. Receptor subtypes mediating facilitation by serotonin of excitability of spinal motoneurons. Neuropharmacology.1990; 29:787–797. DOI: 10.1016/0028-3908(90)90151-G.

[85] Mantilla CB, Bailey JP, Zhan WZ, Sieck G. Phrenic motoneuron expression of serotonergic and glutamatergic receptors following upper cervical spinal cord injury. Exp Neurol. 2012;234:191–199. DOI: 10.1016/j.expneurol.2011.12.036.

[86] el-Yassir N, Fleetwood-Walker SM, Mitchell R. Heterogeneous effects of serotonin in the dorsal horn of rat: the involvement of 5-HT1 receptor subtypes. Brain Res. 1988;456:147–158. DOI: 10.1016/0006-8993(88)90356-3.

[87] Zhang Y, Yang Z, Gao X, Wu G. The role of 5-hydroxytryptamine1A and 5-hydroxytryptamine1B receptors in modulating spinalnociceptive transmission in normal and carrageenan-injected rats. Pain. 2001;92:201–211. DOI: 10.1016/S0304-3959(01)00259-7.

[88] Monroe PJ, Smith DJ. Demonstration of an autoreceptor modulating the release of [3H]5-hydroxytryptamine from a synaptosomal-rich spinal cord tissue preparation. J Neurochem. 1985;45:1886–1894. DOI: 10.1111/j.1471-4159.1985.tb10548.x.

[89] Brown L, Amedro J, Williams G, Smith D. A pharmacological analysis of the rat spinal cord serotonin (5-HT) autoreceptor. Eur J Pharm. 1988;145: 163–171. DOI: 10.1016/0014-2999(88)90227-0.

[90] Murphy RM, Zemlan FP. Selective 5-HT1B agonists identify the 5-HT autoreceptor in lumbar spinal cord of rat. Neuropharmacology. 1988;27:37–42. DOI: 10.1016/0028-3908(88)90198-0.

[91] Allain AE, Ségu L, Meyrand P, Branchereau P. Serotonin controls the maturation of the GABA phenotype in the ventral spinal cord via 5-HT1b receptors. Ann N Y Acad Sci. 2010;1198:208–219. DOI: 10.1111/j.1749-6632.2010.05433.x.

[92] Potrebic S, Ahn AH, Skinner K, Fields HL, Basbaum AI. Peptidergic nociceptors of both trigeminal and dorsal root ganglia express serotonin 1D receptors: implications for the selective antimigraine action of triptans. J Neurosci. 2003;23:10988–10997.

[93] Ahn AH, Basbaum AI. Tissue injury regulates serotonin 1D receptor expression: implications for the control of migraine and inflammatory pain. J Neurosci. 2006;26:8332–8338. DOI: 10.1523/JNEUROSCI.1989-06.2006.

[94] Enjin A, Leão KE, Mikulovic S, Le Merre P, Tourtellotte WG, Kullander K. Sensorimotor function is modulated by the serotonin receptor 1d, a novel marker for gamma motor neurons. Mol Cell Neurosci. 2012;49:322–332. DOI: 10.1016/j.mcn.2012.01.003.

[95] D'Amico JM, Li Y, Bennett DJ, Gorassini MA. Reduction of spinal sensory transmission by facilitation of 5-HT1B/D receptors in noninjured andspinal cord-injured humans. J Neurophysiol. 2013;109:1485–1493. DOI: 10.1152/jn.00822.2012.

[96] Jeong CY, Choi JI, Yoon MH. Roles of serotonin receptor subtypes for the antinociception of 5-HT in the spinal cord of rats. Eur J Pharmacol. 2004;502:205–211. DOI: 10.1016/j.ejphar.2004.08.048.

[97] Honda M, Imaida K, Tanabe M, Ono H. Endogenously released 5-hydroxytryptamine depresses the spinal monosynaptic reflex via 5-HT1D receptors. Eur J Pharmacol. 2004;503:55–61. DOI: 10.1016/j.ejphar.2004.09.045.

[98] Castro ME, Pascual J, Romón T, del Arco C, del Olmo E, Pazos A. Differential distribution of [^{3}H]sumatriptan binding sites (5-HT1B, 5-HT1D and 5-HT1F receptors) in human brain: focus on brainstem and spinal cord. Neuropharmacology. 1997;36:535–542. DOI: 10.1016/S0028-3908(97)00061-0.

[99] Murray KC, Stephens MJ, Rank M, D'Amico J, Gorassini MA, Bennett DJ. Polysynaptic excitatory postsynaptic potentials that trigger spasms after spinal cord injury in rats are inhibited by 5-HT1B and 5-HT1F receptors. J Neurophysiol. 2011;106:925–943. DOI: 10.1152/jn.01011.2010.

[100] Classey JD, Bartsch T, Goadsby PJ. Distribution of 5-HT(1B), 5-HT(1D) and 5-HT(1F) receptor expression in rat trigeminal and dorsal root ganglia neurons: relevance to the selective anti-migraine effect of triptans. Brain Res. 2010;1361:76–85. DOI: 10.1016/j.brainres.2010.09.004.

[101] Agosti RM. 5HT1F- and 5HT7-receptor agonists for the treatment of migraines. CNS Neurol Disord Drug Targets. 2007;6:235–237. DOI: 10.2174/187152707781387242.

[102] Ferrari MD, Färkkilä M, Reuter U, Pilgrim A, Davis C, Krauss M, Diener HC; European COL-144 Investigators. Acute treatment of migraine with the selective 5-HT1F receptor agonist lasmiditan—a randomised proof-of-concept trial. Cephalalgia. 2010;30:1170–1178. DOI: 10.1177/0333102410375512.

[103] Humphrey PP, Hartig P, Hoyer D. A proposed new nomenclature for 5-HT receptors. Trends Pharmacol Sci. 1993;14:233–236. DOI: 10.1016/0165-6147(93)90016-D.

[104] Pompeiano M, Palacios JM, Mengod G. Distribution of the serotonin 5-HT2 receptor family mRNAs: comparison between 5-HT2A and 5-HT2C receptors. Brain Res Mol Brain Res. 1994;23:163–178. DOI: 10.1016/0169-328X(94)90223-2.

[105] Helton LA, Thor KB, Baez M. 5-Hydroxytryptamine2A, 5-hydroxytryptamine2B, and 5-hydroxytryptamine2C receptor mRNA expression in the spinal cord of rat, cat, monkey and human. Neuroreport. 1994;5:2617–2620.

[106] Cornea-Hébert V, Riad M, Wu C, Singh SK, Descarries L. Cellular and subcellular distribution of the serotonin 5-HT2A receptor in the central nervous system of adult rat. J Comp Neurol. 1999;409:187–209. DOI: 10.1002/(SICI)1096-9861(19990628)409:2<187::AID-CNE2>3.0.CO;2-P.

[107] Fonseca MI, Ni YG, Dunning DD, Miledi R. Distribution of serotonin 2A, 2C and 3 receptor mRNA in spinal cord and medulla oblongata. Brain Res Mol Brain Res. 2001;89:11–19. DOI: 10.1016/S0169-328X(01)00049-3.

[108] Doly S, Madeira A, Fischer J, Brisorgueil MJ, Daval G, Bernard R, Verge D, Conrath M. The 5-HT2A receptor is widely distributed in the rat spinal cord and mainly localized at the plasma membrane of postsynaptic neurons. J Comp Neurol. 2004;472:496–511. DOI: 10.1002/cne.20082.

[109] Pineda-Farias JB, Velázquez-Lagunas I, Barragán-Iglesias P, Cervantes-Durán C, Granados-Soto V. 5-HT_{2B} receptor antagonists reduce nerve injury-induced tactile allodynia and expression of 5-HT_{2B} receptors. Drug Dev Res. 2015;76:31–39. DOI: 10.1002/ddr.21238.

[110] Xu C, Giuliano F, Sun XQ, Brisorgueil MJ, Leclerc P, Vergé D, Conrath M. Serotonin 5-HT2A and 5-HT5A receptors are expressed by different motoneuron populations in rat Onuf's nucleus. J Comp Neurol. 2007;502:620–634. DOI: 10.1002/cne.21344.

[111] Eide PK, Hole K. Different role of 5-HT1A and 5-HT2 receptors in spinal cord in the control of nociceptive responsiveness. Neuropharmacology. 1991;30:727–731. DOI: 10.1016/0028-3908(91)90180-J.

[112] Kjørsvik A, Tjølsen A, Hole K. Activation of spinal serotonin(2A/2C) receptors augments nociceptive responses in the rat. Brain Res. 2001;910:179–181. DOI: 10.1016/S0006-8993(01)02652-X.

[113] Nishiyama T. Effects of a 5-HT2A receptor antagonist, sarpogrelate on thermal or inflammatory pain. Eur J Pharmacol. 2005;516:18–22. DOI: 10.1016/j.ejphar.2005.04.026.

[114] Thibault K, Van Steenwinckel J, Brisorgueil MJ, Fischer J, Hamon M, Calvino B, Conrath M. Serotonin 5-HT2A receptor involvement and Fos expression at the spinal level in vincristine-induced neuropathy in the rat. Pain. 2008;140:305–322. DOI: 10.1016/j.pain.2008.09.006.

[115] Xie DJ, Uta D, Feng PY, Wakita M, Shin MC, Furue H, Yoshimura M. Identification of 5-HT receptor subtypes enhancing inhibitory transmission in the rat spinal dorsal horn in vitro. Mol Pain. 2012;8:58. DOI: 10.1186/1744-8069-8-58.

[116] Iwasaki T, Otsuguro K, Kobayashi T, Ohta T, Ito S. Endogenously released 5-HT inhibits A and C fiber-evoked synaptic transmission in the rat spinal cord by the facilitation of

GABA/glycine and 5-HT release via 5-HT(2A) and 5-HT(3) receptors. Eur J Pharmacol. 2013;702:149–157. DOI: 10.1016/j.ejphar.2013.01.058.

[117] Fone KC, Robinson AJ, Marsden CA. Characterization of the 5-HT receptor subtypes involved in the motor behaviours produced by intrathecal administration of 5-HT agonists in rats. Br J Pharmacol. 1991;103:1547–1555. DOI: 10.1111/j.1476-5381.1991.tb09825.x.

[118] Yamazaki J, Fukuda H, Nagao T, Ono H. 5-HT2/5-HT1C receptor-mediated facilitatory action on unit activity of ventral horn cells in rat spinal cord slices. Eur J Pharmacol. 1992;220:237–242. DOI: 10.1016/0014-2999(92)90753-Q.

[119] Mbaki Y, Gardiner J, McMurray G, Ramage AG. 5-HT 2A receptor activation of the external urethral sphincter and 5-HT 2C receptor inhibition of micturition: a study based on pharmacokinetics in the anaesthetized female rat. Eur J Pharmacol. 2012;682:142–152. DOI: 10.1016/j.ejphar.2012.02.010.

[120] Watson NV, Gorzalka BB. DOI-induced inhibition of copulatory behavior in male rats: reversal by 5-HT2 antagonists. Pharmacol Biochem Behav. 1991;39:605–612. DOI: 10.1016/0091-3057(91)90135-O.

[121] Rössler AS, Bernabé J, Denys P, Alexandre L, Giuliano F. Effect of the 5-HT receptor agonist DOI on female rat sexual behavior. J Sex Med. 2006;3:432–441. DOI: 10.1111/j.1743-6109.2006.00240.x.

[122] Wienecke J, Westerdahl AC, Hultborn H, Kiehn O, Ryge J. Global gene expression analysis of rodent motor neurons following spinal cord injury associates molecular mechanisms with development of postinjury spasticity. J Neurophysiol. 2010;103:761–778. DOI: 10.1152/jn.00609.2009.

[123] MacFarlane PM, Vinit S, Mitchell GS. Serotonin 2A and 2B receptor-induced phrenic motor facilitation: differential requirement for spinal NADPH oxidase activity. Neuroscience. 2011;178:45–55. DOI: 10.1016/j.neuroscience.2011.01.011.

[124] Lin SY, Chang WJ, Lin CS, Huang CY, Wang HF, Sun WH. Serotonin receptor 5-HT2B mediates serotonin-induced mechanical hyperalgesia. J Neurosci. 2011;31:1410–1418. DOI: 10.1523/JNEUROSCI.4682-10.2011.

[125] Aira Z, Buesa I, García del Caño G, Salgueiro M, Mendiable N, Mingo J, Aguilera L, Bilbao J, Azkue JJ. Selective impairment of spinal mu-opioid receptor mechanism by plasticity of serotonergic facilitation mediated by 5-HT2A and 5-HT2B receptors. Pain. 2012;153:1418–1425. DOI: 10.1016/j.pain.2012.03.017.

[126] Cervantes-Durán C, Vidal-Cantú GC, Barragán-Iglesias P, Pineda-Farias JB, Bravo-Hernández M, Murbartián J, Granados-Soto V. Role of peripheral and spinal 5-HT2B receptors in formalin-induced nociception. Pharmacol Biochem Behav. 2012;102:30–35. DOI: 10.1016/j.pbb.2012.03.015.

[127] Mbaki Y, Ramage AG. Investigation of the role of 5-HT2 receptor subtypes in the control of the bladder and the urethra in the anaesthetized female rat. Br J Pharmacol. 2008;155:343–356. DOI: 10.1038/bjp.2008.273.

[128] Holohean AM, Hackman JC. Mechanisms intrinsic to 5-HT2B receptor-induced potentiation of NMDA receptor responses in frog motoneurones. Br J Pharmacol. 2004;143:351–360. DOI: 10.1038/sj.bjp.0705935.

[129] Pranzatelli MR, Murthy JN, Pluchino RS. Identification of spinal 5-HT1C binding sites in the rat: characterization of [^{3}H]mesulergine binding. J Pharmacol Exp Ther. 1992;261:161–165.

[130] Bancila M, Vergé D, Rampin O, Backstrom JR, Sanders-Bush E, McKenna KE, Marson L, Calas A, Giuliano F. 5-Hydroxytryptamine 2C receptors on spinal neurons controlling penile erection in the rat. Neuroscience. 1999;92:1523–1537. DOI: 10.1016/S0306-4522(99)00082-2.

[131] Clemett DA, Punhani T, Duxon MS, Blackburn TP, Fone KC. Immunohistochemical localisation of the 5-HT2C receptor protein in the rat CNS. Neuropharmacology. 2000;39:123–132. DOI: 10.1016/S0028-3908(99)00086-6.

[132] Holmes GM. 5-Hydroxytryptamine2C receptors on pudendal motoneurons innervating the external anal sphincter. Brain Res. 2005;1057:65–71. DOI: 10.1016/j.brainres.2005.07.047.

[133] Obata H, Saito S, Sakurazawa S, Sasaki M, Usui T, Goto F. Antiallodynic effects of intrathecally administered 5-HT(2C) receptor agonists in rats with nerve injury. Pain. 2004;108:163–169. DOI: 10.1016/j.pain.2003.12.019.

[134] Machacek DW, Garraway SM, Shay BL, Hochman S. Serotonin 5-HT(2) receptor activation induces a long-lasting amplification of spinal reflex actions in the rat. J Physiol. 2001;537:201–207. DOI: 10.1111/j.1469-7793.2001.0201k.x.

[135] Shay BL, Sawchuk M, Machacek DW, Hochman S. Serotonin 5-HT2 receptors induce a long-lasting facilitation of spinal reflexes independent of ionotropic receptor activity. J Neurophysiol. 2005;94:2867–2877. DOI: 10.1152/jn.00465.2005.

[136] Gajendiran M. In vivo evidence for serotonin 5-HT2C receptor-mediated long-lasting excitability of lumbar spinal reflex and its functional interaction with 5-HT1A receptor in the mammalian spinal cord. Brain Res Bull. 2008;75:674–680. DOI: 10.1016/j.brainresbull.2007.11.003.

[137] Halberstadt AL, van der Heijden I, Ruderman MA, Risbrough VB, Gingrich JA, Geyer MA, Powell SB. 5-HT(2A) and 5-HT(2C) receptors exert opposing effects on locomotor activity in mice. Neuropsychopharmacology. 2009;34:1958–1967. DOI: 10.1038/npp.2009.29.

[138] Conlon K, Miner W, McCleary S, McMurray G. Identification of 5-HT(2C) mediated mechanisms involved in urethral sphincter reflexes in a guinea-pig model of urethral function. BJU Int. 2012;110:E113–117. DOI: 10.1111/j.1464-410X.2011.10756.x.

[139] Thompson AJ, Lummis SC. Discriminating between 5-HT3A and 5-HT3AB receptors. Br J Pharmacol. 2013;169:736–747. DOI: 10.1111/bph.12166.

[140] Kia HK, Miquel MC, McKernan RM, Laporte AM, Lombard MC, Bourgoin S, Hamon M, Vergé D. Localization of 5-HT3 receptors in the rat spinal cord: immunohistochemistry and in situ hybridization. Neuroreport. 1995;6:257–261.

[141] Laporte AM, Doyen C, Nevo IT, Chauveau J, Hauw JJ, Hamon M. Autoradiographic mapping of serotonin 5-HT1A, 5-HT1D, 5-HT2A and 5-HT3 receptors in the aged human spinal cord. J Chem Neuroanat. 1996;11:67–75. DOI: 10.1016/0891-0618(96)00130-5.

[142] Morales M, Battenberg E, Bloom FE. Distribution of neurons expressing immunoreactivity for the 5HT3 receptor subtype in the rat brain and spinal cord. J Comp Neurol. 1998;402:385–401. DOI: 10.1002/(SICI)1096-9861(19981221)402:3<385::AID-CNE7>3.0.CO;2-Q.

[143] Maxwell DJ, Kerr R, Rashid S, Anderson E. Characterisation of axon terminals in the rat dorsal horn that are immunoreactive for serotonin 5-HT3A receptor subunits. Exp Brain Res. 2003;149:114–124. DOI: 10.1007/s00221-002-1339-7.

[144] Glaum SR, Proudfit HK, Anderson EG. 5-HT3 receptors modulate spinal nociceptive reflexes. Brain Res. 1990;510:12–16. DOI: 10.1016/0006-8993(90)90721-M.

[145] Alhaider AA, Lei SZ, Wilcox GL. Spinal 5-HT3 receptor-mediated antinociception: possible release of GABA. J Neurosci. 1991;11:1881–1888.

[146] Khasabov SG, Lopez-Garcia JA, Asghar AU, King AE. Modulation of afferent-evoked neurotransmission by 5-HT3 receptors in young rat dorsal horn neurones in vitro: a putative mechanism of 5-HT3 induced anti-nociception. Br J Pharmacol. 1999;127:843–852. DOI: 10.1038/sj.bjp.0702592.

[147] Fukushima T, Ohtsubo T, Tsuda M, Yanagawa Y, Hori Y. Facilitatory actions of serotonin type 3 receptors on GABAergic inhibitory synaptic transmission in the spinal superficial dorsal horn. J Neurophysiol. 2009;102:1459–1471. DOI: 10.1152/jn.91160.2008.

[148] Guo W, Miyoshi K, Dubner R, Gu M, Li M, Liu J, Yang J, Zou S, Ren K, Noguchi K, Wei F. Spinal 5-HT3 receptors mediate descending facilitation and contribute to behavioral hypersensitivity via a reciprocal neuron–glial signaling cascade. Mol Pain. 2014;10:35. DOI: 10.1186/1744-8069-10-35.

[149] Conte D, Legg ED, McCourt AC, Silajdzic E, Nagy GG, Maxwell DJ. Transmitter content, origins and connections of axons in the spinal cord that possess theserotonin

(5-hydroxytryptamine) 3 receptor. Neuroscience. 2005;134:165–173. DOI: 10.1016/j.neuroscience.2005.02.013.

[150] Huang J, Wang YY, Wang W, Li YQ, Tamamaki N, Wu SX. 5-HT(3A) receptor subunit is expressed in a subpopulation of GABAergic and enkephalinergic neurons in the mouse dorsal spinal cord. Neurosci Lett. 2008;441:1–6. DOI: 10.1016/j.neulet.2008.04.105.

[151] Guertin PA, Steuer I. Ionotropic 5-HT3 receptor agonist-induced motor responses in the hindlimbs of paraplegic mice. J Neurophysiol. 2005;94:3397–3405. DOI: 10.1152/jn.00587.2005.

[152] Espey MJ, Downie JW. Serotonergic modulation of cat bladder function before and after spinal transection. Eur J Pharmacol. 1995;287:173–177. DOI: 10.1016/0014-2999(95)00614-1.

[153] Suwa B, Bock N, Preusse S, Rothenberger A, Manzke T. Distribution of serotonin4(a) receptors in the juvenile rat brain and spinal cord. J Chem Neuroanat. 2014;55:67–77. DOI: 10.1016/j.jchemneu.2013.12.004.

[154] Godínez-Chaparro B, López-Santillán FJ, Orduña P, Granados-Soto V. Secondary mechanical allodynia and hyperalgesia depend on descending facilitation mediated byspinal 5-HT4, 5-HT6 and 5-HT7 receptors. Neuroscience. 2012;222:379–391. DOI: 10.1016/j.neuroscience.2012.07.008.

[155] Grailhe R, Grabtree GW, Hen R. Human 5-HT(5) receptors: the 5-HT(5A) receptor is functional but the 5-HT(5B) receptor was lost during mammalian evolution. Eur J Pharmacol. 2001;418:157–167. DOI: 10.1016/S0014-2999(01)00933-5.

[156] Doly S, Fischer J, Brisorgueil MJ, Vergé D, Conrath M. 5-HT5A receptor localization in the rat spinal cord suggests a role in nociception and control of pelvic floor musculature. J Comp Neurol. 2004;476:316–329. DOI: 10.1002/cne.20214.

[157] Muñoz-Islas E, Vidal-Cantú GC, Bravo-Hernández M, Cervantes-Durán C, Quiñonez-Bastidas GN, Pineda-Farias JB, Barragán-Iglesias P, Granados-Soto V. Spinal 5-HT5A receptors mediate 5-HT-induced antinociception in several pain models in rats. Pharmacol Biochem Behav. 2014;120:25–32. DOI: 10.1016/j.pbb.2014.02.001.

[158] Gérard C, el Mestikawy S, Lebrand C, Adrien J, Ruat M, Traiffort E, Hamon M, Martres MP. Quantitative RT-PCR distribution of serotonin 5-HT6 receptor mRNA in the central nervous system of control or 5,7-dihydroxytryptamine-treated rats. Synapse. 1996;23:164–173. DOI: 10.1002/(SICI)1098-2396(199607)23:3<164::AID-SYN5>3.0.CO;2-6.

[159] Gérard C, Martres MP, Lefèvre K, Miquel MC, Vergé D, Lanfumey L, Doucet E, Hamon M, el Mestikawy S. Immuno-localization of serotonin 5-HT6 receptor-like material in the rat central nervous system. Brain Res. 1997;746:207–219. DOI: 10.1016/S0006-8993(96)01224-3.

[160] Castañeda-Corral G, Rocha-González HI, Araiza-Saldaña CI, Ambriz-Tututi M, Vidal-Cantú GC, Granados-Soto V. Role of peripheral and spinal 5-HT6 receptors according to the rat formalin test. Neuroscience. 2009;162:444–452. DOI: 10.1016/j.neuroscience.2009.04.072.

[161] To ZP, Bonhaus DW, Eglen RM, Jakeman LB. Characterization and distribution of putative 5-ht7 receptors in guinea-pig brain. Br J Pharmacol. 1995;115:107–116. DOI: 10.1111/j.1476-5381.1995.tb16327.x.

[162] Doly S, Fischer J, Brisorgueil MJ, Vergé D, Conrath M. Pre- and postsynaptic localization of the 5-HT7 receptor in rat dorsal spinal cord: immunocytochemical evidence. J Comp Neurol. 2005;490:256–269. DOI: 10.1002/cne.20667.

[163] Viguier F, Michot B, Hamon M, Bourgoin S. Multiple roles of serotonin in pain control mechanisms—implications of 5-HT7 and other 5-HT receptor types. Eur J Pharmacol. 2013;716:8–16. DOI: 10.1016/j.ejphar.2013.01.074.

[164] Yesilyurt O, Seyrek M, Tasdemir S, Kahraman S, Deveci MS, Karakus E, Halici Z, Dogrul A. The critical role of spinal 5-HT7 receptors in opioid and non-opioid type stress-induced analgesia. Eur J Pharmacol. 2015;762:402–410. DOI: 10.1016/j.ejphar.2015.04.020.

[165] Dam LJ, Hai L, Ha YM. Role of the 5-HT(7) receptor in the effects of intrathecal nefopam in neuropathic pain in rats. Neurosci Lett. 2014;566:50–54. DOI: 10.1016/j.neulet.2014.02.021.

[166] Lee HG, Kim WM, Kim JM, Bae HB, Choi JI. Intrathecal nefopam-induced antinociception through activation of descending serotonergic projections involving spinal 5-HT7 but not 5-HT3 receptors. Neurosci Lett. 2015;587:120–125. DOI: 10.1016/j.neulet.2014.12.040.

[167] Liu J, Jordan LM. Stimulation of the parapyramidal region of the neonatal rat brain stem produces locomotor-like activity involving spinal 5-HT7 and 5-HT2A receptors. J Neurophysiol. 2005;94:1392–1404. DOI: 10.1152/jn.00136.2005.

[168] Jordan LM, Liu J, Hedlund PB, Akay T, Pearson KG. Descending command systems for the initiation of locomotion in mammals. Brain Res Rev. 2008;57:183–191. DOI: 10.1016/j.brainresrev.2007.07.019.

[169] Liu J, Akay T, Hedlund PB, Pearson KG, Jordan LM. Spinal 5-HT7 receptors are critical for alternating activity during locomotion: in vitro neonatal and in vivo adult studies using 5-HT7 receptor knockout mice. J Neurophysiol. 2009;102:337–348. DOI: 10.1152/jn.91239.2008.

[170] Cornide-Petronio ME, Fernández-López B, Barreiro-Iglesias A, Rodicio MC. Traumatic injury induces changes in the expression of the serotonin 1A receptor in the spinal cord of lampreys. Neuropharmacology. 2014;77:369–378. DOI: 10.1016/j.neuropharm.2013.10.017.

[171] Cornide-Petronio ME, Ruiz MS, Barreiro-Iglesias A, Rodicio MC. Spontaneous regeneration of the serotonergic descending innervation in the sea lamprey after spinal cord injury. J Neurotrauma. 2011;28:2535–2540. DOI: 10.1089/neu.2011.1766.

[172] Landry ES, Lapointe NP, Rouillard C, Levesque D, Hedlund PB, Guertin PA. Contribution of spinal 5-HT1A and 5-HT7 receptors to locomotor-like movement induced by 8-OH-DPAT in spinal cord-transected mice. Eur J Neurosci. 2006;24:535–546. DOI: 10.1111/j.1460-9568.2006.04917.x.

[173] Gu B, Thor KB, Reiter JP, Dolber PC. Effect of 5-hydroxytryptamine1 serotonin receptor agonists on noxiously stimulated micturition in cats with chronic spinal cord injury. J Urol. 2007;177:2381–2385. DOI: 10.1016/j.juro.2007.01.110.

[174] Honda M, Tanabe M, Ono H. Serotonergic depression of spinal monosynaptic transmission is mediated by 5-HT1B receptors. Eur J Pharmacol. 2003;482:155–161. DOI: 10.1016/j.ejphar.2003.09.070.

[175] Gu B, Olejar KJ, Reiter JP, Thor KB, Dolber PC. Inhibition of bladder activity by 5-hydroxytryptamine1 serotonin receptor agonists in cats with chronicspinal cord injury. J Pharmacol Exp Ther. 2004;310:1266–1272. DOI: 10.1124/jpet.103.063842.

[176] Ung RV, Landry ES, Rouleau P, Lapointe NP, Rouillard C, Guertin PA. Role of spinal 5-HT2 receptor subtypes in quipazine-induced hindlimb movements after a low-thoracic spinal cord transection. Eur J Neurosci. 2008;28:2231–2242. DOI: 10.1111/j.1460-9568.2008.06508.x.

[177] Kao T, Shumsky JS, Jacob-Vadakot S, Himes BT, Murray M, Moxon K. Role of the 5-HT2C receptor in improving weight-supported stepping in adult rats spinalized as neonates. Brain Res. 2006;1112:159–168. DOI: 10.1016/j.brainres.2006.07.020.

[178] Basura GJ, Zhou SY, Walker PD, Goshgarian HG. Distribution of serotonin 2A and 2C receptor mRNA expression in the cervical ventral horn and phrenic motoneurons following spinal cord hemisection. Exp Neurol. 2001;169:255–263. DOI: 10.1006/exnr.2001.7682.

[179] Zhou SY, Basura GJ, Goshgarian HG. Serotonin (2) receptors mediate respiratory recovery after cervical spinal cord hemisection in adult rats. J Appl Physiol. 2001;91:2665–2673.

[180] Majczyński H, Maleszak K, Cabaj A, Sławińska U. Serotonin-related enhancement of recovery of hind limb motor functions in spinal rats after grafting of embryonic raphe nuclei. J Neurotrauma. 2005;22:590–604. DOI: 10.1089/neu.2005.22.590.

[181] Kim D, Murray M, Simansky KJ. The serotonergic 5-HT(2C) agonist m-chlorophenyl-piperazine increases weight-supported locomotion without development of tolerance in rats with spinal transections. Exp Neurol. 2001;169:496–500. DOI: 10.1006/exnr.2001.7660.

[182] Murray KC, Stephens MJ, Ballou EW, Heckman CJ, Bennett DJ. Motoneuron excitability and muscle spasms are regulated by 5-HT2B and 5-HT2C receptor activity. J Neurophysiol. 2011;105:731–748. DOI: 10.1152/jn.00774.2010.

[183] Perrier JF, Hounsgaard J. 5-HT2 receptors promote plateau potentials in turtle spinal motoneurons by facilitating an L-type calcium current. J Neurophysiol. 2003;89:954–959. DOI: 10.1152/jn.00753.2002.

[184] Chen J, Gu B, Wu G, Tu H, Si J, Xu Y, Andersson KE. The effect of the 5-HT2A/2C receptor agonist DOI on micturition in rats with chronic spinal cord injury. J Urol. 2013;189:1982–1988. DOI: 10.1016/j.juro.2012.11.049.

[185] Bos R, Sadlaoud K, Boulenguez P, Buttigieg D, Liabeuf S, Brocard C, Haase G, Bras H, Vinay L. Activation of 5-HT2A receptors upregulates the function of the neuronal K-Cl cotransporter KCC2. Proc Natl Acad Sci USA. 2013;110:348–353. DOI: 10.1073/pnas.1213680110.

[186] Gackière F, Vinay L. Serotonergic modulation of post-synaptic inhibition and locomotor alternating pattern in the spinal cord. Front Neural Circuits. 2014;8:102. DOI: 10.3389/fncir.2014.00102.

[187] Rende M, Morales M, Brizi E, Bruno R, Bloom F, Sanna PP. Modulation of serotonin 5-HT3 receptor expression in injured adult rat spinal cord motoneurons. Brain Res. 1999;823:234–240. DOI: 10.1016/S0006-8993(99)01180-4.

[188] Gang W, Hongjian T, Jasheng C, Jiemin S, Zhong C, Yuemin X, Baojun G, Andersson KE. The effect of the 5-HT7 serotonin receptor agonist, LP44, on micturition in rats with chronic spinal cord injury. Neurourol Urodyn. 2014;33:1165–1170. DOI: 10.1002/nau.22463.

[189] Faden AI, Gannon A, Basbaum AI. Use of serotonin immunocytochemistry as a marker of injury severity after experimental spinal trauma in rats. Brain Res. 1988;450:94–100. DOI: 10.1016/0006-8993(88)91548-X.

[190] Holmes GM, Van Meter MJ, Beattie MS, Bresnahan JC. Serotonergic fiber sprouting to external anal sphincter motoneurons after spinal cord contusion. Exp Neurol. 2005;193:29–42. DOI: 10.1016/j.expneurol.2005.01.002.

[191] Hadjiconstantinou M, Panula P, Lackovic Z, Neff NH. Spinal cord serotonin: a biochemical and immunohistochemical study following transection. Brain Res. 1984;322:245–254. DOI: 10.1016/0006-8993(84)90114-8.

[192] Bregman BS. Development of serotonin immunoreactivity in the rat spinal cord and its plasticity after neonatal spinal cord lesions. Brain Res. 1987;431:245–263. DOI: 10.1016/0165-3806(87)90213-6.

[193] Saruhashi Y, Young W, Perkins R. The recovery of 5-HT immunoreactivity in lumbosacral spinal cord and locomotor function after thoracic hemisection. Exp Neurol. 1996;39:203–213. DOI: 10.1006/exnr.1996.0094.

[194] Filli L, Zörner B, Weinmann O, Schwab ME. Motor deficits and recovery in rats with unilateral spinal cord hemisection mimic the Brown-Sequard syndrome. Brain. 2011;134:2261–2273. DOI: 10.1093/brain/awr167.

[195] Camand E, Morel MP, Faissner A, Sotelo C, Dusart I. Long-term changes in the molecular composition of the glial scar and progressive increase of serotoninergic fibre sprouting after hemisection of the mouse spinal cord. Eur J Neurosci. 2004;20:1161–1176. DOI: 10.1111/j.1460-9568.2004.03558.x.

[196] Magnusson T. Effect of chronic transection on dopamine, noradrenaline and 5-hydroxytryptamine in the rat spinal cord. Naunyn Schmiedebergs Arch Pharmacol. 1973;278:13–22. DOI: 10.1007/BF00501859.

[197] Jaeger CB, Teitelman G, Joh TH, Albert VR, Park DH, Reis DJ. Some neurons of the rat central nervous system contain aromatic-L-amino-acid decarboxylase but not monoamines. Science. 1983;219:1233–1235. DOI: 10.1126/science.6131537.

[198] Ren LQ, Wienecke J, Hultborn H, Zhang M. Production of dopamine by aromatic L-amino acid decarboxylase cells after spinal cord injury. J Neurotrauma. 2016;33:1–11. DOI: 10.1089/neu.2015.4037.

[199] Hou S, Carson DM, Wu D, Klaw MC, Houlé JD, Tom VJ. Dopamine is produced in the rat spinal cord and regulates micturition reflex after spinal cord injury. Exp Neurol. DOI: 10.1016/j.expneurol.2015.12.001.

[200] Bhattacharyya S, Raote I, Bhattacharya A, Miledi R, Panicker MM. Activation, internalization, and recycling of the serotonin 2A receptor by dopamine. Proc Natl Acad Sci USA. 2006;103:15248–15253. DOI: 10.1073/pnas.0606578103.

Chapter 6

Docosahexaenoic Acid Promotes Recovery of Motor Function by Neuroprotection and Neuroplasticity Mechanisms

John V. Priestley and Adina T. Michael-Titus

Additional information is available at the end of the chapter

http://dx.doi.org/10.5772/62709

Abstract

The omega-3 polyunsaturated fatty acid, docosahexaenoic acid (DHA), has been shown to promote recovery of motor function after spinal cord injury. This is likely to be at least partly due to neuroprotective effects of DHA. However, recent studies have shown that DHA also supports neuroplasticity after injury, such as promoting sprouting of spared corticospinal tract (CST) axons. In this chapter, we review the published studies showing that DHA promotes recovery of motor function in rodent models of spinal cord injury (SCI), and consider the available data on the underlying mechanisms. This includes effects on inflammation and on neuronal and oligodendrocyte survival at the injury site, and effects on spared CST axons and serotonergic axons. Current data support the hypothesis that DHA promotes recovery of motor function by both neuroprotection and neuroplasticity mechanisms. The significance of this, and the implications of combining DHA with rehabilitation strategies, will be discussed.

Keywords: thoracic spinal cord injury, cervical spinal cord injury, central pattern generator, V2a interneurons, DHA

1. Introduction

1.1. Polyunsaturated fatty acids and their role in neurology

Polyunsaturated fatty acids (PUFA) of the omega-3 and omega-6 series are lipids with major structural and signalling roles. The long-chain omega-3 PUFA docosahexaenoic acid (DHA) is present in significant concentrations in the central nervous system (CNS), where its synthesis from the dietary precursor alpha-linolenic acid (LNA) occurs through desaturation, elongation and β-oxidation reactions. Its intermediate precursors are eicosapentaenoic acid (EPA) and docosapentaenoic acid (DPA). In humans, the conversion of LNA into DHA is below 5% [1, 2]. Therefore, an adequate dietary supply of DHA is required, especially because due to modern food manufacturing, there has been a significant decrease in the omega-3 intake and the omega-3 to omega-6 PUFA dietary ratio in the Western diet [3]. These changes have been linked to an increase in the incidence and the prevalence of diseases such as cancer, cardiovascular disease, rheumatoid arthritis, osteoporosis and asthma [4]. After absorption, the omega-3 PUFA can cross cellular membranes through specialized fatty acid transporters and interact with fatty acid-binding proteins (FABP). These proteins are a family of lipid chaperones involved in the extracellular and intracellular transport of fatty acids [5]. FABP bind long-chain fatty acids, with different ligand selectivity and binding affinity profiles. Changes in FABP levels have been reported following injury. For example, B-FABP is found in the brain and has very high affinity for DHA; it is detected in plasma as a high specificity and sensitivity biomarker of brain injury [6]. More recently, Figueroa et al. [7] reported increases in tissue levels of FABP-5 after spinal cord injury.

The principal omega-3 PUFA in the brain is DHA, representing 10–20% of the total fatty acid composition. Retinal tissue is also highly enriched in DHA. This fatty acid is a component of phospholipids, in particular phosphatidylethanolamine and phosphatidylserine; it is concentrated in cytoplasmic and synaptosomal membranes, growth cones, microsomal and mitochondrial membranes, and is also a component of myelin [8]. DHA-enriched phospholipids are present in the inner leaflet of the cytoplasmic membrane, and DHA chains are very flexible and transition rapidly between conformational states. This creates a unique microenvironment for the functioning of many proteins embedded in membranes, such as neurotransmitter receptors [9]. After release from membrane phospholipids by phospholipases, long-chain omega-3 PUFA such as DHA can be metabolized and produce a wide range of metabolites, designated with the generic term of "docosanoids", which include protectins, D-series resolvins and maresins. These DHA metabolites have intrinsic biological effects, which are mediated through specific receptors [10, 11]. Therefore, some of the effects induced by DHA may be due not to a direct action of the fatty acid but to specific metabolites which are derived from it, and which could attain significant levels, especially under conditions of chronic DHA supplementation [12].

DHA has an essential role in normal neurodevelopment, in particular for vision and cognition [13]. Supplementation with DHA has been shown to improve various aspects of learning and memory in children [14]. More than two decades ago, Martinez and collaborators [15] carried out seminal studies in children with peroxysomal disorders, which lead to a major DHA deficit, and showed that supplementation with DHA can lead to significant improvement in neurological function, and this is accompanied by improved myelination of the immature brain. At around the same time, studies initiated by Lazdunski and collaborators were providing evidence that omega-3 PUFA had significant neuroprotective potential under conditions which lead to CNS injury, such as seizures and ischaemia [16]. DHA has been increasingly linked to a variety of conditions, such as Alzheimer's disease and Parkinson's disease, and also schizophrenia, depression and attention deficit-hyperactivity disorder [17–19], and this has consolidated the idea that dietary supplementation with DHA could have therapeutic value across a spectrum of major disorders in neurology and psychiatry.

1.2. Pathways controlling movement in the rat and possible strategies for promoting recovery of movement following spinal cord injury (SCI)

Locomotion in rodents is controlled by a central pattern generator (CPG) which generates the basic rhythm of limb flexion and extension and which, for the hindlimbs, is located in the lower thoracic and upper lumbar spinal cord. In recent years, great progress has been made in dissecting the organization of the CPG, by identifying subtypes of neurons based on their developmental expression of specific transcription factors (summarized in [20, 21]). Genetic ablation of specific transcription factors can then be used to probe the functional roles of different neuronal subtypes (see e.g. [22, 23]). **Figure 1** illustrates one possible model of the

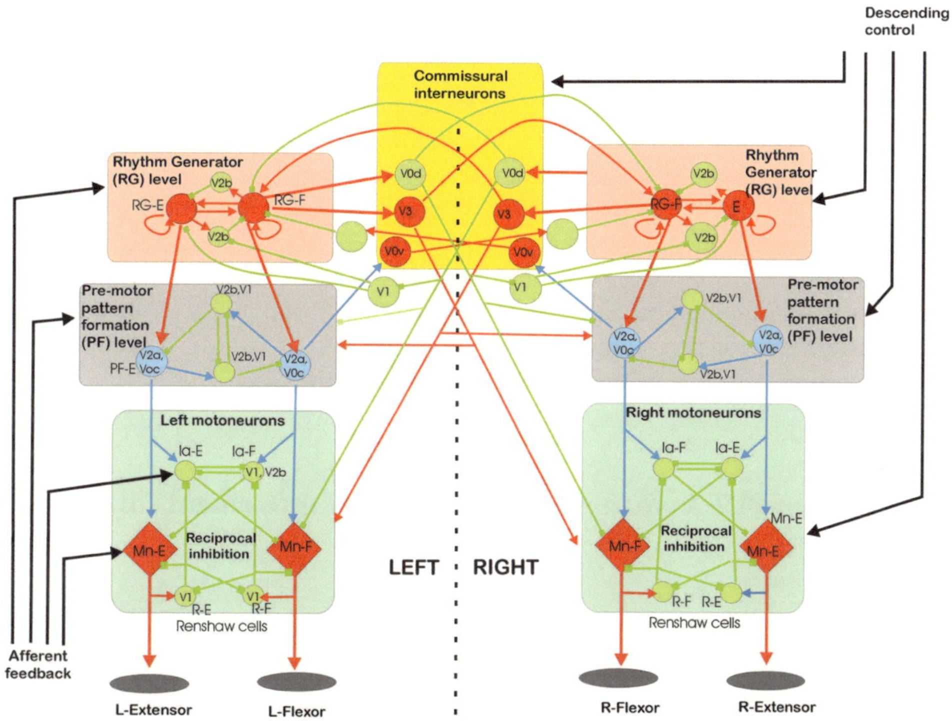

Figure 1. Schematic model of the rodent CPG controlling hind limb movement. Excitatory neurons are shown in red, and inhibitory neurons are shown in green. Rhythm generator (RG), pattern formation (PF) and motoneurons (Mn) are present for both flexion and extension on both sides of the spinal cord. V0d, V0v, V0c, V1, V2a, V2b and V3 are different types of interneurons which in some cases correspond to existing well-characterized neuronal types (e.g. V1 neurons include Renshaw cells). V2a neurons are shown in blue and have direct projections to motoneurons, plus projections to V2b/V1 PF inhibitory interneurons and to V0v excitatory commissural interneurons. Afferent feedback and descending control occur bilaterally, but for simplicity have only been shown ipsilaterally. The diagram is based on diagrams contained in Harris-Warrick [20] and Rybak and colleagues [21].

CPG based on studies reported in [22, 23]. Flexor and extensor motoneurons are thought to have separate rhythm generators (RG) which provide input to a pattern formation (PF) network that controls flexor/extensor alternation. The RG network also connects to commissural interneurons which coordinate left/right hindlimb movement. As an example of the complexity of the system, we have highlighted the V2a class of excitatory interneuron in **Figure 1**. V2a neurons can be identified by their expression of the homeodomain protein Chx10 and receive input from the RG centres. They project to three different targets, namely (1) motoneurons, (2) V2b inhibitory interneurons that are part of the PF centre, and (3) V0v commissural interneurons [21]. They therefore can influence locomotion by direct monosynaptic inputs to motoneurons and by regulating the flexor/extensor and left/right coordinating centres. However, V2a interneurons are not only present in the lumbar CPG, they also occur in the cervical spinal cord and play a key role in skilled forelimb movement, by conveying an internal copy of the premotor signals. This is possible because of their dual innervation of cervical motoneurons and precerebellar interneurons [22].

The CPG can generate alternating hindlimb movements independently, but in the intact animal, the CPG is modulated by afferent feedback and by descending control. The effects of SCI depend on the spinal level of the injury. Rats subject to complete transection above the level of the lumbar locomotor centres show some spontaneous recovery of hindlimb movement [24], and this can be increased by a variety of treatments, including weight supported treadmill training [24], delivery of growth factors [25, 26] and implantation of various exogenous cells [27–29]. At least some of this recovery of function appears to be related to regeneration or sprouting of descending bulbospinal [30, 31] and corticospinal [25] pathways. In contrast, the lasting paraplegia that results from a SCI at lumbar level is thought to result from loss of spinal interneurons, possibly including components of the CPG [32]. An efficacious treatment for SCI might need to preserve and/or restore descending control pathways and repair damage to intrinsic networks such as the CPG.

2. The effects of PUFA treatment on recovery of movement following experimental SCI

2.1. Thoracic hemisection SCI

DHA promotes recovery of quadrupedal locomotion in rats and mice following thoracic hemisection [33], compression [34–36] and contusion [37] SCI, when acutely administered post-injury. Recovery is further improved if an acute injection of DHA is followed by a DHA-supplemented diet (**Figure 2**). The DHA treatment results in increased neuronal and oligodendrocyte survival [34] and decreased macrophage and microglial activation [36, 38] at the injury site. However, since the motoneuron pools that contribute to locomotion are not at thoracic level, it is likely that the effects on locomotion are due to preservation of descending axons passing through the injury site rather than preservation of thoracic neurons themselves. Analysis of axon numbers at the SCI site using generic axonal markers such as neurofilament and myelin basic protein (MBP) reveals that DHA preserves axons in white matter tracts [39] but, with the exception of serotonin (5-hydroxytryptamine, 5-HT), the origin and role of those axons have not been much explored. As outlined above, corticospinal and bulbospinal projections play an important role in motor control but mainly innervate motoneurons indirectly, via interneurons, and so are difficult to analyse (however, see Section 4 on pyramidotomy below). In contrast, 5-HT axons are derived from the medullary raphe nuclei, innervate many motoneurons monosynaptically and play key roles in modulating motoneuron excitability [40]. DHA treatment preserves the number of 5-HT axons at the level of a thoracic compression injury [39], including axons that appear to contact motoneurons (see **Figure 3**). It is therefore likely that at least some of the motor recovery is due to increased preservation of 5-HT axons that pass through the injury site and innervate motoneurons at lumbar level. 5-HT axons have a great capacity to sprout and make new connections [41]. Another possibility is therefore that some 5-HT axons are spared by the SCI but that DHA promotes sprouting and restoration of synaptic circuits by these axons. These possibilities have not been examined directly following thoracic SCI, but the effects of DHA on 5-HT axons have been studied in much more detail following cervical injury.

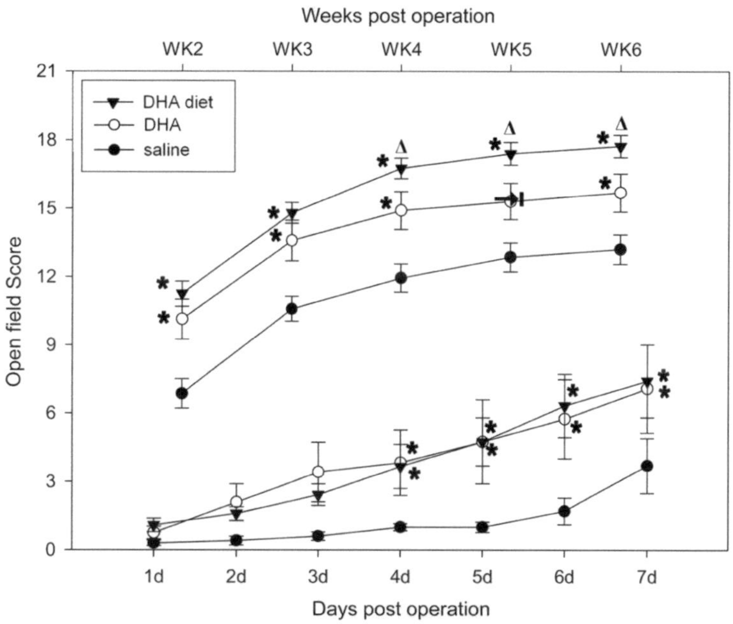

Figure 2. Locomotor performance of thoracic compression SCI rats injected with saline or DHA and of animals injected with DHA and then fed on a DHA-enriched diet. Results for days 1–7 are shown in the bottom half of the graph, plotted against the bottom X-axis. Results for 2–6 weeks are shown in the top half of the graph, plotted against the top X-axis. Both DHA- and saline-treated animals showed similar low levels of locomotor function 1 day after surgery, as assessed on the BBB open field task. During the first week, DHA-treated animals had improved motor function recovery compared with saline-treated animals (days 5, 6 and 7; $*p < 0.05$). Between week 2 and week 6, DHA-treated animals continued to perform better than saline-treated animals ($*p < 0.05$). In addition, from the 4th week onwards, animals injected with DHA followed by maintenance on the DHA-enriched diet, performed better than animals only injected with DHA (weeks 4, 5 and 6; $^{\Delta}p < 0.05$). Error bars represent SEMs. Reproduced from [34] with permission.

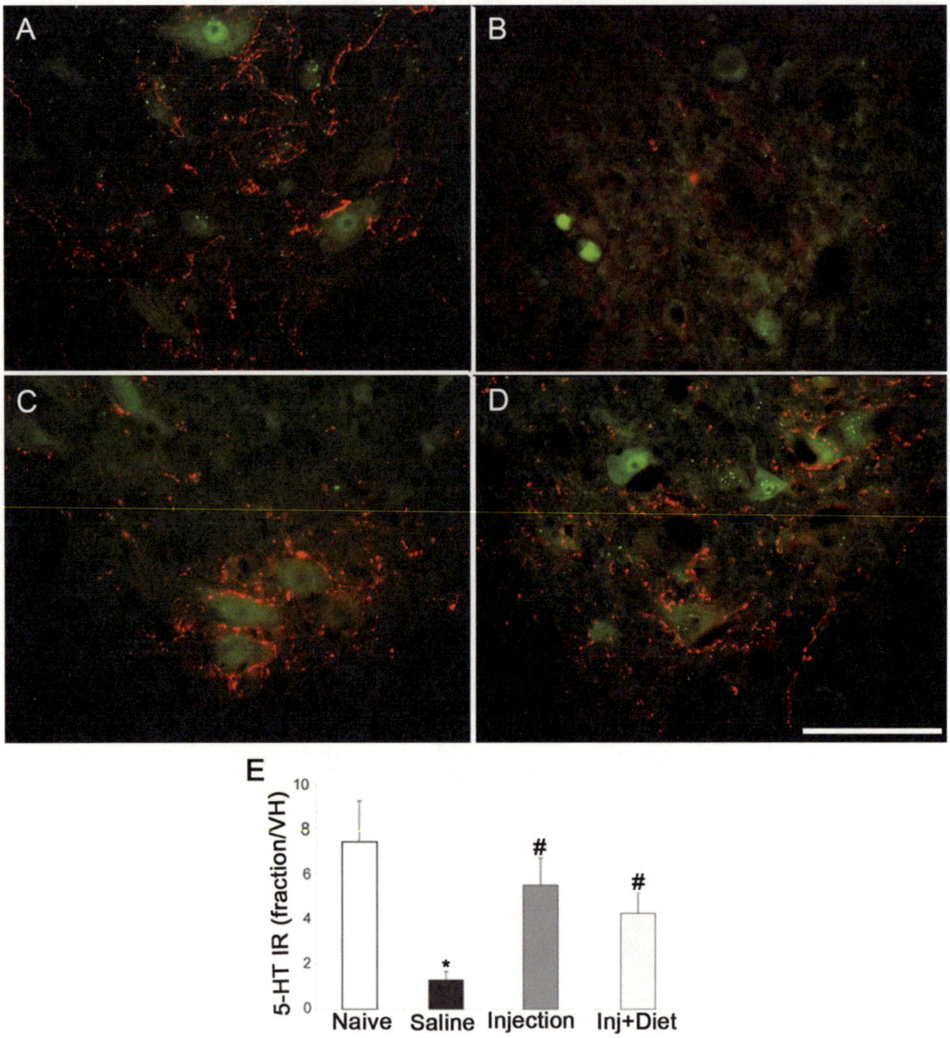

Figure 3. Immunofluorescence micrographs showing thin, 5-HT immunoreactive (IR) axons (red) that innervate NeuN labelled neurons (green) in the ventral horn (VH). In naïve animals (A), a dense network of beaded 5-HT-positive fibres can be seen surrounding large NeuN neurons. At 6 weeks post-thoracic compression injury, a marked loss of 5-HT-positive fibres was seen in saline-treated animals (B) compared with the groups receiving DHA injection alone (C), or in combination with a DHA-enriched diet (D). Quantitative analysis (E) at 6 weeks post-injury revealed a significant loss of 5-HT IR in the VH of saline-treated animals following injury. A significant amelioration in the loss of 5-HT IR was observed in the VH in both DHA-treatment groups (significantly different from *naïve or #saline-treated animals at $p < 0.05$; scale bar = 100 μm). Reproduced from [39] with permission.

2.2. Experimental cervical SCI

The majority of experimental studies have focused on thoracic injury, but the most common clinical injury is at cervical level (57% of SCI). Recently, we have therefore examined the effects

http://dx.doi.org/10.5772/62709

of DHA in a cervical (C5 level) hemisection SCI model [42]. The cervical level of injury also has the advantage of allowing us to examine the effects of DHA treatment on a skilled motor task, namely retrieval of food using the forepaws. Rats are trained to retrieve food by extending a forelimb through a gap in a perspex box and grasping food pellets which are on a staircase [43]. Following SCI at C5 level, rats lose the ability to recover the food pellets, but recover partial function if treated acutely with DHA (**Figure 4**). Following cervical hemisection, 5-HT axons show a remarkable degree of plasticity. Rostral to the hemisection, there is an increase in 5-HT immunoreactivity which is maintained up to 3 weeks. Caudal to the hemisection, there is a transient loss of 5-HT immunoreactivity at 1 week, but levels are restored by 3 weeks (**Figure 5B**). DHA treatment results in an even greater number of 5-HT immunoreactive axons caudal to the injury (**Figure 5B**), and increased density of 5-HT axons contacting motoneurons (**Figure 5C–E**). However, 5-HT axons are not the only ones to sprout in response to DHA treatment. Corticospinal tract (CST) axons on the intact side of the spinal cord were identified by anterograde labelling with the tracer biotinylated dextran amine (BDA). Following hemisection, a small number of these axons sprout across the midline to innervate the denervated side of the spinal cord. However, after DHA treatment, this number doubles [42]. It is therefore possible that the recovery of skilled movement is due to sprouting of 5-HT and CST axons and formation of novel circuits. However, since the increase in axons occurs at the same level as the hemisection, it is possible that the increase in 5-HT and CST axons is due to neuroprotection rather than neuroplasticity. We have therefore examined the effect of DHA treatment in a third model of SCI, namely unilateral pyramidotomy in the mouse [42].

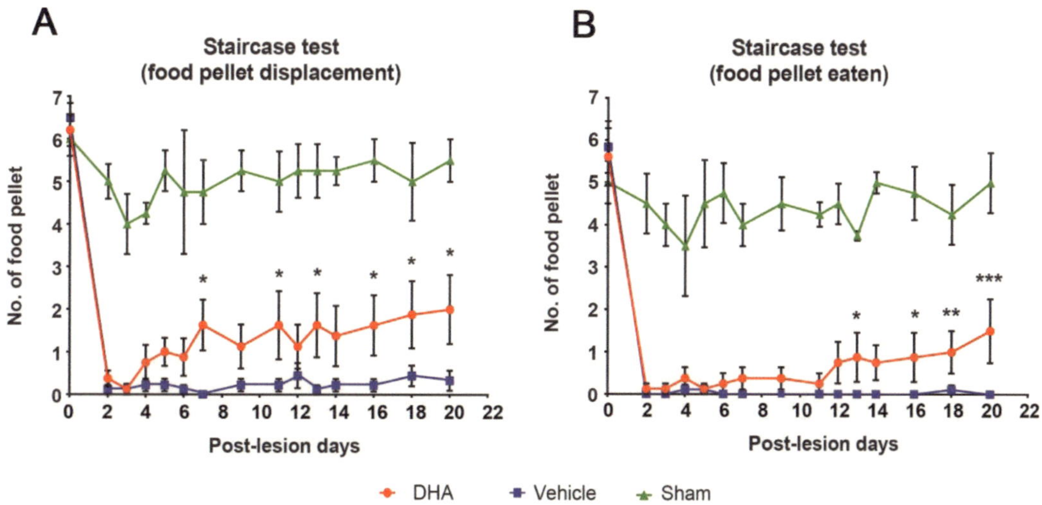

Figure 4. DHA enhances functional recovery following cervical lateral hemisection in the rat. A, B, In the Montoya staircase test, all injured animals lost the ability to displace (gross motor function) or eat (fine motor function) the food pellet after cervical lateral hemisection 2 d after injury. The animals treated with vehicle did not recover any food retrieval ability (blue squares), but DHA-treated animals gradually recovered food retrieval ability (red circles) from around 2 weeks onwards, compared with uninjured sham operated animals (green triangles). $*p < 0.05$, $**p < 0.01$, $***p < 0.001$, compared to vehicle-treated animals. Results represent mean ± SEM. Reproduced from [42] with permission.

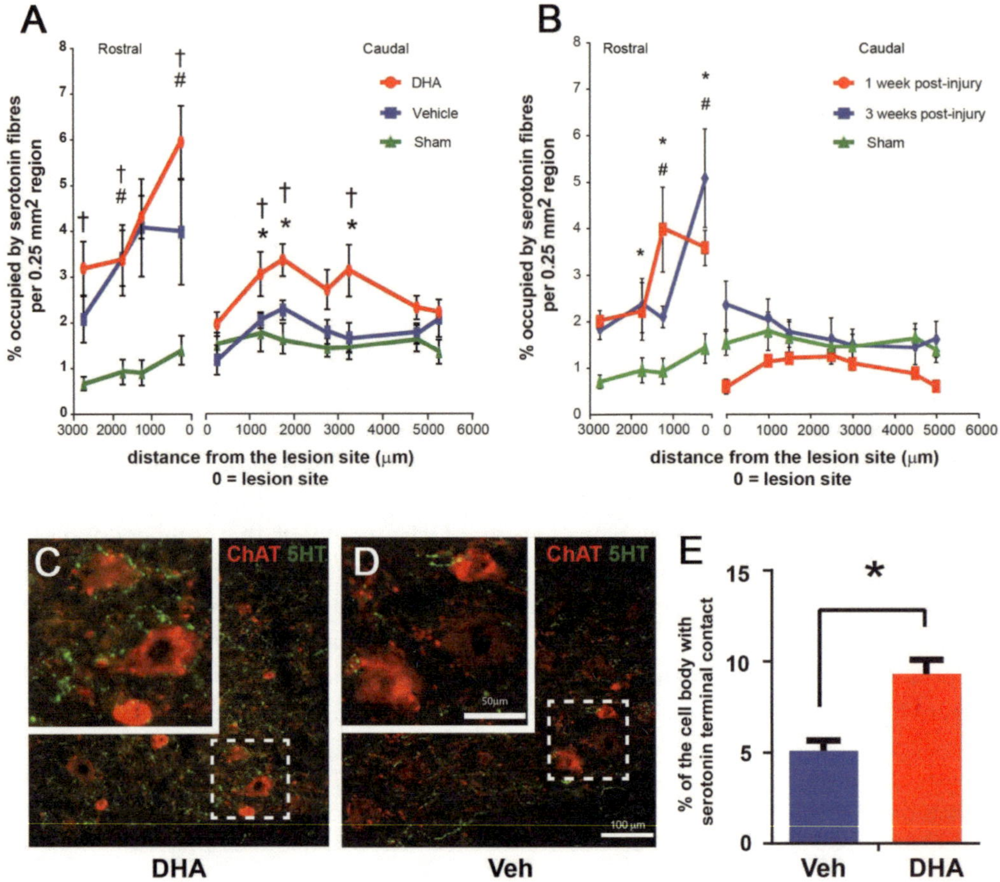

Figure 5. DHA enhances 5-HT (serotonin) fibre regrowth following cervical lateral hemisection in the rat. (*A*) Serotonin fibres in the rostral part of the lesion site were significantly increased in both treatment groups at 3 weeks post-injury, but only the DHA-treated group (red circles), not the vehicle group (blue squares), had significantly increased serotonin in the caudal region compared with the sham operated animals (green triangles). (*B*) Serotonin fibres in the rostral part of the lesion site were significantly increased at 1 week (red square) and 3 weeks (blue circle) compared with the sham operated group after lateral cervical hemisection. However, in the caudal region, 1 and 3 weeks after injury were similar to the sham operated group. 1 week after hemisection, there was a loss of serotonin but by 3 weeks levels had returned to values similar to sham operated animals. *N* = 5 or 6 per group. #$p < 0.05$, 1 week hemisection versus sham group. *$p < 0.05$, 3 week hemisection versus sham group. (*C, D*) The images were captured 1750 μm caudal to the lesion site. Double labelling shows serotonin fibres (green) in contact with ChAT immunoreactive motor neurons (red) in the ventral horn of vehicle- and DHA-treated rats. Insets, dashed boxes at higher magnification. (*E*) Quantitative analysis reveals that there is a significant increase in the density of serotonin fibres contacting motor neurons in the DHA-treated group compared with the control group. N = 5 or 6 per group. *$p < 0.05$, DHA versus vehicle group. †$p < 0.05$, sham versus vehicle group. #$p < 0.05$, DHA versus sham group. Scale bar, 100 μm. Reproduced from [42] with permission.

2.3. Pyramidotomy

The CST axons in rodents run in the medullary pyramids, before decussating and descending at the base of the dorsal columns. Unilateral pyramidotomy transects these CST axons and

http://dx.doi.org/10.5772/62709

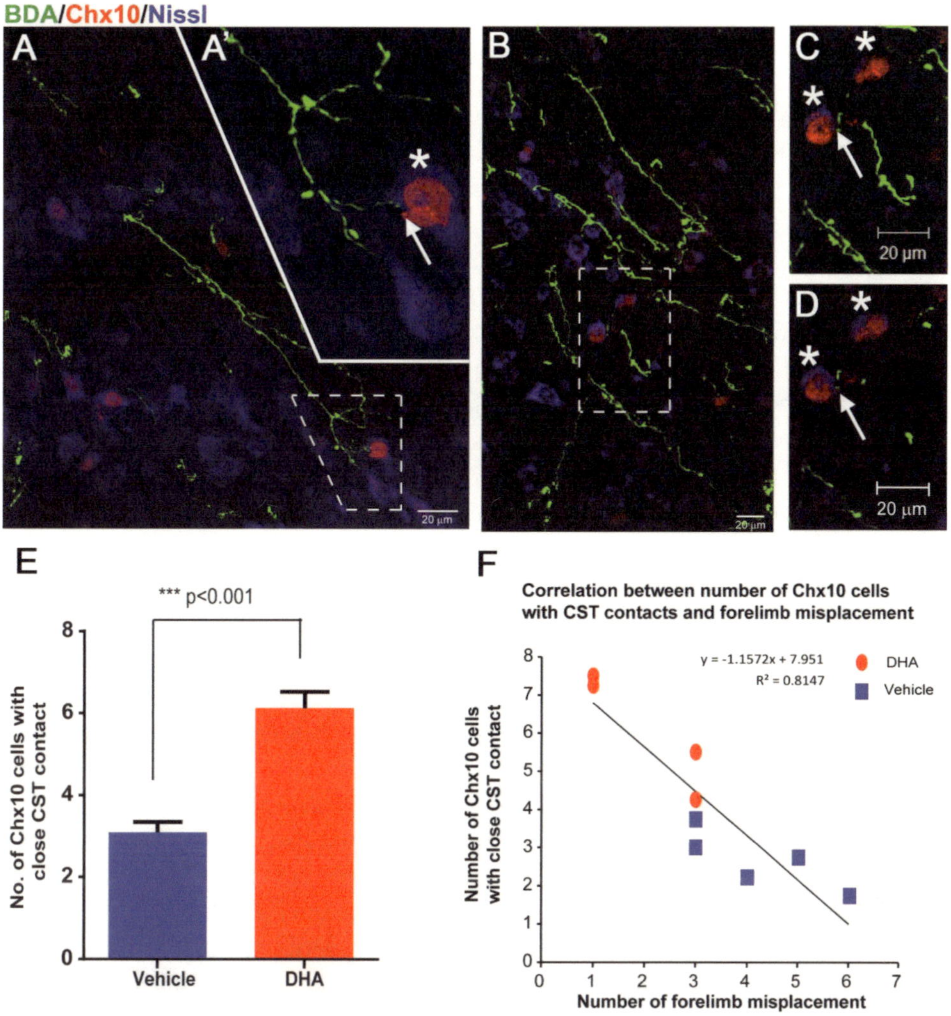

Figure 6. DHA enhances functional recovery via connection with Chx10 interneurons in pyramidotomy mice. (*A–D*), Confocal images of mouse cervical spinal cord transverse sections at the intermediate laminae of the CST-denervated side, showing examples of BDA-labelled CST collaterals (green) in the vicinity of blue fluorescent Nissl-stained cells (Neurotrace 435/455), some of which are V2a interneurons identified by immunostaining for Chx10 (red). (***A, B***) Dashed boxes represent high magnification in ***A'***, and in ***C, D***, which reveal contacts (arrows) between BDA-labelled collaterals and Chx10 interneurons (asterisks). (***A'***) *A Z*-stack comprising 10 × 0.66 μm optical images. (***C***), A stack comprising 25 × 0.72 μm optical images. (***D***, A) Single 0.72 μm optical image. Examination of the single optical image confirms that the BDA-labelled CST fibre contacts (arrow) one of the Chx10 interneurons. (***E***) Quantitative analysis revealed a significant increase in the number of Chx10 interneurons contacted by BDA-labelled CST collaterals following DHA treatment (red bar) compared with vehicle treatment (blue bar). (***F***) A strong negative correlation was observed between the numbers of Chx10 interneurons with BDA-labelled CST contacts and the numbers of forelimb misplacements. Data were taken from DHA-treated (red circle) and vehicle-treated (blue square) animals. ***$p<0.001$, DHA versus vehicle group. Scale bar, 20 μm. Reproduced from [42] with permission.

results in the loss of CST axons in the spinal cord on the contralateral side. Using BDA to label the CST axons on the non-lesioned side, we observed that a small number of CST axons respond to the pyramidotomy by sprouting across the midline to innervate the lesioned side (**Figure 6A**). The number of sprouting CST axons is doubled following DHA treatment [42]. Furthermore, we have shown that the sprouting axons contact a particular class of interneuron, namely the V2a propriospinal neurons described above. V2a neurons were identified by their expression of the Chx10 transcription factor (**Figure 6A–D**). V2a interneurons have been shown to play an important role in skilled reaching [22]. Following DHA treatment and pyramidotomy, an increased number of V2a interneurons receive contacts from CST axons (**Figure 6E**), and the recovery of forelimb movement shows a tight correlation with the number of V2a neurons that receive contacts (**Figure 6F**). It therefore appears that DHA treatment after pyramidotomy results in the formation of a novel circuit (CST to contralateral V2a interneurons) that promotes recovery of skilled reaching. This is in addition to the effects of DHA on sprouting 5-HT axons, and neuroprotective effects on neuronal cell bodies and axons.

3. Discussion

Motor pathways are so complex that it is difficult to establish a direct causal relationship between the effects of a therapeutic agent on spinal circuitry and an improvement in a particular motor task. However, the data reviewed above indicates that there is a strong correlation between the neuroprotective and neuroplasticity effects of DHA and the recovery of motor function. This dual effect of DHA, together with its established safety profile and the recent demonstration of the efficacy in SCI of a multinutrient combination containing DHA and EPA [44], makes DHA a particularly promising candidate for development as a therapeutic agent in SCI. There is a substantial literature on the neuroprotective effects of DHA (reviewed above) but the effects on neuroplasticity are more novel and less studied. We have shown that DHA treatment following SCI upregulates the microRNA miR-21 and suppresses phosphatase and tensin homolog (PTEN), a central negative regulator of the phosphatidylinositol 3-kinase (PI3K) signalling pathway [42]. However, these effects are quite widespread and it is not known how they result in beneficial axon sprouting. Bareyre and colleagues [45] have shown that new connections form after SCI, but inappropriate connections are lost because they are not used. A similar mechanism may mould the sprouting and connections promoted by DHA, in which case, there may be great benefit in combining DHA treatment with rehabilitation and task specific training.

3.1. Therapeutic implications

The magnitude of the effects induced by the acute administration of DHA and reported in various models of SCI is comparable with that described with various other therapeutic approaches which are already being explored in clinical trials in neurotrauma, such as progesterone, erythropoietin, riluzole and minocycline [46]. DHA has clear potential for

http://dx.doi.org/10.5772/62709

clinical translation in SCI; therefore, it is appropriate to consider the issues which remain to be clarified in order to improve the chances of translational success.

It is important to note that in the studies published so far with DHA and reporting beneficial effects of this fatty acid in a variety of conditions, there are two types of administration: DHA administered using a chronic oral supplementation route and DHA administered as an acute bolus, using an injectable route. Are the cellular targets and mechanisms activated by DHA the same in the two types of treatment? When DHA is administered chronically, one of the consequences of this regime is the structural enrichment in DHA in membranes, and because DHA has unique molecular structural characteristics, this influences the dynamics of membrane components, and may change the activity of ion channels and G-protein-coupled receptors (GPCR). DHA incorporation in membranes changes the properties of specialized domains such as the lipid rafts and caveolae, and this can modify signalling [47]. When DHA is administered acutely as a bolus, its half-life in plasma is very short (approximately 2 min), as shown in PET imaging studies carried out in healthy volunteers [48]; therefore, efficacy may be due to the activation of different mechanisms. Long-chain omega-3 PUFA such as DHA and EPA have various specific molecular targets, including ion channels, GPCR and nuclear receptors [17, 47]. They include voltage-sensitive Na^+ and Ca^{2+} channels and two-pore domain background K^+ channels, such as TREK-1 (which is also a target for riluzole), the GPCRs GPR40 and GPR120, and transcription factors such as the retinoid X receptors (RXR) and peroxisome proliferator-activated receptors (PPAR). RXR can heterodimerize with PPAR or with retinoic acid receptors (RAR), and changes in the expression of these receptors have been reported after SCI [49]. Several studies indicate that the activation of retinoid signalling supports axonal regeneration [50].

The spontaneous partial recovery of function which occurs after SCI may be due to neuroplasticity, compensation and repair [51]. Rehabilitation through training is at present the most successful treatment for patients with SCI, to enhance the recovery of some neurological function. Rehabilitation enhances the spontaneous plasticity changes that occur after injury and enhances the activity of sensorimotor pathways, as documented in experimental SCI [52]. Exercise leads to a reconfiguration of cortical representation maps, it modifies the biophysical properties of motoneuron membranes, changes the activity of spinal inhibitory circuits and also increases the levels of neurotrophic factors, such as brain-derived neurotrophic factor (BDNF) and neurotrophin-3 (NT-3) [53]. Liu and collaborators [54] have shown that exercise increases the expression of miR21 and decreases PTEN mRNA levels, a profile of effects similar to our observations with DHA. Considering this similarity of action, a goal of future studies should be the exploration of a combination of DHA and exercise, to establish whether what could be achieved is true synergism or only additivity. The concept of combining treatment with exercise is supported by examples such as the successful combination of exercise with strategies such as the reduction in the glial scar components using chondroitinase ABC [55]. However, not all combinations achieve an optimum effect, as shown by the negative results obtained by combining exercise with antibodies against the myelin-derived inhibitor Nogo A [56]. Therefore, it will be essential to continue to characterize the targets and mode of action of DHA, so that it becomes clear what mechanisms could be harnessed and amplified by combining DHA (acute administration and chronic exposure) and rehabilitation training, to optimize outcome in SCI patients.

Acknowledgements

We acknowledge the generous support of Spinal Research, Corporate Action Trust, Barts Charity and Chang Gung Memorial Hospital (Taiwan) for the DHA studies in the various models of SCI discussed here.

Author details

John V. Priestley* and Adina T. Michael-Titus

*Address all correspondence to: j.v.priestley@qmul.ac.uk

Centre for Neuroscience and Trauma, Blizard Institute, Barts and The London School of Medicine and Dentistry, Queen Mary University of London, London, UK

References

[1] BrennaJT, SalemNJr., SinclairAJ, CunnaneSC. alpha-Linolenic acid supplementation and conversion to n-3 long-chain polyunsaturated fatty acids in humans. Prostaglandins Leukot Essent Fatty Acids. 2009; 80: 85–91.

[2] BrennaJT. Efficiency of conversion of alpha-linolenic acid to long chain n-3 fatty acids in man. Curr Opin Clin Nutr Metab Care. 2002; 5: 127–132.

[3] SimopoulosAP. Evolutionary aspects of omega-3 fatty acids in the food supply. Prostaglandins Leukot Essent Fatty Acids. 1999; 60: 421–429.

[4] SimopoulosAP. The importance of the omega-6/omega-3 fatty acid ratio in cardiovascular disease and other chronic diseases. Exp Biol Med (Maywood). 2008; 233: 674–688.

[5] FuruhashiM, HotamisligilGS. Fatty acid-binding proteins: role in metabolic diseases and potential as drug targets. Nat Rev Drug Discov. 2008; 7: 489–503.

[6] PelsersMM, GlatzJF. Detection of brain injury by fatty acid-binding proteins. Clin Chem Lab Med. 2005; 43: 802–809.

[7] FigueroaJD, IllanMS, LiceroJ, CorderoK, MirandaJD, DeLM. Fatty acid binding protein 5 (FABP5) modulates docosahexaenoic acid (DHA)-induced recovery in rats undergoing spinal cord injury. J Neurotrauma. March 2016, ahead of print.

[8] HorrocksLA, FarooquiAA. Docosahexaenoic acid in the diet: its importance in maintenance and restoration of neural membrane function. Prostaglandins Leukot Essent Fatty Acids. 2004; 70: 361–372.

[9] GawrischK, EldhoNV, HolteLL. The structure of DHA in phospholipid membranes. Lipids. 2003; 38: 445–452.

[10] SerhanCN, KrishnamoorthyS, RecchiutiA, ChiangN. Novel anti-inflammatory—pro-resolving mediators and their receptors. Curr Top Med Chem. 2011; 11: 629–647.

[11] SerhanCN, DalliJ, ColasRA, WinklerJW, ChiangN. Protectins and maresins: new pro-resolving families of mediators in acute inflammation and resolution bioactive metabolome. Biochim Biophys Acta. 2015; 1851: 397–413.

[12] BazanNG, MolinaMF, GordonWC. Docosahexaenoic acid signalolipidomics in nutrition: significance in aging, neuroinflammation, macular degeneration, Alzheimer's, and other neurodegenerative diseases. Annu Rev Nutr. 2011; 31: 321–351.

[13] McNamaraRK, CarlsonSE. Role of omega-3 fatty acids in brain development and function: potential implications for the pathogenesis and prevention of psychopathology. Prostaglandins Leukot Essent Fatty Acids. 2006; 75: 329–349.

[14] KuratkoCN, BarrettEC, NelsonEB, SalemNJr. The relationship of docosahexaenoic acid (DHA) with learning and behavior in healthy children: a review. Nutrients. 2013; 5: 2777–2810.

[15] MartinezM, VazquezE. MRI evidence that docosahexaenoic acid ethyl ester improves myelination in generalized peroxisomal disorders. Neurology. 1998; 51: 26–32.

[16] LauritzenI, BlondeauN, HeurteauxC, WidmannC, RomeyG, LazdunskiM. Polyunsaturated fatty acids are potent neuroprotectors. EMBO J. 2000; 19: 1784–1793.

[17] DyallSC, Michael-TitusAT. Neurological benefits of omega-3 fatty acids. Neuromolecular Med. 2008; 10: 219–235.

[18] DyallSC. Long-chain omega-3 fatty acids and the brain: a review of the independent and shared effects of EPA, DPA and DHA. Front Aging Neurosci. 2015; 7: 52.

[19] RossBM, SeguinJ, SieswerdaLE. Omega-3 fatty acids as treatments for mental illness: which disorder and which fatty acid? Lipids Health Dis. 2007; 6: 21.

[20] Harris-WarrickRM. Locomotor pattern generation in the rodent spinal cord. In: JaegerD, JungR, editors. Encyclopedia of Computational Neuroscience. New York; Springer; 2013. pp. 1–15.

[21] RybakIA, DoughertyKJ, ShevtsovaNA. Organization of the mammalian locomotor CPG: review of computational model and circuit architectures based on genetically identified spinal interneurons. eNeuro. 2015; 2(5) e0069-15.2015 1–21.

[22] AzimE, JiangJ, AlstermarkB, JessellTM. Skilled reaching relies on a V2a propriospinal internal copy circuit. Nature. 2014; 508: 357–363.

[23] CroneSA, QuinlanKA, ZagoraiouL, DrohoS, RestrepoCE, LundfaldL, EndoT, SetlakJ, JessellTM, KiehnO, SharmaK. Genetic ablation of V2a ipsilateral interneurons disrupts left-right locomotor coordination in mammalian spinal cord. Neuron. 2008; 60: 70–83.

[24] ZhangY, JiSR, WuCY, FanXH, ZhouHJ, LiuGL. Observation of locomotor functional recovery in adult complete spinal rats with BWSTT using semiquantitative and qualitative methods. Spinal Cord. 2007; 45: 496–501.

[25] FernandezE, PalliniR, LaurettiL, MercantiD, SerraA, CalissanoP, PiepmeierJM, TatorCH. Spinal cord transection in adult rats—effects of local infusion of nerve growth factor on the corticospinal tract axons. Neurosurgery. 1993; 33: 889–893.

[26] BoyceVS, ParkJ, GageFH, MendellLM. Differential effects of brain-derived neurotrophic factor and neurotrophin-3 on hindlimb function in paraplegic rats. Eur J Neurosci. 2012; 35: 221–232.

[27] KubasakMD, JindrichDL, ZhongH, TakeokaA, McFarlandKC, Munoz-QuilesC, RoyRR, EdgertonVR, Ramon-CuetoA, PhelpsPE. OEG implantation and step training enhance hindlimb-stepping ability in adult spinal transected rats. Brain. 2008; 131: 264–276.

[28] RapalinoO, LazarovSpieglerO, AgranovE, VelanGJ, YolesE, FraidakisM, SolomonA, GepsteinR, KatzA, BelkinM, HadaniM, SchwartzM. Implantation of stimulated homologous macrophages results in partial recovery of paraplegic rats. Nat Med. 1998; 4: 814–821.

[29] SlawinskaU, MajczynskiH, DjavadianR. Recovery of hindlimb motor functions after spinal cord transection is enhanced by grafts of the embryonic raphe nuclei. Exp Brain Res. 2000; 132: 27–38.

[30] FouadK, SchnellL, BungeMB, SchwabME, LiebscherT, PearseDD. Combining Schwann cell bridges and olfactory-ensheathing glia grafts with chondroitinase promotes locomotor recovery after complete transection of the spinal cord. J Neurosci. 2005; 25: 1169–1178.

[31] Lopez-ValesR, ForesJ, NavarroX, VerduE. Chronic transplantation of olfactory ensheathing cells promotes partial recovery after complete spinal cord transection in the rat. Glia. 2007; 55: 303–311.

[32] HadiB, ZhangYP, BurkeDA, ShieldsCB, MagnusonDS. Lasting paraplegia caused by loss of lumbar spinal cord interneurons in rats: no direct correlation with motor neuron loss. J Neurosurg. 2000; 93: 266–275.

[33] KingVR, HuangWL, DyallSC, CurranOE, PriestleyJV, Michael-TitusAT. Omega-3 fatty acids improve recovery, whereas omega-6 fatty acids worsen outcome, after spinal cord injury in the adult rat. J Neurosci. 2006; 26: 4672–4680.

[34] HuangWL, KingVR, CurranOE, DyallSC, WardRE, LalN, PriestleyJV, Michael-TitusAT. A combination of intravenous and dietary docosahexaenoic acid significantly improves outcome after spinal cord injury. Brain. 2007; 130: 3004–3019.

[35] LimSN, HuangW, HallJC, Michael-TitusAT, PriestleyJV. Improved outcome after spinal cord compression injury in mice treated with docosahexaenoic acid. Exp Neurol. 2013; 239: 13–27.

[36] PaternitiI, ImpellizzeriD, DiPR, EspositoE, GladmanS, YipP, PriestleyJV, Michael-TitusAT, CuzzocreaS. Docosahexaenoic acid attenuates the early inflammatory response following spinal cord injury in mice: in-vivo and in-vitro studies. J Neuroinflamm. 2014; 11: 6.

[37] BaskervilleTA, PriestleyJV, Michael-TitusAT. The effect of docosahexaenoic acid in a rat model of spinal cord injury by contusion. Soc Neurosci Abstr. 2012; 658.26/P15.

[38] HallJC, PriestleyJV, PerryVH, Michael-TitusAT. Effect of docosahexaenoic acid and eicosapentaenoic acid on the early inflammatory response following compression spinal cord injury in the rat. J Neurochem. 2012; 121: 738–750.

[39] WardRE, HuangW, CurranOE, PriestleyJV, Michael-TitusAT. Docosahexaenoic acid prevents white matter damage after spinal cord injury. J Neurotrauma. 2010; 27: 1769–1780.

[40] LiX, MurrayK, HarveyPJ, BallouEW, BennettDJ. Serotonin facilitates a persistent calcium current in motoneurons of rats with and without chronic spinal cord injury. J Neurophysiol. 2007; 97: 1236–1246.

[41] SaruhashiY, YoungW, PerkinsR. The recovery of 5-HT immunoreactivity in lumbosacral spinal cord and locomotor function after thoracic hemisection. Exp Neurol. 1996; 139: 203–213.

[42] LiuZH, YipPK, AdamsL, DaviesM, LeeJW, MichaelGJ, PriestleyJV, Michael-TitusAT. A single bolus of docosahexaenoic acid promotes neuroplastic changes in the innervation of spinal cord interneurons and motor neurons and improves functional recovery after spinal cord injury. J Neurosci. 2015; 35: 12733–12752.

[43] MontoyaCP, Campbell-HopeLJ, PembertonKD, DunnettSB. The "staircase test": a measure of independent forelimb reaching and grasping abilities in rats. J Neurosci Methods. 1991; 36: 219–228.

[44] PallierPN, PoddigheL, ZbarskyV, KostusiakM, ChoudhuryR, HartT, BurguillosMA, MusbahiO, GroenendijkM, SijbenJW, deWildeMC, QuartuM, PriestleyJV, Michael-TitusAT. A nutrient combination designed to enhance synapse formation and func-

tion improves outcome in experimental spinal cord injury. Neurobiol Dis. 2015; 82: 504–515.

[45] BareyreFM, KerschensteinerM, RaineteauO, MettenleiterTC, WeinmannO, SchwabME. The injured spinal cord spontaneously forms a new intraspinal circuit in adult rats. Nat Neurosci. 2004; 7: 269–277.

[46] PriestleyJV, Michael-TitusAT, TetzlaffW. Limiting spinal cord injury by pharmacological intervention. Handb Clin Neurol. 2012; 109: 463–484.

[47] CalderPC. Mechanisms of action of (n-3) fatty acids. J Nutr. 2012; 142: 592S–599S.

[48] UmhauJC, ZhouW, CarsonRE, RapoportSI, PolozovaA, DemarJ, HusseinN, BhattacharjeeAK, MaK, EspositoG, MajchrzakS, HerscovitchP, EckelmanWC, KurdzielKA, SalemNJr. Imaging incorporation of circulating docosahexaenoic acid into the human brain using positron emission tomography. J Lipid Res. 2009; 50: 1259–1268.

[49] Van NeervenS, MeyJ. RAR/RXR and PPAR/RXR signaling in spinal cord injury. PPAR Res. 2007; 2007: 29275.

[50] PuttaguntaR & DiGS. Retinoic acid signaling in axonal regeneration. Front Mol Neurosci. 2011; 4: 59.

[51] CurtA, van HedelHJ, KlausD, DietzV. Recovery from a spinal cord injury: significance of compensation, neural plasticity, and repair. J Neurotrauma. 2008; 25: 677–685.

[52] IchiyamaRM, CourtineG, GerasimenkoYP, YangGJ, van den BrandR, LavrovIA, ZhongH, RoyRR, EdgertonVR. Step training reinforces specific spinal locomotor circuitry in adult spinal rats. J Neurosci. 2008; 28: 7370–7375.

[53] FouadK & TetzlaffW. Rehabilitative training and plasticity following spinal cord injury. Exp Neurol. 2012; 235: 91–99.

[54] LiuG, DetloffMR, MillerKN, SantiL, HouleJD. Exercise modulates microRNAs that affect the PTEN/mTOR pathway in rats after spinal cord injury. Exp Neurol. 2012; 233: 447–456.

[55] Garcia-AliasG, FawcettJW. Training and anti-CSPG combination therapy for spinal cord injury. Exp Neurol. 2012; 235: 26–32.

[56] MaierIC, IchiyamaRM, CourtineG, SchnellL, LavrovI, EdgertonVR, SchwabME. Differential effects of anti-Nogo-A antibody treatment and treadmill training in rats with incomplete spinal cord injury. Brain. 2009; 132: 1426–1440.

Chapter 7

Role of JAK-STAT Signalling on Motor Function Recovery after Spinal Cord Injury

Victor S. Tapia and Juan Larrain

Additional information is available at the end of the chapter

http://dx.doi.org/10.5772/63418

Abstract

JAK-STAT signalling is a main transduction pathway of cytokines and growth factors, which is involved in several biological processes including cell proliferation, cell differentiation, axon regeneration, apoptosis and inflammation. After spinal cord injury several cytokines activate the JAK-STAT pathway, thereby modulating several cell responses. In this chapter we discuss how regulation of this signalling pathway could improve motor recovery after injury by modulation of axon regeneration, neuroprotection, glial scar formation, demyelination and inflammatory response. Studies with gene over-expression, gene deletion and *in vitro* approaches will be discussed for understanding the cell-specific response to JAK-STAT signalling, with a focus on preclinical treatment with IL6-family cytokines, hematopoietic cytokines and IL10.

Keywords: cytokine, JAK-STAT, STAT3, axon regeneration, glial scar, inflammation

1. Introduction

Worldwide, an estimate of 180,000 cases of spinal cord injuries (SCI) occur yearly [1]. SCI results in the complete or partial loss of motor and sensory functions below the lesion site. This type of injury causes irreversible paralysis, chronic pain, loss of bladder, bowel and sexual function, amongst others dysfunctions, impairing quality and increasing the cost of life [2, 3].

The pathology of SCI in mammals starts with an acute phase during the first days of injury, which includes massive cell death and inflammatory response. The acute response is followed by a second phase during the first week after injury consisting of tissue replacement, where the loss of cells is replaced by a glial scar. After the second week it finalizes with a third phase which continues for months involving chronic tissue remodelling, remyelination and circuit remodelling [4]. Although some spontaneous repair after SCI has been described in mammals including humans, it contributes poorly to motor and functional recovery. Progenitor cells proliferate and differentiate but mostly to glial cells while no neurogenesis occurs [5, 6]. Besides there is only a partial axon regeneration and circuit remodelling response that contribute to a limited compensatory recovery [2].

Several reviews have been published describing growth factors and cytokines that regulate cell response in SCI [2, 7, 8]. Advancements using these factors to improve spinal cord repair are being made, and preclinical treatments have been achieved by local delivery of growth factors and by physiological delivery with i.v. or i.p. injections (intravenous or intraperitoneal, respectively) [2]. Between the plethora of signalling pathways activated in response to tissue injury, the JAK-STAT signalling pathway is one of the main pathways that has been extensively studied because of its broad effect on the response to injury. In this chapter, we discuss the activation and role of JAK-STAT signalling in response to SCI and studies focused on modulating JAK-STAT to improve motor recovery. First, we briefly describe the JAK-STAT pathway components, followed by a discussion of its role in different cellular processes including: axonal regeneration, neuroprotection, glial response and its effects on the inflammatory response.

2. JAK-STAT signalling pathway

The JAK-STAT signalling pathway is involved in transmitting information from the extracellular milieu to gene promoters in the nucleus. The basic components of the JAK-STAT pathway are depicted in **Figure 1**. Several cytokines, growth factors and even hormones signal through the JAK-STAT pathway. Currently, there are 38 protein ligands and 36 cell surface receptor combinations have been described [9]. Besides the several combinations of protein ligands and receptor complexes, in mammals there are four JAK (Janus kinase) tyrosine kinases: JAK1, JAK2, JAK3 and Tyk2 (Non-receptor tyrosine-protein kinase TYK2); and seven STAT (Signal transducer and activator of transcription) transcription factors: STAT1, STAT2, STAT3, STAT4, STAT5a, STAT5b and STAT6 [9].

Activation of the JAK-STAT pathway begins after ligand binding to the receptor subunits, which forms homodimers, heterodimers or heteromultimers depending on the family receptor (**Table 1** presents ligands and receptors related to SCI). After multimerization, intracellular transduction is initiated through the recruitment of JAK kinases. JAKs phosphorylate receptor subunits and STAT transcription factors. After tyrosine phosphorylation, cytosolic STATs dimerize and are translocated to the nucleus to bind specific DNA regulatory sequences and regulate gene expression [10].

The JAK-STAT signalling pathway has different negative inhibitors. The most important inhibitor for preclinical studies is the classical negative feedback loop of suppressor of cytokine signalling (SOCS) proteins, which are target genes for STATs proteins and switch off JAK

http://dx.doi.org/10.5772/63418

proteins. Over-expression or deletion of SOCS3, one of the eight mammalian SOCS proteins, has been extensively used to modulate endogenous pathway activation [11–13].

Although it will not be discussed in this chapter, it has to be considered that ligands binding to receptor complexes also activate other intracellular signalling cascades besides the JAK-STAT pathway [10]. Phosphorylation of receptors induces activation of ERK1/2 and AKT pathways. Moreover, STATs can also be activated independently to the canonical JAK-STAT signalling pathway. Growth factor activation of RTKs (receptor tyrosine kinases) and NRTKs (non-receptor tyrosine kinases) can activate STATs. Hormone and chemokine binding to G protein–coupled receptors can also activate JAKs proteins to phosphorylate STATs [10].

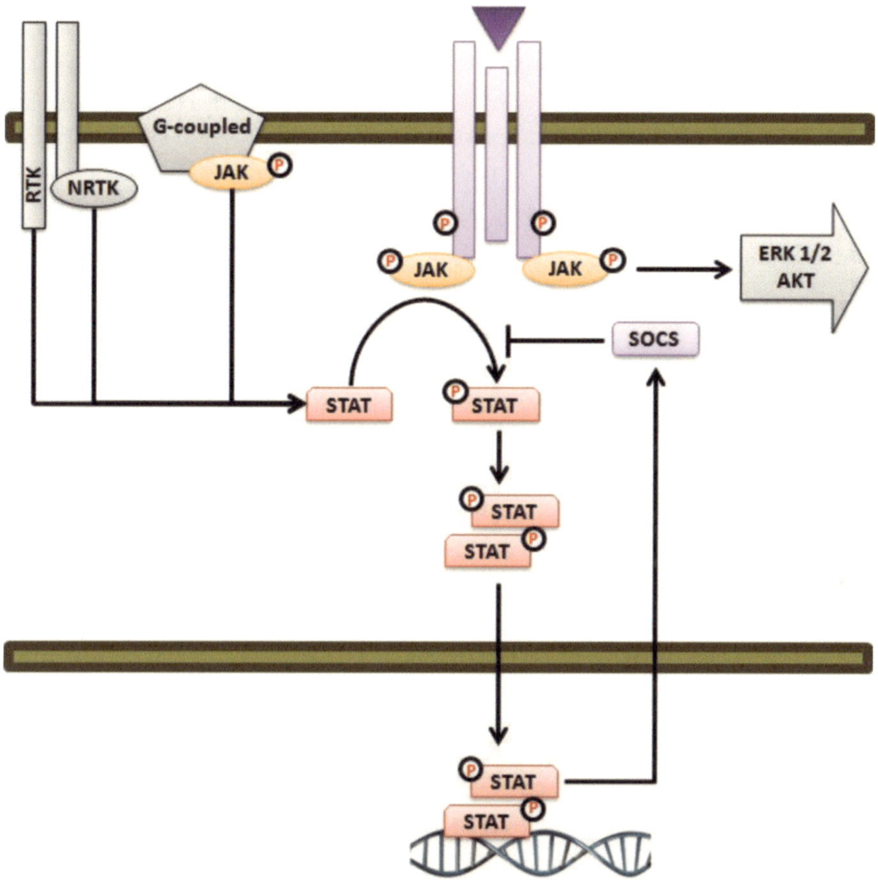

Figure 1. Basic components of the JAK-STAT signaling pathway. After binding of cytokines, receptors multimerize (violet boxes) recruiting to the membrane and activating JAK kinases (orange boxes) that initiate substrate phosphorylation (letter P). STAT transcription factors (pink boxes) are phosphorylated, dimerized and transported to the nucleus. STAT dimers regulate gene transcription. Among others, a classic target is SOCS that forms a negative feedback loop inhibiting JAK function. Alternative signaling pathways (grey boxes) for JAK-STAT are JAK-receptor complex activation of ERK1/2 and AKT pathways; STATs phosphorylation by RTKs, NRTKs or JAKs associated to G-coupled protein receptors.

3. JAK-STAT pathway activation in response to SCI

3.1. Cytokine expression in response to SCI

Before discussing the role of the JAK-STAT pathway in motor recovery, we will discuss the endogenous expression of cytokines and activation of STAT proteins in response to SCI. The upregulation of the IL6 family cytokines, IL6 (Interleukin 6), LIF (Leukemia inhibitory factor), OSM (Oncostatin M), IL11 (Interleukin 11) and CNTF (Ciliary neurotrophic factor) have been well characterized in response to SCI. Early IL6 and LIF upregulation has been detected in the acute phase after SCI, with a peak of expression around 6–12 hpi (hours post-injury) and basal levels at 4 dpi (days post-injury) [14, 15]. Different neural cell types contribute to IL6 and LIF expression. It has been shown that IL6 has a broad cell type expression, being detected in neurons, astrocytes and macrophages, while LIF is mainly expressed in meningeal astrocytes [14]. IL6 mRNA expression correlates with IL6 protein levels analyzed in another study, which detected an increase in IL6 concentration from 3 hours to 3 dpi [16]. In these studies the upregulation of cytokines occurs in the surrounding area of the lesion site, around 1 or 2 mm from the epicentre.

Early upregulation of OSM is also detected after SCI, with a strong peak at 6 hpi, but on the contrary to IL6 and LIF, upregulation of OSM is still detected until 1 mpi (months post-injury) [15]. IL11 and CNTF protein upregulation has also been detected after the acute phase. A steady increase in protein levels has been detected during the first week of injury for IL11 and during the first month for CNTF. In both cases no later times were analyzed to determine when the cytokines reached basal levels, therefore there is a possibility that they had an extended upregulation [17, 18]. IL11 cell expression has not been analyzed; on the contrary, it has been shown that CNTF has a chronic expression in glial cell types after spinal cord injury. CNTF has been detected in oligodendrocytes during the first month and in astrocytes up to 4 mpi [18, 19]. This chronic expression of CNTF is more spatially restricted than the early expressed cytokines IL6 and LIF, being detected only in the lesion borders [19].

Cytokine family	Cytokine	Receptors	JAKs	STATs	Endogenous levels, preclinical or clinical trials
IL6	IL6	Gp130 – IL6R	Jak1	STAT1-3	U/P
	LIF	Gp130 – LIFR	Jak2	STAT3	U/P
	CNTF	Gp130 – LIFR – CNTFR	Tyk2	STAT3	U/P
	IL11	Gp130 – IL11R		STAT3	U
	OSM	Gp130 –		STAT3	U/P

Cytokine family	Cytokine	Receptors	JAKs	STATs	Endogenous levels, preclinical or clinical trials
		LIFR			
Hematopoietic	G-CSF	CSF3R	Jak2	STAT3	P/C
	GM-CSF	CSF2Ra – βcR	Jak2	STAT5a/b	P/C
	EPO	EpoR or EpoR-βcR	Jak2	STAT5a/b	P/C
IL10	IL10	IL10Rα – IL10Rβ	Jak1 – Tyk2	STAT1-3	P

Table 1. JAK-STAT ligands, receptors and transducers involved in spinal cord injury. Cytokines are shown with associated receptors and JAK-STAT components. It is shown if cytokines are up-regulated in response to SCI (U) or if they have been used in preclinical (P) or clinical (C) studies for spinal cord recovery.

3.2. JAK-STAT signalling in response to SCI

In concordance with the upregulation of cytokines in response to SCI, several studies have characterized JAK-STAT pathway activation in spinal cord cells. Consistent with the transient increase of IL6 concentration, in the same study it was detected an increase in gp130 dimerization and JAK1 phosphorylation [16]. As expected for the activation of the gp130/JAK1 axis, STAT1 and STAT3 are phosphorylated in response to SCI. pSTAT1 has an acute increase which reach basal levels at 2 dpi [20]. On the contrary, pSTAT3 has an extended increase which differs between studies. An increase in pSTAT3 has been detected up to 7 dpi in some studies [12, 16], while in another no basal levels were reached even after 2 weeks post-injury (wpi) [21]. Nevertheless, all studies agree that STAT3 has a longer activation than STAT1. Together with the temporal difference, protein localization suggests that STAT3 has a more prominent role in regulating gene expression than STAT1 in cell response. While pSTAT3 has been detected in neuron nuclei after spinal cord injury, pSTAT1 has been only detected in the cytoplasm [16, 20].

STAT3 activation has been characterized in several spinal cord cell types. In the acute injury, nuclear pSTAT3 is observed in neurons of the anterior horns [16] and transcriptional activity is also supported by the detection of SOCS3+ neurons [21]. Nuclear pSTAT3 and SOCS3 has been also detected in microglia/macrophage during the acute phase of injury [16, 21] and nuclear pSTAT3 in oligodendrocytes and astrocytes during the first week near the lesion site [12, 22]. Due to a prominent role in glial scar formation, spatial STAT3 activation on astrocytes has also been highly defined. It has been determined that during the first week pSTAT3+ astrocytes appear at the border of the lesion with elevated predominance on the first 500 μm near the injury [12, 22].

After the first week of injury, contusion models show chronic pSTAT3 signalling in glial cell types located in the lesion borders. pSTAT3 has been detected in oligodendrocyte precursor cells (OPCs) and oligodendrocytes at 2 wpi [18, 19]. This activation decreases from 1 to 5 wpi, but at that time is still higher than on uninjured spinal cords [19]. pSTAT3+ astrocytes have been detected even further, at 12 wpi in the lesion borders [19].

4. Role of JAK-STAT in axon regeneration and collateral sprouting

To recover motor function after SCI, new connections have to be established after neuron death and axon degeneration [2]. These circuits can be established by two different cellular responses that should not be confused: Axon regeneration is the process where axons from severed neurons regrow from the injured tip or from a lateral growth distant to the injury (**Figure 2a-b**). On the contrary, collateral sprouting is a compensatory growth from undamaged axons initiated in response to injury (**Figure 2c**) [23].

While there is limited axon regeneration through the lesion area in response to complete SCI (**Figure 2a**), there is a compensatory remodelling on brain and spinal circuits when the spinal

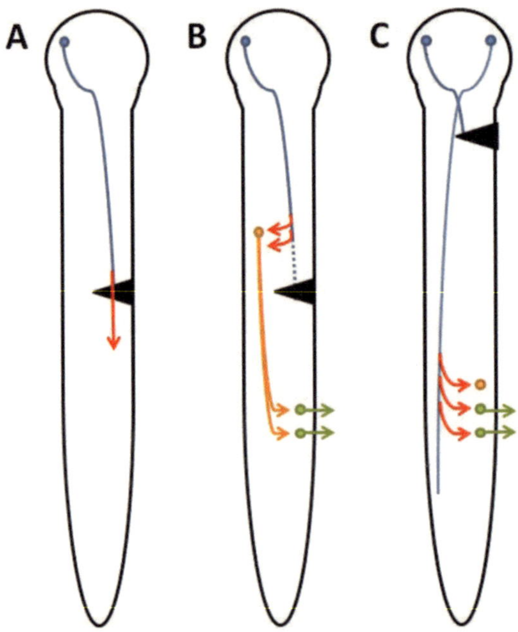

Figure 2. Axonal regeneration and collateral sprouting in spinal cord injury. Models used to evaluate axon regeneration and circuit remodeling, showing corticospinal tract (CST, in blue) as an example. Remodeling can be evaluated by axonal regeneration or collateral sprouting (both in red arrows) and new innervations can be connected to propiospinal neurons (PSNs, interneurons in orange) or motor neurons (in green). CNS injury is indicated as a darkened triangle in every model. **A**, In SCI models (usually contusion and hemisection) axonal regeneration of injured CSTs can be evaluated through and beyond the lesion area. **B**, in a hemisection model, innervation of new targets by injured CSTs can be evaluated. Regenerative axons from CSTs can innervate PSNs, which then connect to denervated motoneurons. **C**, in a unilateral pyramidotomy injury paradigm, collateral sprouting of uninjured CSTs to denervated PSNs and motor neurons can be measured. Anterograde, retrograde or retrograde trans-synaptic labelling are used depending of the injury model.

cord lesion is incomplete [2]. The corticospinal tract (CST) has been used as a model to study this recovery process. CST starts in the motor cortex and connects to spinal motor neurons, controlling voluntary motor function [23]. After spinal cord injury, CST circuit remodelling can be achieved by axon regeneration innervating long descendent interneurons that increase connection to motoneurons (**Figure 2b**) [24] or by collateral sprouting of uninjured axons to denervated motoneurons (**Figure 2c**) [25]. In this section we will discuss the role of JAK-STAT pathway on the promotion of axon regeneration and collateral sprouting after SCI. Briefly, we will discuss the results involving dorsal root ganglion (DRG) and optic nerve injury, to follow with studies of axon growth and collateral sprouting of the CSTs after SCI.

4.1. Role of JAK-STAT pathway in axon regeneration in SCI and other nerve injury models

4.1.1. Axon regeneration after dorsal root ganglion or optic nerve axotomy

The DRG model has been useful to study axon regeneration due to regenerative and non-regenerative branches. Sensory neurons from DRG target peripheral tissue with branches (i.e. sciatic nerve) that regenerate after axotomy. On the contrary, DRG neurons also target the dorsal column of the spinal cord, which do not regenerate after injury. This difference in the regenerative capacity has been partially related to the JAK-STAT pathway activation by studies on cytokine deficient mice, but conclusive results have been obtained in a study assessing the role of STAT3 in axon regeneration. While STAT3 deletion reduced axon growth of the severed sciatic nerve, STAT3 viral over-expression in the DRG improves axon regeneration of the non-regenerative nerve [26].

Similar to the activation of the JAK-STAT pathway in the DRG model, axon growth has been also promoted in the non-regenerative optic nerve. JAK-STAT activation by CNTF treatment or deletion of the SOCS3 negative feedback improved axon regeneration in optic nerve injury [11]. The studies in both injury models demonstrate that the JAK-STAT pathway, specifically the axis of STAT3/SOCS3, promotes axon regeneration. Therefore, a possible mechanism to improve motor recovery after SCI is through modulation of the JAK-STAT pathway to induce axon regeneration.

4.1.2. Axon regeneration after the spinal cord injury

A hemisection study showed that only a small subset of cortical neurons presented an increment in STAT3 and pSTAT3 levels after SCI, suggesting that on the contrary of peripheral nerves, in the spinal cord there is a lack of retrograde JAK-STAT activation [27]. As in DRG and optic nerve injury models, insufficient JAK-STAT activation could be related to the lack of axon regeneration. Several studies have shown that improvement of local extrinsic factors, such as cytokines administration, or improvement of intrinsic factors, such as the genetic modulation of the JAK-STAT pathway in neurons, improves axon regeneration after SCI, suggesting that modulation of JAK-STAT can be a bona fide target for designing novel therapies for spinal cord repair.

Administration of CNTF, G-CSF (granulocyte-colony stimulating factor), IL6 and LIF by intrathecal or i.p. injections results in improved axon regeneration through the lesion site and motor recovery after SCI. CNTF intrathecal injections during the first 10 days or administration in sodium-hyaluronate particles placed in the transection site have improved functional recovery after SCI [28, 29]. Although CST axon regeneration has not been assessed in CNTF treatment, a study showed increased retrograde labelling of the rubrospinal tracts [28]. Another study showed improved axonal sprouting through the lesion site, although it was not evaluated if these axons were from local neurons or descended from the brain [29].

Axon regeneration has also been assessed after spinal cord administration of G-CSF during 2 weeks after a hemisection [30]. CST axon regeneration was improved in the lesion site although no axon growth caudal to the injury was detected. The local G-CSF delivery also results in improvement of motor function and a similar result was observed in a transgenic mice line expressing G-CSF under the control of the MapKII promoter that is specifically activated in cortical and spinal cord neurons [30].

On the contrary to CNTF and G-CSF treatments, LIF has been administered daily by intraperitoneal injection since it is actively transported through the BBB with a mechanism involving the LIFRα receptor [31, 32]. LIF treatment for 14 days in a hemisection injury model improved the number of retrograde labelled CST and rubrospinal neurons. Improvement in motor recovery was assessed by RotaRod and Platform hang tests [32].

Although CNTF, G-CSF and LIF treatments showed an improvement in axon regeneration and motor function in rodents, in these studies the activation of the JAK-STAT pathway in cortical neurons was not assessed. Besides, these studies cannot distinguish if the improvement in axon regeneration and functional recovery is due to the modulation of the intrinsic program of cortical neurons or due to the modulation of other spinal cord cell types. Contrary to these studies, local IL6 administration has been shown to activate the JAK-STAT pathway in spinal and cortical neurons [33, 34]. IL6 intrathecal administration during the first week after a hemisection injury increased pSTAT3 levels in the spinal cord and in cortical neurons, while up-regulated the regeneration associated gene GAP-43 mRNA [34]. Although no motor recovery analyses were assessed, anterograde labelling showed an increase in the number of synapsin1+ CST axons near the lesion site [33].

The IL6 treatment suggests that cytokine delivery can promote the regenerative response of motoneurons by JAK-STAT pathway activation. In addition, specific STAT3 over-expression in the cortex has shown that this pathway can promote axon regeneration. After over-expression mediated by adenovirus injection in the cortex, pSTAT3 levels increased in cortical neurons and CST axonal regeneration improved through and beyond the lesion site of a hemisection [27].

4.2. Role of JAK-STAT in circuit remodelling by collateral sprouting

Although improvement in axon regeneration (**Figure 2a**) and motor recovery has been achieved by cytokine delivery, no relation has been established between the observed axon regeneration in the lesion site and the motor recovery. On the contrary, studies involving JAK-

STAT pathway and circuit remodelling by collateral sprouting (**Figure 2c**) have suggested that motor recovery is accomplished by innervation of uninjured axons to denervated motoneurons and interneurons.

Cytokine	Treatment	Cell response	Motor recovery	References
Il6	Acute by i.t.	Axon regeneration	Not assessed	[33, 34]
	Acute i.p., MR16-1	Immune modulation	Improved	[66, 84, 85]
LIF	10-14 days by i.p.	Axon regeneration Glial modulation	Improved	[32, 60, 61]
CNTF	10 days by i.p. or Hyaluronate	Axon regeneration Glial modulation	Improved	[28, 29]
	SC viral expression	Collateral sprouting	Not assessed	[13]
OSM	Gel foam	Glial modulation	Improved	[15]
G-CSF	2 weeks by i.t.	Axon regeneration Neuroprotection	Improved	[30]
	Acute by subcutaneous, i.v. or i.t.	Neuroprotection Glial modulation Immune modulation	Improved	[40, 54-57, 81]
GM-CSF	Acute by i.v., i.t. or i.p.	Glial modulation	Improved	[54, 55, 64]
EPO	Acute by i.p.	Collateral sprouting Glial modulation	Improved	[35, 58, 59]
IL10	Acute by i.p.	Glial modulation Immune modulation	Improved Not improved	[77, 78]
	SC viral expression	Neuroprotection	Improved	[48, 49]
IL12	Gel foam	Glial modulation Immune modulation	Not improved	[82]

Table 2. Pre-clinical studies with cytokine for motor recovery of SCI. Summary of JAK-STAT cytokine preclinical studies, for any cytokine it is shown administration timing and method. Time indicated as acute means a single dose at the moment of injury or daily doses from 1 to 5 dpi. Methods of administration are indicated as intrathecal (i.t.), intraperitoneal (i.p.), intravenous (i.v.) or subcutaneous injection; embedded on hyaluronate or gel foam placed in the lesion site; and by SC (spinal cord) viral expression. Contrary to the other studies, MR16-1 indicates a treatment with a neutralizing antibody against IL6 receptor.

Promotion of collateral sprouting by the hematopoietic cytokine EPO (Erythropoietin) has been assessed in a model of traumatic brain injury that results in denervation of the CST circuit. EPO i.p. injections during the acute phase resulted in increased collateral sprouting of uninjured CST fibers in the cervical and lumbar area and improved motor function [35]. Although it has not been shown that EPO activate the JAK-STAT signalling pathway in neurons, cortical viral infection has been useful to determine the role of the pathway in collateral sprouting. STAT3 viral over-expression in uninjured mice induced collateral sprouting and innervations to propiospinal neuron (PSN, a type of interneuron) [27]. This viral expression was also assessed in a unilateral pyramidotomy model, which is an injury at the level of the medulla oblongata that severs half of the CST (**Figure 2c**) and it is useful to evaluate how collateral sprouting connects to spinal neurons. In this approach it was shown that STAT3 induced collateral sprouting, innervation of PSNs and motoneurons, and improvement in motor recovery which was assessed by behavioural and electrophysiological tests [27]. Cortical SOCS3 deletion also induced collateral sprouting in the pyramidotomy paradigm [13], suggesting that an endogenous JAK-STAT pathway activation promotes circuit remodelling. After finding a transient CNTF expression in denervated neurons caudal to injury, the same study showed that combination of cortical SOCS3 deletion and spinal cord CNTF over-expression improved collateral sprouting [13].

5. Role of JAK-STAT in local neuron response

In response to SCI the number of local motor and interneurons decrease with no neurogenesis to generate new neurons [2]. To improve motor recovery, promotion of axon regeneration and collateral sprouting should be accompanied by neuroprotective strategies, since number and dendrite distribution of local spinal neurons would be beneficial for circuit remodelling. We will start this section discussing *in vitro* studies related to the neuroprotective role of the JAK-STAT pathway, following *in vivo* studies with cytokine delivery and knockdown treatments after SCI.

5.1. Role of JAK-STAT in neuron survival

At a molecular level, studies in non-neural cells have shown that STAT transcription factors have different roles in apoptosis regulation. A comparative *in vitro* study of STAT1 and STAT3 showed that while STAT1 inhibits the expression of the anti-apoptotic genes Bcl-2 and Bcl-X, STAT3 promoted their expression [36]. STAT5 proteins, which are activated by a different set of cytokines (Table 1), also promote cell survival by Bcl-X upregulation [37].

In vitro studies have shown that the neuroprotective role of JAK-STAT cytokines is partly associated to STAT3 activation and expression of anti-apoptotic genes. IL10 activated STAT3 and promoted Bcl-2 and Bcl-xl expression in embryonic spinal cord neurons [38]. IL6 and OSM cytokines also activated STAT3 and promoted anti-apoptotic gene expression in cortical neurons and neuroblastoma cells [39]. In cultured cerebellar granule neurons, G-CSF also promoted STAT3 activation while increased Bcl-2 levels [40]. It should be considered that theses cytokines also activate the AKT pathway [39, 40]. Both inhibition of the JAK and AKT pathway decreased the neuroprotective effect, suggesting that probably both pathways contribute to the anti-apoptotic response [38, 40].

Related to the previous *in vitro* studies, *in vivo* studies in CNS injury suggest a protective role of STAT3 while an opposite role for STAT1. On a focal cerebral ischemia model, it was shown that STAT1 deficient mice presented a reduced infarct size and apoptotic cell number [41]. On the contrary, on a permanent cerebral ischemia model the IL6/STAT3 axis has been associated to positive outcomes. While the neutralization with an anti-IL6R antibody resulted in decreased STAT3 activation and increased lesion area, IL6 administration reduced the lesion size [42, 43]. Although these studies indicate a neuroprotective role of STAT3, specific cell type modulation should be assessed to differentiate the direct modulation on neuron response from indirect neuroprotection by modulation of glial and inflammatory cell types. At this moment, there is only one study where specific STAT3 deletion in neurons is analyzed in an *in vivo* CNS injury model. Mice with STAT3 deletion in neurons (using the Neurofilament L promoter) showed a decrease in motoneuron number after facial nerve injury and diminished expression of anti-apoptotic genes [44].

5.2. JAK-STAT modulation of neuronal protection in SCI

G-CSF and IL10 are cytokines with several studies showing beneficial outcomes in neuroprotection, inflammatory response and motor recovery after SCI [45, 46]. It has been shown that a pro-inflammatory response is negative for neuron survival [47]; therefore, in these cytokine treatments it is difficult to differentiate a direct modulation on neuronal survival and the effect on neuro-inflammation. Since it has been shown that spinal cord neurons express G-CSF and IL10 receptors [40, 48], we will discuss a small set of studies that focused in neuroprotection and in a following section we will discuss the modulation of the immune response in SCI.

G-CSF has been locally administrated to evaluate neuroprotection in SCI. Subcutaneous G-CSF treatment during the first five days after compression improved motor recovery, decreased apoptotic neurons in the acute phase and improved neuron number in the remodelling phase (6 wpi) [40]. Other studies with intrathecal administration of G-CSF for 2 weeks, commented before for assessing axonal regeneration, also showed neuroprotective results. This long-term treatment reduced apoptotic cell number and increased Bcl-xL expression in the spinal cord [30]. Two independent IL10 viral over-expression studies also improved motor function [48, 49] and one of these studies showed decreased pro-apoptotic protein levels and increased Bcl-2 levels, resulting in a higher neuron number [48]. Although it was shown by *in vitro* studies that G-CSF and IL10 treatments activate STAT3 in spinal neurons [40, 48], it has not been demonstrated that this activation occurs on *in vivo* treatments. *In vivo* analyses of IL10 over-expression only focused in neuronal NF-κβ activation [48]. Therefore, it is an open question if these cytokines promotes neuron survival by JAK-STAT activation or by other signalling pathway, as NF-κβ gene regulation.

Although by results of cytokine treatments the role of STAT3 in neuroprotection remains inconclusive, knockdown of the inhibitory protein SOCS3 has contributed to this proposition [21]. Local over-expression of shSOCS3 diminished SOCS3 mRNA levels. This knockdown increased pSTAT3 levels in a transection model and it decreased the Bax/Bcl-2 protein ratio, while improving neuron number near the lesion site [21]. A following study of the same group showed that SOCS3 knockdown increased dendrite growth in dorsal and ventral horns near the injury site [50].

Finally, consistent with the pro-apoptotic role of STAT1 on *in vitro* studies [36], STAT1 knockdown has shown positive outcomes after SCI. Administration of STAT1 siRNA reduced STAT1 protein levels in the spinal cord. Although no analysis of neuronal survival was assessed, 1 day post-contusion the STAT1 knockdown mice had increased its Bcl-2 levels. siRNA treated mice also improved motor function assessed by BMS open-field score.

6. Role of JAK-STAT in glial response

In response to SCI, apoptosis of astrocytes and oligodendrocytes occurs in the acute phase of injury and then glial cells dynamically respond during weeks and months after injury. A glial hallmark of CNS injury is the glial scar, formed by reactive astrocytes, OPCs and meningeal cells [51]. This compact scar gathers around damaged tissue, inflammatory cells and fibroblasts. The glial scar is necessary to contain secondary injury, as disruption of the astrocyte scar with different transgenic models leads to increased cell death, demyelination and reduced functional motor recovery [12, 52, 53]. Although the glial scar is necessary for the containment of the lesion, reactive astrocytes express and secrete inhibitory molecules for axonal growth and sprouting, as chondroitin sulfate proteoglycans (CSPGs) [51]. Altogether with the glial scar formation, a demyelination process occurs during weeks after injury by oligodendrocyte apoptosis. Although mature oligodendrocytes do not proliferate to recover cell number, OPCs start to proliferate and differentiate and remyelination proceeds near the lesion area [6]. Accordingly to the glial response commented above, in this section we will discuss the following topics: Cytokine modulation of the glial response to reduce secondary damage, the regulation of reactive astrocyte and the neural stem progenitor cells (NSPCs) by the STAT3/SOCS3 axis.

6.1. Cytokines modulate glial response in SCI

Several studies with the hematopoietic and IL6-family cytokines have assessed astrocyte and oligodendrocyte responses with positive outcomes on tissue preservation and motor recovery. Acute administration of GM-CSF or G-CSF by i.p. or i.v. injections during the acute phase reduced lesion area, while increasing the spared myelin area and improving motor recovery after SCI [54–56]. Both cytokine treatments reduced NG2 levels (OPC marker) during the first week of injury [54, 55]. In one of these studies it was also shown that G-CSF up-regulated Bcl-xL and reduced apoptosis in oligodendrocytes [56]. Therefore, these results suggest that these cytokines maintain spared myelin by a protective mechanism and not by promotion of OPC proliferation.

GM-CSF and G-CSF also modulate the reactive astrocyte response during the first month after SCI, as seen by the reduction of GFAP levels and the CSPG neurocan [54, 55]. Another study with improvement in motor recovery by G-CSF intrathecal administration during the first day of injury also showed a reduction in the CSPG proteins neurocan and phosphocan [57]. Altogether with the previous studies, this last study suggest that G-CSF decrease the reactive gliosis because the treatment reduced TGF-β levels, a growth factor that promotes reactive gliosis; reduced vimentin levels, an astrocyte filament induced in glial scar; and presented less astrocyte proliferation [57]. Acute EPO i.p. injection also has similar results in astrocyte regulation after SCI. EPO treatment reduced lesion area and GFAP levels, while improving preservation of myelin and motor recovery at 2 wpi [58]. A following study showed possible differences with GM-CSF and G-CSF on the OPC response. Although these cytokines reduce NG2 levels, it was shown that EPO treatment increased it at 4 wpi [59].

The IL6-family of cytokines also regulates glial response. LIF i.p. administration has been shown to reduce oligodendrocyte apoptosis [60, 61], although *in vivo* LIF signalling on oligodendrocyte is not clear. On one hand, one study found that SCI induced LIFRβ expression on oligodendrocytes and that LIF treatment induced pSTAT3 and pAKT in these cells [60]. On the contrary, an alternative study did not find LIFRβ expression on oligodendrocytes and suggested a LIF positive modulation of microglia [61]. Although studies with LIF i.p. treatment have not assessed the astrocyte response in SCI, it has been shown that this treatment incremented Nestin+ cell number near the lesion site [32]. CNTF treatment, previously commented for improved motor recovery and axon regeneration, also increased the density of astrocytes [28]. Finally, gel foam administration of OSM reduced the lesion area and preserved MBP (myelin basic protein), but on the contrary to the other IL6-family cytokines, it reduced GFAP levels near the lesion site. This glial modulation was accompanied by improved serotonergic fiber outgrowth and motor recovery [15].

6.2. STAT modulation of reactive astrocytes

Contrary to motoneuron response in SCI, astrocyte response has been studied with cell-specific deletions of STAT3 and SOCS3. Deletions on Nestin or GFAP expressing cells, two genes up-regulated in reactive astrocytes, have elucidated the role of the JAK-STAT signalling pathway on reactive gliosis. Mice with Nestin:STAT3KO or GFAP:STAT3KO had an increased lesion area and decreased glial scar after 2 weeks of a contusive SCI [12, 22]. Consistent with the protective role of the glial scar, this was accompanied by increased demyelination and inflammatory response, altogether with a lack of motor recovery after injury. On the contrary, the deletion of the negative feedback in a Nestin:SOCS3KO mice had prolonged and increased pSTAT3 levels in response to SCI, resulting in reduced lesion area, early and increased glial scar surrounding this area, and improved motor recovery [12].

These *in vivo* studies demonstrated that the glial JAK-STAT signalling is necessary for secondary damage contention and further studies have elucidated the cellular mechanisms modulated by this pathway. First, it seems that JAK-STAT pathway is necessary for astrocyte survival in response to injury, as an *in vitro* study showed that GFAP:STAT3KO astrocytes had increased necrosis and protein release after a mechanical injury [62]. Besides cell survival, JAK-STAT controls gene expression associated to reactive gliosis. STAT3 controls the expression of glial filaments, as it is known that GFAP is a target gene for STAT3 [63] and in GFAP:STAT3KO mice, reduced levels of GFAP and vimentin were detected [22]. Cell morphology is also modulated by JAK-STAT pathway. In response to SCI, astrocytes near the lesion site change their cell morphology and orientation to form the glial scar. In GFAP:STAT3KO mice, astrocytes failed to change orientation and did not form the closed boundaries of the glial scar [53].

Another STAT transcription factor that controls astrocyte response is STAT5, which is activated by GM-CSF. As commented before, this cytokine reduced GFAP and CSPG levels with an increase in motor recovery [55]. An *in vitro* study with astrocytes activated with TGF-β3, which up-regulates CSPG proteins, found that GM-CSF increased pSTAT5, pAKT and pRaf levels [64]. The cytokine also reduced TGF-β signalling and CSPGs expression. GM-CSF effects were blocked by JAK and PI3K inhibitors, suggesting that STAT5 and PI3K signalling could reduce the levels of axon inhibitory proteins secreted by reactive astrocytes [64]. Following studies should clarify if STAT5 has a similar role *in vivo*.

6.3. JAK-STAT modulation of neural stem progenitor cells

Adult neural stem progenitor cells (NSPCs) can generate new astrocytes and oligodendrocytes in homeostasis and in response to injury [5, 6]. NSPCs can also generate new neurons but only in some CNS specific areas, the dentate gyrus and the subventricular zone (SVZ) [65]. The role on the JAK-STAT pathway to modulate neurogenesis and gliogenesis is not clear and probably depends on the specific context, the cytokine types and cellular phenotype. At one hand, *in vitro* studies show that the JAK-STAT pathway induces gliogenesis in opposition to neurogenic differentiation, as seen in the blocking of IL6/STAT3 axis in NSPCs [66, 67]. On the other hand, there are some *in vivo* studies that have shown a JAK-STAT role for specific cytokines in adult NSPC proliferation and neurogenesis. In the dentate gyrus, CNTF and STAT3 deficient mice had reduced NSPC proliferation and neurogenesis [68]. Using cytokine injections and deficient mice it has been also shown that IL15 and IL10 regulate NSPC proliferation in the SVZ [69, 70].

Contrary to the neurogenesis of the dentate gyrus and the SVZ, in the spinal cord there is only gliogenesis. This cell differentiation occurs in three main cell types that proliferate in response to injury: ependymal cells, astrocytes and OPCs [6]. The role of the JAK-STAT pathway on proliferation and differentiation of ependymal cells and astrocytes has not been assessed, as transgenic mice with specific cell type deletion has been done only for Nestin and GFAP promoters, which are markers for both NSPCs and mature astrocytes. On the contrary, understanding on OPCs modulation has been done *in vivo* by NG2 knockout cells [71]. In response to injury, NG2+ cells proliferate and increase in number near the lesion site. NG2 proliferation is incremented in a NG2:SOCS3KO mice. On the contrary, in the NG2:STAT3KO mice no differences in NG2 cell number and proliferation were detected [71]. This could be explained by the modulation of OPC proliferation by other STAT transcription factors or by other pathways activated by JAK proteins (**Figure 1**), which are inhibited by SOCS3. JAK-STAT modulation of NG2 cell differentiation was also assessed in this study. Although STAT3 did not regulate OPC proliferation, in the same study it was shown that NG2:STAT3KO mice had reduced differentiation to mature oligodendrocytes during the first week of injury, but not at chronic phases (1mpi) [71].

7. Role of JAK-STAT in the inflammatory response

In response to injury neutrophils, macrophages and lymphocytes infiltrate to the spinal cord [72]. There are several studies where reduction of cell infiltration improves motor recovery and tissue sparing [73, 74]. Even so, the reduction of functional recovery after SCI in mice with total ablation of infiltrated macrophages indicates that the inflammatory response is also necessary for proper recovery [75]. These differences could be explained taking into account that immune cells have different and opposite phenotypes. Microglia and macrophages, the main effectors during spinal cord inflammation, are capable of polarization that leads to either pro-inflammatory (M1 type) or anti-inflammatory cells (M2 type). While M1 macrophages participate in secondary damage as well as in axonal retraction observed after SCI, M2 macrophages are proposed to be protective and promote axonal growth [47]. Considering the role of cytokines in the regulation of the immune response, in this section we discuss studies where JAK-STAT signalling has been shown to reduce the inflammatory response or change macrophage phenotype for improvement in spinal cord functional recovery.

7.1. Anti-inflammatory cytokines

IL10 is a cytokine that has been studied in SCI for anti-inflammatory modulation and neuroprotection [46]. Endogenous IL10 expression has not been assessed in detail after SCI and it is only known that M2 infiltrated macrophages express Il10 surrounding the glial scar [75]. Using IL10 deficient mice it has been found that this cytokine is necessary for controlling the inflammatory response and apoptosis. After SCI, IL10 deficient mice have an increased expression of pro-inflammatory genes, increased levels of the pro-apoptotic proteins and decreased motor recovery [76]. Another study which replaced normal monocytes with IL10 deficient monocytes also resulted in reduced motor recovery, suggesting that this cytokine is necessary for the positive macrophage anti-inflammatory response [75]. IL10 treatments in SCI has resulted in motor recovery improvement by inflammatory and neuroprotective regulation. Acute i.p. administration of IL10 reduced lesion volume in two independent studies [77, 78]. But while one study showed that IL10 improved motor recovery and reduced TNFα expression in the injured spinal cord and in infiltrated macrophages [77], the other study did not find any functional recovery [78]. Although we previously commented other studies with motor recovery improvement by local viral over-expression of IL10 [48, 49], on those studies the inflammatory response was not assessed.

Another important anti-inflammatory cytokine is IL4, which signals by the STAT6 transcription factor. Although the neutralization of this cytokine by anti-IL4 antibody administration increased the inflammatory response, neither the IL4-neutralization treatment nor a study with STAT6 deficient mice found differences in motor recovery after SCI [79, 80]. These results indicate that Il4 signalling is not necessary for motor recovery. Further studies should test this cytokine in the promotion of the anti-inflammatory response in SCI.

In addition, there are some G-CSF studies which have shown immune modulation upon SCI. Previously commented studies for G-CSF modulation on glial cells also assessed immune response. Daily intravenous administration of G-CSF during the first 4 dpi showed that treatment not only improved motor recovery and oligodendrocyte protection, but also suppressed upregulation of the pro-inflammatory cytokines TNFα and IL1β and reduced IL1β + neutrophils infiltration [56]. Another treatment with G-CSF intrathecal injection during the first day reduced macrophage/microglia cell number and TNFα levels during the first 2 wpi

[57]. Although G-CSF is well known for neuroprotective modulation [45], only one study has elucidated a biological mechanism for G-CSF inflammatory modulation on SCI. While in this study was found an increase in microglial number at 7dpi in the G-CSF treated mice, *in vitro* analyses indicated that this cytokine induced a M2 microglial phenotype, reducing pro-inflammatory genes while inducing IL10 expression [81]. A further characterization should be done to demonstrate that G-CSF induces a M2 phenotype *in vivo*.

7.2. Pro-inflammatory cytokines

IL12 is a pro-inflammatory cytokine produced by macrophages and dendritic cells which signals via STAT4 [82]. Although it was shown that gel foam administration of IL12 regulated immune and OPC response, this treatment slightly improved motor recovery in C57BL/6 mice and did not improve function in BALB/c strain [83]. A similar result was found after SCI in STAT4 deficient mice, no improvement was found in comparison WT mice [79]. These studies suggest that IL12 signalling is not functionally important for motor recovery.

The IL6-cytokine family has shown different effects in inflammatory response after spinal cord injury. IL11 deficient mice have been assessed in SCI, with no significant differences in motor recovery or macrophage infiltration [17]. LIF treatment incremented Mac1 levels, a marker for macrophage/microglial, and IGF-1 expression on these cells [61], while gel foam administration of OSM reduced T-cell infiltration [15]. Although we previously discussed IL6 intrathecal administration for axon regeneration modulation [33, 34], IL6 is a pro-inflammatory cytokine which can be blocked to decrease inflammatory response. To avoid Il6 mediated immune response, a single i.p. administration of MR16-1, an anti-mouse IL6 receptor antibody, has been tested with positive outcomes. MR16-1 improved motor recovery after a contusive SCI [66, 84]. This treatment also reduced the lesion area, astrocyte proliferation and increased spared myelin area and neurofilament and serotonergic fibers near the lesion area [66, 85]. The mechanism underlying the MR16-1 improvement in tissue and functional recovery has been associated to microglial and infiltrated macrophage function. MR16-1 accelerated inflammatory resolution, as number of total macrophage/microglial began to decrease earlier in the treated group [85]. Further phenotypic characterization of immune cells lead to the discovery that in MR16-1 treated mice, the microglial cells had an increased phagocytic phenotype. It was also shown that macrophages had a predominant M2 phenotype and that anti-inflammatory cytokines were up-regulated while pro-inflammatory cytokines were down-regulated [84, 85].

8. Conclusion and clinical implications

Cytokine upregulation and JAK-STAT signalling activation are endogenous mechanism that are activated in response to SCI and can be used to improve motor recovery. Cell type specific and *in vitro* studies have identified the role of STATs modulation in spinal cord cells. STAT3 has been the most extensively studied STAT transcription factor in SCI, but promising results have been found in other STATs and further studies should continue to determine the roles of

STAT1 and STAT5 in SCI. Moreover, further studies with transgenic models should focus in other specific cell responses not studied up to now, like motoneuron and NSPC responses.

Several preclinical studies have shown positive outcomes for motor recovery and tissue sparing in JAK-STAT cytokine treatments (**Table 2**). Thus, modulation of the JAK-STAT signalling presents an opportunity to modulate neuron and glial response after an SCI in clinical settings. The hematopoietic cytokines have been already used in clinical studies for several pathologies, therefore are advanced in comparison with other JAK-STAT cytokines. Discussion of G-CSF and EPO treatments for SCI can be found in previous chapters [45, 86], while for GM-CSF there is one SCI clinical study finished which consisted in cytokine administration with transplant of bone marrow cells [87]. Although clinical studies have not been assessed for other cytokines in CNS trauma, there are clinical studies involving other pathologies that could be translated to SCI. The anti-inflammatory and neuroprotective mechanism of IL10 could also be assessed with a recombinant human IL10 that has been used for HIV infection and other several pathologies [46]. Emfilermin is a recombinant human LIF that has been tested, although with a lack of effectiveness, in clinical trials for embryo implantation and peripheral neuropathy [88, 89] that could also be used in SCI or other CNS diseases. Finally, tocilizumab, an anti-human IL6R, has shown positive outcomes in clinical studies for rheumatoid arthritis [90] and could be used for anti-inflammatory treatment in the spinal cord acute response.

Acknowledgements

Special thanks to Daniel Guzmán for critical reading and valuable suggestions. This work was supported by ICM (P07/011-F, P09/016-F) and FONDECYT (1141162).

Author details

Victor S. Tapia and Juan Larrain*

*Address all correspondence to: jlarrain@bio.puc.cl

Center for Aging and Regeneration, Millennium Nucleus in Regenerative Biology, Faculty of Biological Sciences, Pontifical Catholic University of Chile, Santiago, Chile

References

[1] Lee B.B., Cripps R.A., Fitzharris M., Wing P.C. The global map for traumatic spinal cord injury epidemiology: update 2011, global incidence rate. Spinal Cord. 2014;52:110–116. DOI: 10.1038/sc.2012.158

[2] Thuret S., Moon L.D.F., Gage F.H. Therapeutic interventions after spinal cord injury. Nature Reviews Neuroscience. 2006;7(8):628–643. DOI: 10.1038/nrn1955

[3] Cannon B. Sensation and loss. Nature. 2013;503(7475):S2–3. DOI: 10.1038/503S2a

[4] Burda J.E., Sofroniew M.V. Reactive gliosis and the multicellular response to CNS damage and disease. Neuron. 2014;81(2):229–248. DOI: 10.1016/j.neuron.2013.12.034

[5] Horky L., Galimi F. Fate of endogenous stem/progenitor cells following spinal cord injury. Journal of Comparative Neurology. 2006;498(4):525–538. DOI: 10.1002/cne. 21065.Fate

[6] Barnabé-Heider F., Göritz C., Sabelström H., Takebayashi H., Pfrieger F.W., Meletis K., et al. Origin of new glial cells in intact and injured adult spinal cord. Cell Stem Cell. 2010;7(4):470–482. DOI: 10.1016/j.stem.2010.07.014

[7] Bastien D., Lacroix S. Cytokine pathways regulating glial and leukocyte function after spinal cord and peripheral nerve injury. Experimental Neurology. 2014;258:62–77. DOI: 10.1016/j.expneurol.2014.04.006

[8] Kundi S., Bicknell R., Ahmed Z. The role of angiogenic and wound-healing factors after spinal cord injury in mammals. Neuroscience Research. 2013;76:1–9. DOI: 10.1016/ j.neures.2013.03.013

[9] Murray P. The JAK-STAT signaling pathway: input and output integration. The Journal of Immunology. 2007;178:2623–2629. DOI: 10.4049/jimmunol.178.5.2623

[10] Rawlings J.S., Rosler K.M., Harrison D. The JAK/STAT signaling pathway. Journal of Cell Science. 2004;117:1281–1283. DOI: 10.1242/jcs.00963

[11] Smith P., Sun F., Park K., Cai B., Wang C. SOCS3 deletion promotes optic nerve regeneration in vivo. Neuron. 2009;64(5):617–623. DOI: 10.1016/j.neuron. 2009.11.021.SOCS3

[12] Okada S., Nakamura M., Katoh H., Miyao T., Shimazaki T., Ishii K., et al. Conditional ablation of Stat3 or Socs3 discloses a dual role for reactive astrocytes after spinal cord injury. Nature Medicine. 2006;12(7):829–834. DOI: 10.1038/nm1425

[13] Jin D., Liu Y., Sun F., Wang X., Liu X., He Z. Restoration of skilled locomotion by sprouting corticospinal axons induced by co-deletion of PTEN and SOCS3. Nature Communications. 2015;6:8074. DOI: 10.1038/ncomms9074

[14] Pineau I., Lacroix S. Proinflammatory cytokine synthesis in the injured mouse spinal cord: multiphasic expression pattern and identification of the cell types involved. Journal of Comparative Neurology. 2007;500(2):267–285. DOI: 10.1002/cne

[15] Slaets H., Nelissen S., Janssens K., Vidal P.M., Lemmens E., Stinissen P., et al. Oncostatin M reduces lesion size and promotes functional recovery and neurite outgrowth after spinal cord injury. Molecular Neurobiology. 2014;50(3):1142–1151. DOI: 10.1007/ s12035-014-8795-5

[16] Yamauchi K., Osuka K., Takayasu M., Usuda N., Nakazawa A., Nakahara N., et al. Activation of JAK/STAT signalling in neurons following spinal cord injury in mice. Journal of Neurochemistry. 2006;96(4):1060–1070. DOI: 10.1111/j.1471-4159.2005.03559.x

[17] Cho N., Nguyen D.H., Satkunendrarajah K., Branch D.R., Fehlings M.G. Evaluating the role of IL-11, a novel cytokine in the IL-6 family, in a mouse model of spinal cord injury. Journal of Neuroinflammation. 2012;9:134. DOI: 10.1186/1742-2094-9-134

[18] Tripathi R.B., McTigue D.M. Chronically increased ciliary neurotrophic factor and fibroblast growth factor-2 expression after spinal contusion in rats. Journal of Comparative Neurology. 2008;510(2):129–144. DOI: 10.1002/cne.21787

[19] Hesp Z.C., Goldstein E.Z., Goldstein E., Miranda C.J., Kaspar B.K., et al. Chronic oligodendrogenesis and remyelination after spinal cord injury in mice and rats. Journal of Neuroscience. 2015;35(3):1274–1290. DOI: 10.1523/JNEUROSCI.2568-14.2015

[20] Osuka K., Watanabe Y., Usuda N., Atsuzawa K., Yasuda M., Aoshima C., et al. Activation of STAT1 in neurons following spinal cord injury in mice. Neurochemical Research. 2011;36(12):2236–2243. DOI: 10.1007/s11064-011-0547-6

[21] Park K., Lin C., Lee Y. Expression of suppressor of cytokine signaling-3 (SOCS3) and its role in neuronal death after complete spinal cord injury. Experimental Neurology. 2014;0:65–75. DOI: 10.1016/j.expneurol.2014.06.013

[22] Herrmann J.E., Imura T., Song B., Qi J., Ao Y., Thu K., et al. STAT3 is a critical regulator of astrogliosis and scar formation after spinal cord injury. Journal of Neuroscience. 2009;28(28):7231–7243. DOI: 10.1523/JNEUROSCI.1709-08.2008.

[23] Tuszynski M.H., Steward O. Concepts and methods for the study of axonal regeneration in the CNS. Neuron. 2012;74(5):777–791. DOI: 10.1016/j.neuron.2012.05.006

[24] Bareyre F.M., Kerschensteiner M., Raineteau O., Mettenleiter T.C., Weinmann O., Schwab M.E. The injured spinal cord spontaneously forms a new intraspinal circuit in adult rats. Nature Neuroscience. 2004;7(3):269–277. DOI: 10.1038/nn1195

[25] Weidner N., Ner A. Spontaneous corticospinal axonal plasticity and functional recovery after adult central nervous system injury. Proceedings of the National Academy of Sciences of the United States of America. 2001;98(6):3513–3518. DOI: 10.1073/pnas.051626798

[26] Bareyre F.M., Garzorz N., Lang C., Misgeld T., Büning H., Kerschensteiner M. In vivo imaging reveals a phase-specific role of STAT3 during central and peripheral nervous system axon regeneration. Proceedings of the National Academy of Sciences of the United States of America. 2011;108(15):6282–62787. DOI: 10.1073/pnas.1015239108

[27] Lang C., Bradley P.M., Jacobi A., Kerschensteiner M., Bareyre F.M. STAT3 promotes corticospinal remodelling and functional recovery after spinal cord injury. EMBO Reports. 2013;14(10):931–937. DOI: 10.1038/embor.2013.117

[28] Ye J., Cao L., Cui R., Huang A., Yan Z., Lu C., et al. The effects of ciliary neurotrophic factor on neurological function and glial activity following contusive spinal cord injury in the rats. Brain Research. 2004;997(1):30–39. DOI: 10.1016/j.brainres.2003.10.036

[29] Wang N., Zhang S., Zhang F., Yang Z.Y., Li X.G. Sodium hyaluronate-CNTF gelatinous particles promote axonal growth, neurogenesis and functional recovery after spinal cord injury. Spinal Cord. 2014;52(7):517–523. DOI: 10.1038/sc.2014.54

[30] Pitzer C., Klussmann S., Krüger C., Letellier E., Plaas C., Dittgen T., et al. The hematopoietic factor granulocyte-colony stimulating factor improves outcome in experimental spinal cord injury. Journal of Neurochemistry. 210;113(4):930–942. DOI: 10.1111/j.1471-4159.2010.06659.x

[31] Pan W., Cain C., Yu Y., Kastin A.J. Receptor-mediated transport of LIF across blood-spinal cord barrier is upregulated after spinal cord injury. Journal of Neuroimmunology. 2006;174:119–125. DOI: 10.1016/j.jneuroim.2006.02.006

[32] Li Y., Zang D. The neuron regrowth is associated with the proliferation of neural precursor cells after leukemia inhibitory factor administration following spinal cord injury in mice. PloS One. 2014;9(12):e116031. DOI: 10.1371/journal.pone.0116031

[33] Yang P., Wen H., Ou S., Cui J., Fan D. IL-6 promotes regeneration and functional recovery after cortical spinal tract injury by reactivating intrinsic growth program of neurons and enhancing synapse formation. Experimental Neurology. 2012;236:19–27. DOI: 10.1016/j.expneurol.2012.03.019

[34] Yang P., Qin Y., Bian C., Zhao Y., Zhang W. Intrathecal delivery of IL-6 reactivates the intrinsic growth capacity of pyramidal cells in the sensorimotor cortex after spinal cord injury. PloS One. 2015;10(5):e0127772. DOI: 10.1371/journal.pone.0127772

[35] Zhang Y., Xiong Y., Mahmood A., Meng Y., Liu Z. Sprouting of corticospinal tract axons from the contralateral hemisphere into the denervated side of the spinal cord is associated with functional recovery in adult rat. Brain Research. 2010;1353:249–257. DOI: 10.1016/j.brainres.2010.07.046

[36] Stephanou A., Brar B. Opposing actions of STAT-1 and STAT-3 on the Bcl-2 and Bcl-x promoters. Cell Death and Differentiation. 2000;7(3):329–330.

[37] Silva M., Benito A., Sanz C., Prosper F. Erythropoietin can induce the expression of bcl-xLthrough stat5 in erythropoietin-dependent progenitor cell lines. Journal of Biological Chemistry. 1999;274(32):22165–22169.

[38] Zhou Z., Peng X., Insolera R. Interleukin-10 provides direct trophic support to neurons. Journal of Neurochemistry. 2009;110(5):1617–1627. DOI: 10.1111/j.1471-4159.2009.06263.x.

[39] Park K.W., Nozell S.E., Benveniste E.N. Protective role of STAT3 in NMDA and glutamate-induced neuronal death: negative regulatory effect of SOCS3. PloS One. 1012;7(11):e50874. DOI: 10.1371/journal.pone.0050874

[40] Nishio Y., Koda M., Kamada T. Granulocyte colony-stimulating factor attenuates neuronal death and promotes functional recovery after spinal cord injury in mice. Journal of Neuropathology and Experimental Neurology. 2997;66(8):724–731.

[41] Takagi Y., Harada J., Chiarugi A., Moskowitz M. STAT1 is activated in neurons after ischemia and contributes to ischemic brain injury. Journal of Cerebral Blood Flow and Metabolism. 2002;22(11):1311–1318. DOI: 10.1097/01.WCB.0000034148.72481.F4

[42] Loddick S., Turnbull A., Rothwell N. Cerebral interleukin-6 is neuroprotective during permanent focal cerebral ischemia in the rat. Journal of Cerebral Blood Flow and Metabolis. 1998;18:176–17.

[43] Yamashita T., Sawamoto K., Suzuki S., Suzuki N., Adachi K., Kawase T., et al. Blockade of interleukin-6 signaling aggravates ischemic cerebral damage in mice: possible involvement of Stat3 activation in the protection of neurons. Journal of Neurochemistry. 2005;94(2):459–68. DOI: 10.1111/j.1471-4159.2005.03227.x

[44] Schweizer U., Gunnersen J., Karch C., Wiese S., Holtmann B., Takeda K., et al. Conditional gene ablation of Stat3 reveals differential signaling requirements for survival of motoneurons during development and after nerve injury in the adult. Journal of Cell Biology. 2002;156(2):287–97. DOI: 10.1083/jcb.200107009

[45] Wallner S., Peters S., Pitzer C., Resch H., Bogdahn U., Schneider A. The granulocyte-colony stimulating factor has a dual role in neuronal and vascular plasticity. Frontiers in Cell and Developmental Biology. 2015;3:48. DOI: 10.3389/fcell.2015.00048

[46] Thompson C.D., Zurko J.C., Hanna B.F., Hellenbrand D.J., Hanna A. The therapeutic role of interleukin-10 after spinal cord injury. Journal of Neurotrauma. 2013;30:1311–1324. DOI: 10.1089/neu.2012.2651

[47] David S., Kroner A. Repertoire of microglial and macrophage responses after spinal cord injury. Nature Reviews Neuroscience. 2011;12(7):388–399. DOI: 10.1038/nrn3053

[48] Zhou Z., Peng X., Insolera R., Fink D., Mata M. IL-10 promotes neuronal survival following spinal cord injury. Experimental Neurology. 2009;220(1):183–190. DOI: 10.1016/j.expneurol.2009.08.018

[49] Jackson C., Messinger J., Peduzzi J.D., Ansardi D.C., Morrow C.D. Enhanced functional recovery from spinal cord injury following intrathecal or intramuscular administration of poliovirus replicons encoding IL-10. Virology. 2005;336(2):173–183. DOI: 10.1016/j.virol.2005.03.025

[50] Park K.W., Lin C.Y., Li K., Lee Y.S. Effects of reducing suppressors of cytokine signaling-3 (SOCS3) expression on dendritic outgrowth and demyelination after spinal cord injury. PloS One. 2015;10(9):e0138301. DOI: 10.1371/journal.pone.0138301

[51] Yiu G., He Z. Glial inhibition of CNS axon regeneration. Nature Reviews Neuroscience. 2006;7(8):617–627. DOI: 10.1038/nrn1956.

[52] Faulkner J.R., Herrmann J.E., Woo M.J., Tansey K.E., Doan N.B., Sofroniew M.V. Reactive astrocytes protect tissue and preserve function after spinal cord injury. Journal of Neuroscience. 2004;24(9):2143–2155. DOI: 10.1523/JNEUROSCI.3547-03.2004

[53] Wanner I.B., Anderson M., Song B., Levine J., Fernandez A., Gray-Thompson Z., et al. Glial scar borders are formed by newly proliferated, elongated astrocytes that interact to corral inflammatory and fibrotic cells via STAT3-dependent mechanisms after spinal cord injury. Journal of Neuroscience. 2013;33(31):12870–12886. DOI: 10.1523/JNEUROSCI.2121-13.2013

[54] Huang X., Kim J.M., Kong T.H., Park S.R., Ha Y., Kim M.H., et al. GM-CSF inhibits glial scar formation and shows long-term protective effect after spinal cord injury. Journal of the Neurological Science. 2009;277:87–97. DOI: 10.1016/j.jns.2008.10.02

[55] Chung J., Kim M., Yoon Y., Kim K. Effects of granulocyte colony–stimulating factor and granulocyte-macrophage colony–stimulating factor on glial scar formation after spinal cord injury in rats. Journal of Neurosurgery: Spine. 2014;21(6):966–973. DOI: 10.3171/2014.8.SPINE131090

[56] Kadota R., Koda M., Kawabe J., Hashimoto M., Nishio Y., Mannoji C., et al. Granulocyte colony-stimulating factor (G–CSF) protects oligodendrocyte and promotes hindlimb functional recovery after spinal cord injury in rats. PloS One. 2012;7(11):e50391. DOI: 10.1371/journal.pone.0050391

[57] Chen W.F., Chen C.H., Chen N.F., Sung C.S., Wen Z.H. Neuroprotective effects of direct intrathecal administration of granulocyte colony-stimulating factor in rats with spinal cord injury. CNS Neuroscience & Therapeutics. 2015;21(9):698–707. DOI: 10.1111/cns.12429

[58] Gorio A., Madaschi L. Methylprednisolone neutralizes the beneficial effects of erythropoietin in experimental spinal cord injury. Proceedings of the National Academy of Sciences of the United States of America. 2005;102(45):16379–16384. DOI: 10.1073/pnas.0508479102

[59] Vitellaro-Zuccarello L., Mazzetti S., Madaschi L., Bosisio P., Gorio A., De Biasi S. Erythropoietin-mediated preservation of the white matter in rat spinal cord injury. Neuroscience. 2007;144(3):865–877. DOI: 10.1016/j.neuroscience.2006.10.023

[60] Azari M., Profyris C. Leukemia inhibitory factor arrests oligodendrocyte death and demyelination in spinal cord injury. Journal of Neuropathology and Experimental Neurology. 2006;65(6):914–929. DOI: 10.1097/01.jnen.0000235855.77716.25

[61] Kerr B.J., Patterson P.H. Leukemia inhibitory factor promotes oligodendrocyte survival after spinal cord injury. Glia. 2005;51:73–79. DOI: 10.1002/glia.20177

[62] Levine J., Kwon E., Paez P., Yan W., Czerwieniec G., Loo J., et al. Traumatically injured astrocytes release a proteomic signature modulated by STAT3-dependent cell survival. Glia. 2015; 64(5):668-694. DOI: 10.1002/glia.22953

[63] Takizawa T., Nakashima K., Namihira M. DNA methylation is a critical cell-intrinsic determinant of astrocyte differentiation in the fetal brain. Developmental Cell. 2001;1(6):749–758. DOI: 10.1016/S1534-5807(01)00101-0

[64] Choi J., Park S., Kim K., Park S. GM-CSF reduces expression of chondroitin sulfate proteoglycan (CSPG) core proteins in TGF-β-treated primary astrocytes. BMB Reports. 2014;47(12):679–684. DOI: 10.5483/BMBRep.2014.47.12.018

[65] Alvarez-Buylla A., Seri B., Doetsch F. Identification of neural stem cells in the adult vertebrate brain. Brain Research Bulletin. 2002;57(6):751–758. DOI: 10.1016/S0361-9230(01)00770-5

[66] Okada S., Nakamura M., Mikami Y., Shimazaki T., Mihara M., Ohsugi Y., et al. Blockade of interleukin-6 receptor suppresses reactive astrogliosis and ameliorates functional recovery in experimental spinal cord injury. Journal of Neuroscience Research. 2004;76(2):265–276. DOI: 10.1002/jnr.20044

[67] Gu F., Hata R., Ma Y.J., Tanaka J., Mitsuda N., Kumon Y., et al. Suppression of Stat3 promotes neurogenesis in cultured neural stem cells. Journal of Neuroscience Research. 2005;81(2):163–171. DOI: 10.1002/jnr.20561

[68] Müller S., Chakrapani B.P.S., Schwegler H., Hofmann H.D., Kirsch M. Neurogenesis in the dentate gyrus depends on ciliary neurotrophic factor and signal transducer and activator of transcription 3 signaling. Stem Cells. 2009;27(2):431–441. DOI: 10.1634/stemcells.2008-0234

[69] Gómez-Nicola D., Valle-Argos B., Pallas-Bazarra N., Nieto-Sampedro M. Interleukin-15 regulates proliferation and self-renewal of adult neural stem cells. Molecular Biology of the Cell. 2011;22:1960–1970. DOI: 10.1091/mbc.E11-01-0053

[70] Pereira L., Font-Nieves M., Van den Haute C., Baekelandt V., Planas A.M., Pozas E. IL-10 regulates adult neurogenesis by modulating ERK and STAT3 activity. Frontiers in Cellular Neuroscience. 2015;9:57. DOI: 10.3389/fncel.2015.00057

[71] Hackett A.R., Lee D.H., Dawood A., Rodriguez M., Funk L., Tsoulfas P., et al. STAT3 and SOCS3 regulate NG2 cell proliferation and differentiation after contusive spinal cord injury. Neurobiology of Disease. 2016;89:10–22. DOI: 10.1016/j.nbd.2016.01.017

[72] Prüss H., Kopp M., Brommer B., Gatzemeier N., Laginha I., Dirnagl U., et al. Non-resolving aspects of acute inflammation after spinal cord injury (SCI): indices and resolution plateau. Brain Pathology. 2011;21(6):652–660. DOI: 10.1111/j.1750-3639.2011.00488.x

[73] Popovich P.G., Guan Z., Wei P., Huitinga I., van Rooijen N., Stokes B.T. Depletion of hematogenous macrophages promotes partial hindlimb recovery and neuroanatomical repair after experimental spinal cord injury. Experimental Neurology. 1999;158:351–365. DOI: 10.1006/exnr.1999.7118

[74] Saville L.R., Pospisil C.H., Mawhinney L.A., Bao F., Simedrea F.C., Peters A.A., et al. A monoclonal antibody to CD11d reduces the inflammatory infiltrate into the injured

spinal cord: A potential neuroprotective treatment. Journal of Neuroimmunology. 2004;156:42–57. DOI: 10.1016/j.jneuroim.2004.07.002

[75] Shechter R., London A., Varol C., Raposo C., Cusimano M., Yovel G., et al. Infiltrating blood-derived macrophages are vital cells playing an anti-inflammatory role in recovery from spinal cord injury in mice. PLoS Medicine. 2009;6(7):e1000113. DOI: 10.1371/journal.pmed.1000113

[76] Genovese T., Esposito E., Mazzon E., Di Paola R., Caminiti R., Bramanti P., et al. Absence of endogenous interleukin-10 enhances secondary inflammatory process after spinal cord compression injury in mice. Journal of Neurochemistry. 2009;108(6):1360–1372. DOI: 10.1111/j.1471-4159.2009.05899.x

[77] Bethea J.R., Nagashima H., Acosta M.C., Briceno C., Gomez F., Marcillo A.E., et al. Systemically administered interleukin-10 reduces tumor necrosis factor-alpha production and significantly improves functional recovery following traumatic spinal cord. Journal of Neurotrauma. 1999;16(10):851–863. DOI: 10.1089/neu.1999.16.851

[78] Takami T., Oudega M., Bethea J.R., Wood P.M., Kleitman N., Bunge M.B. Methylprednisolone and interleukin-10 reduce gray matter damage in the contused Fischer rat thoracic spinal cord but do not improve functional outcome. Journal of Neurotrauma. 2002;19(5):653–666. DOI: 10.1089/089771502753754118

[79] Fraidakis M., Kiyotani T., Pernold K. Recovery from spinal cord injury in tumor necrosis factor-alpha, signal transducers and activators of transcription 4 and signal transducers and activators of transcription 6 null mice. Neuroimmunology. 2007;18(2): 185–189.

[80] Lee S.I., Jeong S.R., Kang Y.M., Han D.H., Jin B.K., Namgung U., et al. Endogenous expression of interleukin-4 regulates macrophage activation and confines cavity formation after traumatic spinal cord injury. Journal of Neuroscience Research. 2010;88:2409–2419. DOI: 10.1002/jnr.22411

[81] Guo Y., Zhang H., Yang J., Liu S., Bing L., Gao J., et al. Granulocyte colony-stimulating factor improves alternative activation of microglia under microenvironment of spinal cord injury. Neuroscience. 2013;238:1–10. DOI: 10.1016/j.neuroscience.2013.01.047

[82] Vignali D., Kuchroo V.K. IL-12 family cytokines: immunological playmakers. Nature Immunology. 2012;13(8):722–728. DOI: 10.1038/ni.2366

[83] Yaguchi M., Ohta S., Toyama Y., Kawakami Y., Toda M. Functional recovery after spinal cord injury in mice through activation of microglia and dendritic cells after IL-12 administration. Journal of Neuroscience Research. 2008;86(9):1972–1980. DOI: 10.1002/jnr.21658

[84] Guerrero A.R., Uchida K., Nakajima H., Watanabe S., Nakamura M., Johnson W.E., et al. Blockade of interleukin-6 signaling inhibits the classic pathway and promotes an

alternative pathway of macrophage activation after spinal cord injury in mice. Journal of Neuroinflammation. 2012;9:40. DOI: 10.1186/1742-2094-9-40

[85] Mukaino M., Nakamura M., Yamada O., Okada S., Morikawa S., Renault-Mihara F., et al. Anti-IL-6-receptor antibody promotes repair of spinal cord injury by inducing microglia-dominant inflammation. Experimental Neurology. 2010;224:403–414. DOI: 10.1016/j.expneurol.2010.04.020

[86] Carelli S., Marfia G., Di Giulio A.M., Ghilardi G., Gorio A. Erythropoietin: recent developments in the treatment of spinal cord injury. Neurology Research International. 2011;2011:453179. DOI: 10.1155/2011/453179

[87] Yoon S.H., Shim Y.S., Park Y.H., Chung J.K., Nam J.H., Kim M.O., et al. Complete spinal cord injury treatment using autologous bone marrow cell transplantation and bone marrow stimulation with granulocyte macrophage-colony stimulating factor: Phase I/II clinical trial. Stem Cells. 2007;25(8):2066–2073. DOI: 10.1634/stemcells.2006-0807

[88] Davis I.D., Kiers L., MacGregor L., Quinn M., Arezzo J., Green M., et al. A randomized, double-blinded, placebo-controlled phase II trial of recombinant human leukemia inhibitory factor (rhuLIF, emfilermin, AM424) to prevent chemotherapy-induced peripheral neuropathy. Clinical Cancer Research. 2005;11:1890–1898. DOI: 10.1158/1078-0432.CCR-04-1655

[89] Brinsden P.R., Alam V., de Moustier B., Engrand P. Recombinant human leukemia inhibitory factor does not improve implantation and pregnancy outcomes after assisted reproductive techniques in women with recurrent unexplained implantation failure. Fertility and Sterility. 2009;91:1445–1447. DOI: 10.1016/j.fertnstert.2008.06.047

[90] Hashizume M., Tan S.L., Takano J., Ohsawa K., Hasada I., Hanasaki A., et al. Tocilizumab, a humanized anti-IL-6R antibody, as an emerging therapeutic option for rheumatoid arthritis: molecular and cellular mechanistic insights. International Reviews of Immunology. 2015;34(3):265–279. DOI: 10.3109/08830185.2014.938325

Section 3

Surgical Approaches for Repair and Regeneration Following Spinal Cord Injury

Chapter 8

Bridging Defects in Chronic Spinal Cord Injury Using Peripheral Nerve Grafts: From Basic Science to Clinical Experience

Sherif M. Amr

Additional information is available at the end of the chapter

Abstract

Nerve grafting of the injured spinal cord should pursue a sixfold attack: lysing the fibrosis/gliosis to an extent that allows settling of the basal lamina preventing meanwhile collapse of the neural tissue matrix; supplying the tissue matrix with a suitable scaffold, on which the basal lamina can settle; basal lamina synthesis; seeding the basal lamina with cell adhesion molecules; providing the axonal growth cone with neurite outgrowth promoting factors that allow its distal progression; supplying the axonal growth cone with neurotrophic factors that power its continued growth. In addition to this, the intrinsic properties of the neurons should be stimulated, possibly through modulating the function of astrocytes by heparin, aspirin and other factors. Nerve side grafting of the cord increases the incidence of nerve regeneration by applying additional grafts extending from the side of the donor end of the cord to the side of the recipient end. Also, it allows the surgeon to enhance regeneration through a partially regenerated cord. During surgery, after establishment of CSF circulation, a long-lasting indwelling catheter has to be inserted for postoperative drug and cell delivery. This allows for continual lysis of the gliosis by chondroitinase ABC, sialidase and other factors.

Keywords: spinal cord injury, nerve grafting, indwelling intrathecal catheter implantation, lysis of the gliosis, chondroitinase ABC

1. Introduction

Since 1903, when Tello and Cajal demonstrated that the central nervous system (CNS) could regenerate [1, 2], experimental neuroscience has advanced our knowledge repairing the injured spinal cord. Several cellular transplantation strategies have been recommended with some clinical success [3–6]. Clinically, however, the injured spinal cord is usually extensively gliotic, cystic, even disrupted, necessitating bridging the injury zone first before contemplating cellular transplantation. Placing peripheral nerve grafts to bridge the injury zone has been successful experimentally [7–13], yet only anecdotal clinical evidence supports it [14, 15]. In a review article on bridging spinal cord injuries, Fawcett [16] commented on this disparity between experimental and clinical neuroscience: 'Sadly, we have yet to achieve a treatment that is licensed for this purpose in human patients'. The aim of this review is to enable clinicians to put the findings made by neuroscientists into clinical practice and to provide neuroscientists with upcoming ideas investigating the clinical issues physicians face.

2. Changing concepts of nerve grafting

2.1. Basic concepts of nerve grafting

Autogenous nerve grafting is the standard for repair of irreducible nerve gaps [17]. The basic principles of nerve grafting include the following (**Figure 1**):

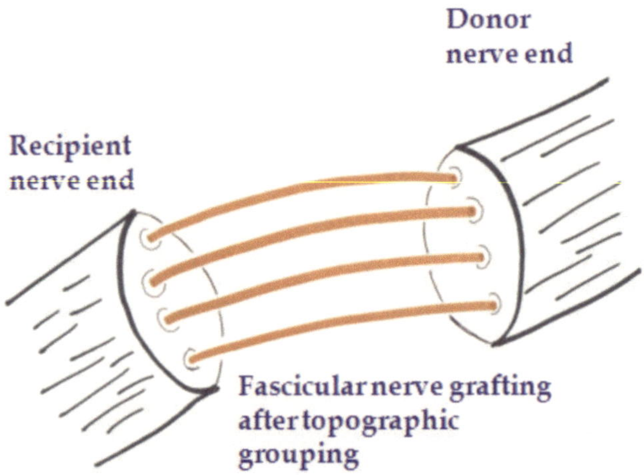

Figure 1. The basic principles of conventional end-to-end grafting include trimming both proximal and distal nerve ends up to healthy nerve fascicles; avoiding any tension at the repair site, avoiding any shearing stress at the repair site, fascicular grafting, end-to-end grafting suturing fascicles at proximal nerve ends to their counterparts at distal nerve ends after grouping them topographically, using small caliber sutures (9/0 or 10/0 sutures), and healthy vascular bed.

- trimming both proximal and distal nerve ends up to healthy nerve fascicles;

- avoiding any tension at the repair site, for even minimal tension, can end up with fibrosis, hampering progression of regeneration;

- avoiding any shearing stress at the repair site because this incites an inflammatory reaction ending up with fibrosis and hampering progression of regeneration;

- fascicular grafting because autogenous nerve grafts derive their nutrition from the extracellular matrix; using large diameter grafts instead of small diameter fascicles can produce central necrosis of the graft;

- end-to-end grafting suturing fascicles at proximal nerve ends to their counterparts at distal nerve ends after grouping them topographically, in order to avoid aberrant nerve sprouting;

- using small caliber sutures (9/0 or 10/0 sutures) because large caliber sutures may produce fibrosis;

- healthy vascular bed because a fibrotic bed may prevent progression of regeneration through the grafts.

In the absence of a proximal nerve end, such as in brachial plexus avulsions, nerve transfer (neurotisation) refers to using an expendable nearby donor nerve as a substitute, grafting it to the original recipient. The principles of nerve transfer include:

- donor nerve of high axonal load,

- single donor to single recipient to prevent cocontractions.

Autogenous grafts act as immunogenically inert scaffolds, providing appropriate neurotrophic factors and viable Schwann cells for axonal regeneration [17].

2.2. Molecular aspects of peripheral nerve regeneration

Advances in the understanding of molecular pathways and their physiological role have provided us with new insights as to the mechanism of axonal (peripheral nerve) regeneration [18, 19].

Fibrous tissue and chondroitin sulphate proteoglycans secreted by astrocytes provide the necessary scaffold for settling of the basal lamina and subsequent basement membrane synthesis. *Neurite outgrowth promoting factors* are basement membrane-related extracellular matrix proteins (such as laminin (LN), fibronectin (FN), heparin sulphate proteoglycans (HSP) and tenascin), which pave the proper path by supplying orientation and adhesiveness for axons. *Neurotrophic factors* are specific trophic agents that power peripheral nerve regeneration. They include (a) the neurotrophins (nerve growth factor (NGF), brain-derived neurotrophic factor (BDNF), neurotrophin-3 (NT-3) and neurotrophin-4/5(NT-4/5)); (b) the neurokines (ciliary neurotrophic factor (CNTF) and leukaemia inhibitory factor (LIF)); (c) the transforming growth factor (TGF)-b family (TGF-b1, TGF-b2, TGF-b3, glial cell line¦derived neurotrophic factor (GDNF)). *Schwann cells* secrete (a) cell adhesion molecules (CAMs), such as N-CAM, Ng-CAM/L1, N-cadherin and L2/HNK-1; (b) produce basement membrane that contains many extracellular matrix proteins, such as laminin (LN), fibronectin (FN), heparin sulphate proteoglycans (HSP) and tenascin; (c) secrete neurotrophic factors and their receptors. In addition to this, axonal regeneration is determined by trophic factors from activated perineural glial cells (astrocytes), trophic factors from efferent axons by anterograde transport, gene-induced trophic factors by intracrine or autocrine transport, trophic factors from retrograde target cell support, trophic factors from retroaxonal transport and trophic factors from recruited macrophages (secretory products, cytokines). Activated mesenchymal cells contribute to repair and vascularisation (**Figure 2**).

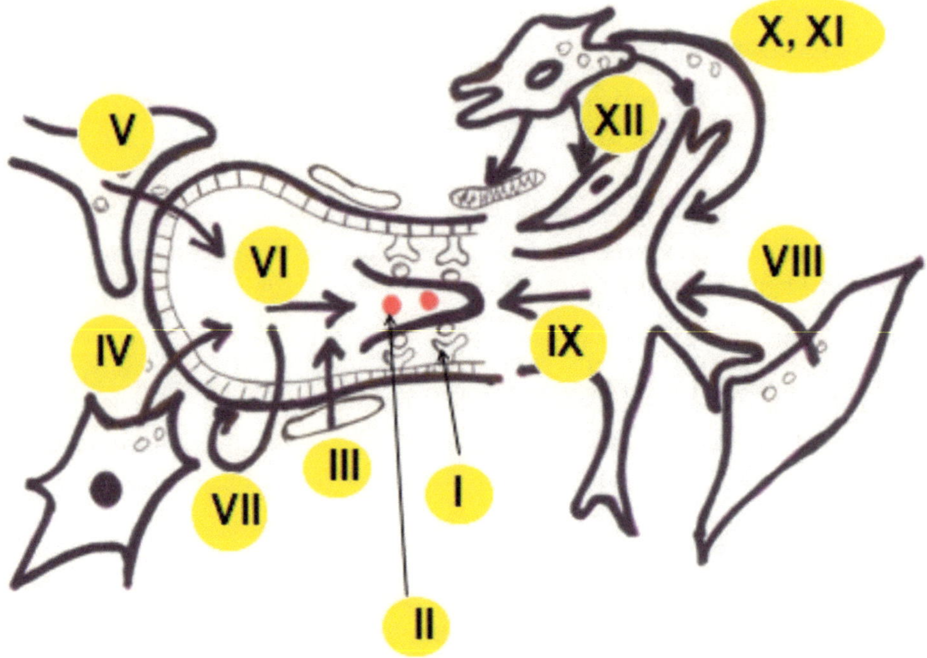

Figure 2. Molecular aspects of axonal regeneration. (I) *Neurite outgrowth promoting factors* [such as laminin (LN), fibronectin (FN), heparin sulphate proteoglycans (HSP) and tenascin] pave the proper path by supplying orientation and adhesiveness for axons. (II) *Neurotrophic factors* are the specific trophic agents that power peripheral nerve regeneration. They include (a) neurotrophins (NGF, BDNF, NT-4/5); (b) neurokines (CNTF, LIF); (c) (TGF)-β family (TGF-β1, TGF-β2, TGF-β3, GDNF). (III) *Schwann cells* secrete (a) cell adhesion molecules (CAMs), such as N-CAM, Ng-CAM/L1, N-cadherin, andL2/HNK-1; (b) basement membrane that contains many extracellular matrix proteins, such as laminin (LN), fibronectin (FN), heparin sulphate proteoglycans (HSP) and tenascin; (c) neurotrophic factors and their receptors. In addition to this, axonal regeneration is determined by trophic factors from activated perineural glial cells (astrocytes) (IV), trophic factors from efferents by anterograde transport (V), gene-induced trophic factors by intracrine (VI) or autocrine (VII) transport, trophic factors from retrograde target cell support (VIII), trophic factors from retroaxonal transport (IX), trophic factors from recruited macrophages (secretory products X, cytokines XI). Activated mesenchymal cells contribute to repair and vascularisation (XII). Among other molecules, heparin and aspirin modulate astrocytic function stimulating them to secrete axonal trophic factors (IV).

Based on the previous considerations, axonal sprouting and nerve grafting are based on a sixfold attack (**Figure 3**):

– lysing the fibrosis/gliosis in the injury zone to an extent that allows settling of the basal lamina preventing meanwhile collapse of the neural tissue matrix; or excision of the fibrotic segment and replacing it with nerve grafts;

– supplying the tissue matrix with a suitable scaffold, on which the basal lamina can settle,

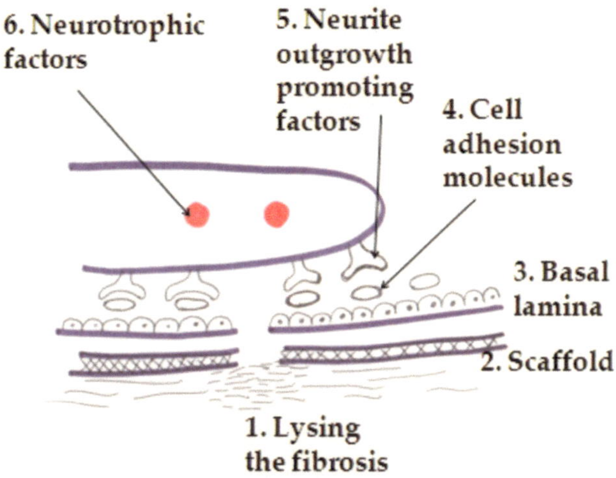

Figure 3. The sixfold attack: lysing the fibrosis/gliosis to an extent that allows settling of the basal lamina preventing meanwhile collapse of the neural tissue matrix; supplying the tissue matrix with a suitable scaffold, on which the basal lamina can settle; basal lamina synthesis; seeding the basal lamina with cell adhesion molecules; providing the axonal growth cone with neurite outgrowth promoting factors (FGF) that allow its distal progression; supplying the axonal growth cone with neurotrophic factors that allow its continued growth.

– basal lamina synthesis;

– seeding the basal lamina with cell adhesion molecules;

– providing the axonal growth cone with neurite outgrowth promoting factors that allow its distal progression;

– supplying the axonal growth cone with neurotrophic factors that power its continued growth.

2.3. Changing concepts of nerve grafting: side grafting

The previous conditions prevailing, if the side of a motor nerve is injured, the axonal growth cone may be enticed to grow off motor nerve side to the injured end of another motor nerve, the so-called recipient end to donor side coaptation. Described independently by Balance and Harris over a century ago (in 1903), interest in end-to-side coaptation has been rekindled by Viterbo et al. [17]. In its essence, it involves grafting donor side to recipient end after stimulating donor side collateral sprouting by mechanical trauma or axotomy (**Figure 4(a)**). An indirect application of it is increasing the incidence of nerve regeneration after conventional end-to-end grafting by applying additional grafts extending from the side of the donor end to the side of the recipient end [20] (**Figure 4(b)**). In nerve transfer, the latter technique allows the surgeon to use a single high axonal load donor for multiple recipients without producing cocontractions (e.g., major brachial plexus root to several peripheral nerves and caudal cord to cauda equina) [20] (**Figure 4(c)**). Also, partially regenerated nerves cannot be surgically cut and nerve grafted leading to loss of already regained function; the latter technique allows the surgeon to enhance regeneration through them (**Figure 4(d)**).

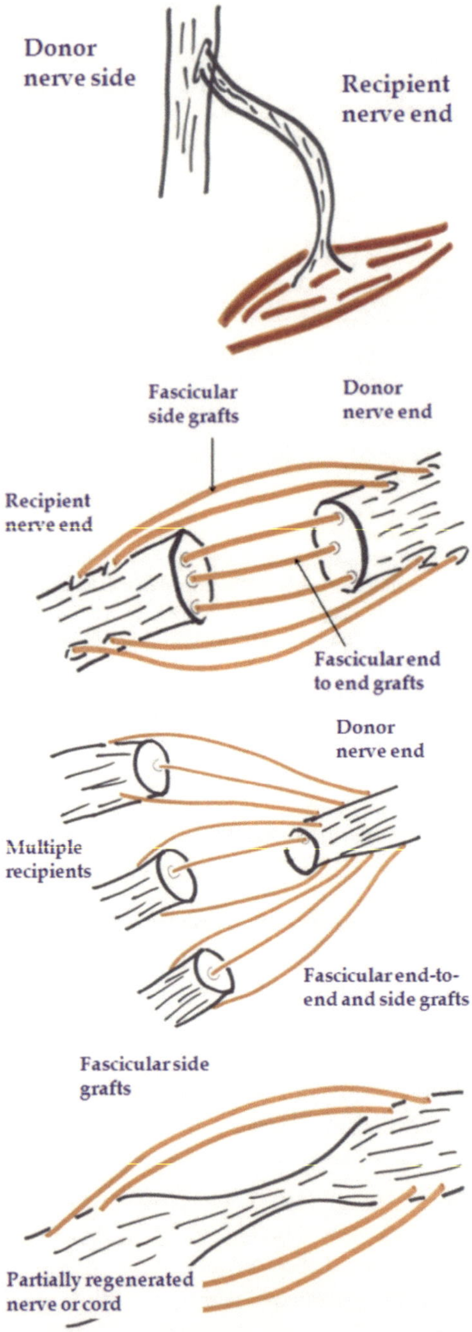

Figure 4. (a) End-to-side grafting involves grafting donor side to recipient end after stimulating donor side collateral sprouting by mechanical trauma or axotomy. (b) An indirect application of side grafting is increasing the incidence of nerve regeneration after conventional end-to-end grafting by applying additional grafts extending from the side of the donor end to the side of the recipient end. (c) Side grafting allows the surgeon to use a single high axonal load donor for multiple recipients without producing cocontractions. (d) Partially regenerated nerves cannot be surgically cut and nerve grafted sacrifying already regained function; side grafting allows the surgeon to enhance regeneration through them.

2.4. Mathematical modelling and channel-carrying capacity applied to nerve grafting: necessary concepts for subsequent computer-assisted fabrication of artificial nerve grafts

Can we manipulate the molecular mechanisms of the sixfold attack to increase neurite outgrowth into the side grafts? Manipulating molecular mechanisms is based on the sensitivity of the axonal growth cone to spatial molecular concentration gradients [21, 22]. In a study by Rosoff et al. [21], axonal growth has been shown to be enhanced by a steep nerve growth factor (NGF) spatial concentration gradient. There is a narrow range, however, between the lowest NGF concentration necessary for axonal growth stimulation and the highest NCF concentration beyond which axonal growth is competitively blocked. As the lower and upper limits of the concentration gradient should fall within this narrow range, the maximal distance for axonal growth cone progression guided by that gradient would be far less than the length of the neural defect. Utilising synthetic nerve graft scaffolds and observing the sixfold attack, axonal growth can be hypothetically made to bridge the whole length of the neural gap by seeding the scaffolds with multiple NGF spatial concentration gradients [22]. Neurite outgrowth has been modelled as a non-linear partial differential equation, that is solved by an iterative mathematical process suitable for numerical analysis and for subsequent computer-assisted fabrication of artificial nerve grafts [22]. By diffusion, these NGF spatial concentration gradients might also enhance axonal growth within the adjacent natural nerve side grafts.

Alternatively, and also to increase neurite outgrowth into the side grafts and decrease aberrant neural sprouting, multiple microspheres embedding chemical attractive and repulsive cues and placed along nerve side grafts may be used to guide axonal growth [23]. Preliminary experiments conducted with embryonic rat hippocampal neurons and calcium alginate microspheres have been encouraging [24]. A mathematical model has been developed based on the diffusion gradient of the implanted microspheres; a genetic algorithm has been used to study its proper spatial implementation [23].

A more accurate mathematical model for axonal growth cone progression has been provided based on sensory pinch test data [25]. Disadvantages of this model, however, include the assumptions that the initial delay is the major cause of variability, and that delay to scarring of the neural bed lies within the initial delay and that the regeneration rate is linear (constant).

Can we quantify the molecular mechanisms of the sixfold attack so that nearly 100% of all axons sprouting from the proximal spinal cord reach the distal spinal cord through the side grafts and simultaneously minimise the probability of aberrant neural sprouting to nearly 0%? Unless incorporated in information theory, which is a theory based on mathematical probability [26, 27], the mathematical models mentioned above do not provide a numerical solution for this problem. This is imperative, however, for subsequent computer-assisted fabrication of artificial nerve grafts. The Shannon-Hartley channel-carrying capacity principle, a central concept in information theory, refers to the intrinsic property of any information channel to accept all information from the donor and transmit it noiseless to the recipient. Applied to nerve grafting, the channel-carrying capacity of a nerve graft scaffold is its ability to transmit all axons sprouting from the proximal cord to the distal cord and simultaneously minimise the probability of aberrant neural sprouting.

3. Peripheral nerve grafting of the injured spinal cord as an application of the concept of side grafting and the sixfold attack

3.1. Technical aspects of peripheral nerve grafting and repair of the injured spinal cord

An indirect application of side grafting, as mentioned previously, is, first, increasing the incidence of nerve regeneration after conventional end-to-end grafting by applying additional grafts extending from the side of the donor end to the side of the recipient end; and, second, preserving partially regenerated nerves which cannot be surgically cut and nerve grafted leading to loss of already regained function [20]. Both of these apply to the spinal cord; compared to its high axonal load, the cross-sectional area of the spinal cord is too small for efficient end-to-end grafting. In addition, some kind of regeneration may have occurred in a contused cord in a completely paraplegic patient; this may take the form of less than Grade 3 motor power improvement, which, according to ASIA standards, is not enough to be considered motor or neurological level progression [28]. Third, side grafting produces less trauma to the spinal cord. In fact, the glial tissue secreted by astrocytes provides the necessary supporting tissue for axons and neurons [2, 29]. In side grafting, fine pial incisions are used. This process is far less traumatic than freshening of the cord ends during end-to-end grafting, a procedure which would lead to excessive glial tissue secretion and subsequent blocking of regeneration.

3.2. Donor nerves

Clinically, the sural nerve is the most commonly used donor nerve, other suitable donor nerves include the medial and lateral cutaneous nerves of the forearm, dorsal cutaneous branch of the ulnar nerve, superficial and deep peroneal nerves, intercostal nerves, and the posterior and lateral cutaneous nerves of the thigh [17].

Pre-degenerated (segments of nerve cut and left in situ for 7–10 days prior to harvesting) peripheral nerves are infiltrated by regenerating axons to a greater extent (both in number and distance) than freshly cut and harvested nerves [30]. The use of pre-degenerated nerves has been contested by other authors, however [31].

3.3. Experimental applications of side grafting

Based on the work of David and Aguayo [5, 7], numerous studies have confirmed axonal outgrowth after nerve grafting of the injured spinal cord [30, 32–38]; axons growing within peripheral nerve grafts have not only retained their physiological properties [39] but have synapsed with neurons near the point of central nervous system re-entry as well [40].

3.4. Re-evaluation of the use of peripheral nerve grafts to bridge spinal cord defects

Nerve grafts supply the injured spinal cord with five factors of the sixfold attack: a suitable scaffold, on which the basal lamina can settle; basal laminae; cell adhesion molecules; neurite outgrowth promoting factors; and neurotrophic factors. Nevertheless, the use of peripheral nerve grafts has been challenged [5, 16, 35, 41, 42]. According to experimental observation, damaged spinal cord axons might grow from the cranial cord into peripheral nerve grafts but would not leave them to enter the caudal cord [5]. Schwann cells might even promote gliosis [16, 41].

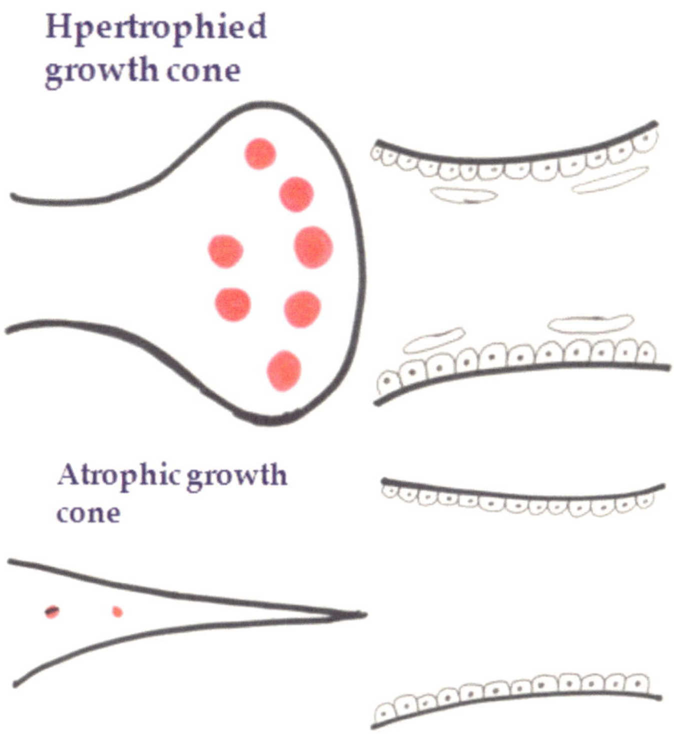

Figure 5. (a) Excessive fibrosis in the presence of neurotophic factors and adequate neuron growth potential leads to hypertrophy of both donor and recipient ends of the damaged neural tissue (excessive neuroma formation; dystrophic growth cones). (b) Excessive fibrosis in the absence of neurotophic factors and adequate neuron growth potential leads to atrophy of both donor and recipient ends of the damaged neural tissue (atrophic neuroma formation; atrophic growth cones).

It might be assumed that failure of growth cone progression is due to missing of the sixth factor in the sixfold attack (lysing the fibrosis/gliosis to an extent that allows settling of the basal lamina preventing meanwhile collapse of the neural tissue matrix). However, failure of axons to regenerate following peripheral nerve grafting may also result from intrinsic properties of the neurons and the absence of neurotrophic factors [43–46]. These considerations help us assess neural tissue during surgery. Excessive fibrosis in the presence of neurotophic factors and adequate neuron growth potential leads to hypertrophy of both donor and recipient ends of the damaged neural tissue (excessive neuroma formation and dystrophic growth cones) [47, 48] (**Figure 5(a)**), whereas excessive fibrosis in the absence of neurotophic factors and adequate neuron growth potential leads to atrophy of both donor and recipient ends of the damaged neural tissue (atrophic neuroma formation; atrophic growth cones) (**Figure 5(b)**). In conclusion, in addition to the sixfold attack, the intrinsic properties of the neurons should be stimulated to produce neurites.

4. Lysing the gliosis in conjunction with nerve grafting

4.1. The gliosis: blocking of regeneration mechanically and through the activation of RhoA

Injured axons encounter a series of inhibitory factors that are non-permissive for growth [4, 29, 41, 49]. These include myelin inhibitors (Nogo-A ,MAG108 (myelin-associated glycoprotein) and OMgp109 (oligodendrocyte myelin glycoprotein)); chondroitin sulphate proteoglycans (neurocan, versican, aggrecan, brevican, phosphacan and NG2); and semaphorins and ephrins. Upregulated in response to spinal cord injury [50–52], they act not only by mechanical blocking of neural regeneration but by inhibiting axon outgrowth neuronal receptors and subsequent activation of signalling pathways known to be involved in the activation of RhoA and the rise in intracellular calcium.

4.2. Lysing the gliosis by chondroitinase ABC

Chondroitinase ABC cleaves the inhibitory chondroitin sulphate glycosaminoglycan chains from the core protein, reducing the inhibition by chondroitin sulphate proteoglycans [53, 54]. Houle et al. [55] have demonstrated CNS axons regenerating through a peripheral nerve graft and entering the caudal spinal cord following chondroitinase ABC treatment.

4.2.1. Chondroitinase ABC in combination with growth factors and scaffolds

Combined with glial-derived neurotrophic factor (GDNF) delivery, chondroitinase ABC promotes axon extension through peripheral nerve bridges [50, 56]. Combined with growth factors, chondroitinase ABC enhances the activation and oligodendrocyte differentiation of endogenous precursor cells after spinal cord injury and attenuates astrogliosis. When added to polycaprolactone or poly (acrylonitrile)/poly(vinyl chloride) (PAN/PVC) scaffolds, chondroitinase ABC allows regenerating axons to exit the distal end of the scaffold and continue on to distal targets [57–60].

4.2.2. Chondroitinase ABC in combination with cell therapies

Chondroitinase ABC has improved recovery of function in synergy with mesenchymal stromal cells [D43], or a Schwann cell bridge and olfactory ensheathing cells or in combination with transplanted neural precursor cells and a growth factor (GF) cocktail containing EGF, FGF2 and platelet-derived growth factor (PDGF)-AA [61, 62].

4.2.3. Thermostabilisation, delivery, dosage and complications of chondroitinase ABC: chondroitinase ABC might be a weak enzyme

Thermostabilisation of chondroitinase ABC with the sugar trehalose can reduce its temperature-dependent loss of activity [50, 63]. Delivery of chondroitinase ABC is predominantly

http://dx.doi.org/10.5772/64211

intrathecal using osmotic minipumps [30, 55, 64]. Nevertheless, the enzyme can also be loaded into lipid microtubes or possibly poly (lactic-co-glycolic acid) (PLGA), providing a means for its gradual release over 1–2 weeks [65]. It can also be loaded into fibrin gel scaffolds before injecting it intrathecally; this ensures its continuous release for at least 3 weeks [66].

The effect of chondroitinase ABC is dose-dependent [67]. Injected intrathecally in acute injuries at a low dose (1 or 5 IUs), chondroitinase ABC may enhance axonal progression; injected at a high dose (50 IU), it may produce subarachnoid haemorrhage. In subacute or chronic injuries, low-dose injection produces no or limited functional recovery, whilst high-dose injection (50 or 100 IUs) produce lysis of the gliosis [68, 69].

Single-dose chondroitinase ABC is not considered enough. Therefore, multiple single injections at 0, 1, 2 and 4 weeks have been recommended [70]. Daily injections for 2 weeks at 0.06 Units per dose have also been recommended [71]. Four weeks of treatment have promoted recovery more than 2 weeks [72]. One way to ensure the continued release of chondroitinase ABC is neuron transfection with a vector containing the gene encoding chondroitinase ABC [73]. Another way is loading scaffolds with chondroitinase ABC.

Although chondroitinase ABC allows substantial structural plasticity in the spinal cord, it is not sufficient to enhance locomotor recovery unless combined with neural precursor cell transplantation and in vivo infusion of growth factors [74]. In a rat spinal cord injury model, Wilems et al. [62] have used fibrin scaffolds loaded with neurotrophic factors (item I), anti-inhibitory molecules (item II) and encapsulated embryonic stem-cell-derived progenitor motor neurons (pMNs) (item III). Fibrin scaffolds containing items I and II but not item III have had lower chondroitin sulphate proteoglycan levels compared to scaffolds containing items II and III. This shows the importance of combining neurotrophic factors with chondroitinase ABC and cellular transplants. Scaffolds containing item III, but not item II, have shown differentiation into neuronal cell types, axonal extension and the ability to integrate into host tissue. However, the combination of items II and III have led to reduced cell survival and increased macrophage infiltration. This shows that cellular transplants not only claim priority over chondroitinase ABC, but that chondroitinase ABC may be a weak enzyme as well. Because of this fact, a combination treatment of zymosan and chondroitinase ABC has been recommended [75]. Lastly, adipose-derived stem cell transplantation has been found to produce the same effect as chondroitinase ABC administration [76]. Thus, chondroitinase ABC might be a weak enzyme.

4.3. Sialidase as an alternative

In a rat model of spinal cord contusion injury the effects of sialidase (Vibrio cholerae) and chondroitinase ABC (ChABC, Proteus vulgaris) have been tested [77]. Immunohistochemistry has revealed that infused sialidase has acted robustly throughout the spinal cord grey and white matter, whereas ChABC activity has been more intense superficially. Sialidase treatment alone has resulted in improved behavioural and anatomical outcomes.

4.4. Anti-Nogo

Blocking myelin-associated inhibitors with Nogo-A monoclonal antibodies or with Nogo-receptor competitive agonist peptide, NEP1-40 has been shown to increase axonal regeneration [50]. Combination therapies, such as cross-linking the Nogo-66 receptor antibody into a hyaluronic acid hydrogel [50], a combination of methylprednisolone and NEP1-40 and Nogo-receptor vaccination combined with neural stem cell transplantation have improved neural fibre regeneration.

4.5. Rho inhibition

Many of the inhibitory signals described above (ephrins, Nogo) converge on the intracellular molecule Rho-A, which is a key mediator of actin depolymerisation and hence inhibition of axonal elongation. Blocking Rho-A with Rho inhibitor 'cethrin' might overcome its effect. A synthetic membrane-permeable peptide mimetic of the protein tyrosine phosphatase σ (PTPσ), wedge domain can bind to PTPσ and relieve chondroitin sulphate proteoglycan-mediated inhibition [78].

4.6. Reversing the inhibition of phosphoinositide 3-kinase (PI3K) by cell permeable phosphopeptide (PI3Kpep)

Phosphoinositide 3-kinase (PI3K) is a lipid kinase activated by axon growth promoting signals. Chondroitin sulphate proteoglycans inhibit phosphoinositide 3-kinase signalling in axons and growth cones, an effect that can be reversed by cell permeable phosphopeptide (PI3Kpep). The latter acts by R-Ras-PI3K signalling [79].

4.7. Rolipram

Increased intracellular levels of cyclic adenosine monophosphate (cAMP) and protein kinase A have been associated with CNS ability to overcome the gliosis [50]. Rolipram, a phosphodiesterase4 inhibitor, can increase intracellular cAMP levels [50].

4.8. Improving blood vessel formation

Improving blood vessel formation might reduce cell death and promote angiogenesis within the injury zone. Neural stem cells modified to express vascular endothelial growth factor have improved white matter sparing following thoracic contusion spinal cord injury [50]. Biomaterial poly-lactic-co-glycolic acid (PLGA) scaffolds loaded with neural stem cells and endothelial cells have shown increased vessel and neurofilament density at the injury centre [50].

5. Modulating astrocyte function enhances the intrinsic properties of neurons to stimulate neurite outgrowth into peripheral nerve grafts

In addition to the sixfold attack, the intrinsic properties of the neurons have to be stimulated to produce neurites. This can take place by modulating astrocyte function (**Figure 2**).

5.1. Endogenous inhibitors of axonal regeneration (intrinsic properties of neurons)

Endogenous inhibitors of axonal regeneration include the molecule phosphatase and tensin homologue (PTEN), loss of neuronal cAMP and deactivation/activation of certain transcription factors [46].

The molecule phosphatase and tensin homologue (PTEN) on chromosome 10 is a tumour suppressor. Its deletion has been shown to increase post-embryonic neural regeneration after injury. Its inhibition–mediated regeneration is partly mediated by the inhibitor of the mechanistic target of rapamycin (mTOR) pathway; it is also mediated by glycogen synthesis kinase GSK-3β.

When levels of cAMP at the growth cone are high, the effect on the growth cone is chemoattraction, whereas when they are low, the effect is chemorepulsion.

Certain transcription factors are positive regulators of axonal growth (e.g., members of the Krüppel-like factors (KLFs) present in retinal ganglion cells (RGCs); STAT3 a transcription factor, part of the JAK-STAT signaling pathway; members of the Jun and Fos families, components of the transcription factor AP-1 and ATF3). Other transcription factors are negative regulators of axonal growth. Nuclear factor IL-3 (NFIL3) represses CREB-mediated transcription and expression of regeneration-associated genes such as arginase and GAP-43.

It follows that combatting endogenous inhibitors of axonal regeneration include the following:

– Inactivation of GSK-3β by neurotrophins. This increases collapsin response mediator protein-2 (CRMP-2) stabilisation of microtubules and increases axon elongation in developing neurites.

– Local administration of taxol. Microtubules and actin microfilaments are critical for regeneration [80]. They potentiate the effect of GAP-43. Thus, local administration of taxol, a microtubule-stabilising agent, increases neurite outgrowth [81].

– Elevating cAMP levels by local injection of a phosphodiesterase inhibitor. This improves axonal regeneration.

– Conditioning lesions. Conditioning lesions [46] are based on the observation that double level nerve lesions regenerate better than single level nerve lesions. Thus sciatic nerve transection prior to a spinal cord lesion improves regeneration within the injured spinal cord.

– Cell adhesion molecules. Their synthesis is increased after peripheral nerve injury but not after CNS injury [82, 83]. Expression of cell adhesion molecules by neurons can be induced by virally mediated vectors or by injecting them into the CNS injury site [84, 85].

Many of these functions can be activated by modulating astrocyte function.

5.2. Astrocyte trophic effects on neurite outgrowth and neurogenesis

Astrocytes release a variety of trophic factors [86–88]. These trophic factors include nerve growth factor, basic fibroblast growth factor, transforming growth factor-β, platelet-derived growth factor, brain-derived neurotrophic factor, ciliary neurotrophic factor and others.

Reactive astrocytes increase the expression of several of these, notably nerve growth factor, basic fibroblast growth factor, brain-derived neurotrophic factor and neuregulins, which can stimulate neurite outgrowth. Reactive astrocytes also overexpress neuropilin-1 and vascular endothelial growth factor, which act in concert to promote angiogenesis after cerebral ischemia. Hevin (SPARC-like protein 1), a synaptogenic protein released by astrocytes, forms a relay between a neurexin (pre-synaptic) and a neuroligin (post-synaptic); this relay is crucial for the synaptogenesis [89].

5.3. Modulating the function of astrocytes and heparin

5.3.1. Role of heparin in lysing the gliosis

Both unfractionated and low molecular weight heparins inhibit thrombin activation [90]. In addition, they have a fibrolytic (gliolytic) effect and can modulate astrocyte function.

Clinically, perineural application of condensed polytetrafluoroethylene-extractum cepae-heparin-allantoin gel during peripheral nerve surgery improves functional recovery [91]. The anti-fibrotic effects of heparin are well documented after flexor tendon surgery of the hand [92], in the resolution of intraperitoneal fibrosis [93, 94] and in improving various scar types [95].

Among other actions, heparan sulphate/heparin influences fibroblast growth factor responsible for cell proliferation, differentiation, signal transduction and angiogenesis [96, 97]. Heparin is known to inhibit fibroblast growth factor (FGF)-2-stimulated DNA synthesis as well as gene expression of FGF-2 and its receptor in AT2 pneumocytes [98]. Probably via syndecan-1, the presence of heparin at high concentrations reduces the activity of FGF-7, which is responsible for enhancement of keratinocytes migration and proliferation. Heparin enhances the action of FGF-1, which regulates the proliferation of fibroblasts, endothelial and epithelial cells, and influences angiogenesis via effect on the activity of endothelial cells. Heparin can enhance the stability of FGF-1 and might determine the formation of FGF1-FGFR (fibroblast growth factor receptor) active complex.

5.3.2. Possible role of heparin in modulating astrocyte function

Astrocyte stress response and trophic effects are mediated by the FGF family member, on which heparin exerts a profound influence [96, 99]. Fibroblast growth factor 1 (FGF1) has been shown to maintain the survival of neurons and induce neurite outgrowth [100]. Basic fibroblast growth factor (FGF-2) has been found to increase neuronal survival and neurite extension in foetal rat hippocampal neurons when bound to heparin substrates [101]. The length and sulphated position of heparin regulate FGF-2-dependent astrocytic transformation (stellation), native heparin significantly promoting FGF-2-dependent astrocytic transformation, whereas heparin hexasaccharide and 2-O-, 6-O- and N-desulphated heparins inhibit it [102]. Heparin affin regulatory peptide (HARP, pleiotrophin, heparin-binding growth-associated molecule) promotes neurite outgrowth and synaptic development. High levels of heparin affin regulatory peptide HARP mRNA and protein are induced in transformed astrocytes [103, 104].

Glypican-1 is a major high-affinity ligand of the Slit proteins, both of which are strongly upregulated in reactive astrocytes, suggesting their possible role in the inhibitory environment preventing axonal regeneration after injury. Heparins inhibit glypican-Slit interactions [105, 106].

5.4. Possible role of aspirin in modulating astrocyte function

Ciliary neurotrophic factor (CNTF) is a promyelinating trophic factor. Acetylsalicylic acid (aspirin) increases mRNA and protein expression of CNTF in primary mouse and human astrocytes in a dose- and time-dependent manner. Aspirin-induced astroglial CNTF is also functionally active; supernatants of aspirin-treated astrocytes of wild type, but not Cntf null, mice increase myelin-associated proteins in oligodendrocytes and protected oligodendrocytes from TNF-α insult [107].

5.5. Possible role of hyaluronic acid salts in modulating astrocyte function

The presence of high molecular weight hyaluronic acid (hyaluronic acid with limited degradation) after spinal cord injury decreases glial scarring. High molecular weight hyaluronic acid stabilised against degradation mitigates astrocyte activation in vitro and in vivo. Therefore, hyaluronic-acid-based hydrogel systems hold great potential for minimising undesired scarring as part of future repair strategies after spinal cord injury [108].

6. Combining peripheral nerve grafts with scaffolds: the scaffold as a drug release system

The defect within the spinal cord is too large to be bridged by nerve grafts alone; besides, the myelin sheath within them is inhibitory to axonal growth. The rationale for polymer implants is twofold, to replace a damaged area of the cord with just such a structural matrix [109] and to provide it with a synthetic scaffold, in which myelin is absent. Combining peripheral nerve grafts with scaffolds has gained more acceptance because of the importance of seeding the scaffolds with multiple nerve growth factor (NGF) spatial concentration gradients in order to promote axonal growth both within the scaffolds and the nerve grafts [22].

Biomaterial scaffolds in spinal cord injury have been reviewed by Madigan et al. [109] and Straley et al. [110]. Commonly used scaffolds include natural polymers (in vivo extracellular matrix polymers, polymers derived from blood, and polymers from marine life) and synthetic polymers (poly-hydroxy acid polymers and synthetic hydrogels). Examples for in vivo extracellular matrix polymers are collagen solutions and the glycosaminoglycan hyaluronic acid. Examples for polymers derived from blood are plasma-derived polymers, fibronectin and fibrin. Examples for polymers from marine life are agarose, alginate and chitosan. Synthetic polymers include poly-hydroxy acid polymers and synthetic hydrogels. Compared to natural polymers, they offer wider scope to design and control the characteristics of the material. Poly-hydroxy acid polymers are biodegradable materials based on polyesters of lactic and glycolic acid (PLA and PGA) and their co-polymer PLGA. Synthetic hydrogels are based on polyethylene glycol, a biodegradable synthetic polymer of ethylene oxide units. Poly(2-hydroxyethyl methacrylate) (pHEMA) compounds and pHEMA-co-methyl methacrylate (pHEMA-MMA) are used as spinal cord scaffolds.

Whatever macroengineering and microengineering procedures scaffolds are subjected to allow for axonal growth, this will not occur unless the scaffold is seeded with basal lamina and supplied with neurite outgrowth promoting factors and neurotrophic factors (**Figure 3**). These factors can be released from the scaffold material itself, from integrated micro- or nano-spheres or tubules of a different material, or by means of a scaffold's capacity to support a genetically modified cell line in vivo [58, 109, 110].

7. Augmentation of peripheral nerve grafts with cellular transplants

Nearly half of the spinal cord injuries occur at the thoracolumbar junction (D12-L1), the site of the conus medullaris. We could potentially nerve graft the spinal cord (part of the CNS) directly to the cauda equina (part of the peripheral nervous system) without resorting to cellular transplants to restitute the neuronal and astrocytic components of the CNS. There is mounting evidence, however, that cellular transplants potentiate the effect of other factors and might even recruit endogenous neural precursor cells [62, 76].

7.1. Types of cellular transplants used to augment peripheral nerve grafts

In a meta-analysis reviewing cellular transplantation strategies in spinal cord injury, Tetzlaff et al. [111], have come to the following conclusions. Schwann cells are the most extensively studied cell type. They are reported both to remyelinate-injured spinal cord axons and to form a permissive substrate for their regeneration [112]. However, compared to neural precursors such as oligodendrocyte precursors or neural precursor/stem cells, they provoke a more robust astrocytic reaction, resulting in less effective integration into the host spinal cord [113]. Olfactory ensheathing cells demonstrate good integration into host spinal cord [114]. However, there is no robust evidence of improvement after their transplantation [115]. They also appear to require adjuvant treatment to increase efficacy (e.g., Schwann cells, Matrigel, rolipram, cAMP and neurotrophic factors) [116,117]. Neural stem/progenitor cells appear to integrate well into the host spinal cord with improved outcomes [118]. They differentiate mostly into astroglial cells, less so oligodendrocytes seen but rarely into neurons [119]. Suspicion has been raised as to their role in axonal regeneration [120, 121]. Fate-restricted neural and glial precursor have the potential to remyelinate injured axons [122]. More evidence is needed, however, to confirm this observation [123]. Bone marrow stromal cells have some bridging capacity in sharp transaction models [124]. However, their integration in the injured spinal cord is very limited. There is no convincing differentiation into neural cells despite claims to the contrary [125]. They are reported to stimulate neurite outgrowth over neural proteoglycans, myelin-associated glycoprotein and Nogo-A [126, 127].

7.2. Cellular transplants in combination strategy

Because of the previous controversies, the use of a combination strategy including Schwann cells has been recommended by Bunge [128]. The following combination strategy has been suggested [128]: Schwann cells, neuroprotective agents and growth factors administered in various ways, such as, olfactory ensheathing cell (OEC) implantation, chondroitinase addition or elevation of cyclic AMP. A targeted approach has been proposed by Kadoya et al. [43]. It includes the following: a peripheral conditioning lesion (bilateral sciatic nerve crush), mesenchymal stem cell transplantation mixed with neurotrophin-3 (NT-3) and creating a neurotrophic factor gradient by injection of lentivirus expressing neurotrophin-3 (NT-3) just proximal to the site of the lesion.

7.3. Number of cellular transplant injections

A third unresolved issue is the number of injections that the patient has to receive. Mackay-Sim et al. [129] have used a single intraoperative injection. Multiple injections have been recorded by other authors [130, 131].

7.4. Inducing mobilisation of neural precursor cells

Stem cell transplantation has the potential to recruit endogenous neural stem cells [132]. Neural stem cells exist in the mammalian developing and adult nervous system (mainly in the hippocamous and subventricular area). Multiple cell-intrinsic regulators coordinate neural stem cell maintenance, self-renewal and migration into injured areas. Essential intracellular regulators include the orphan nuclear receptor TLX, the high-mobility-group DNA binding protein Sox2, the basic helix-loop-helix transcription factor Hes, the tumour suppressor gene Pten, the membrane-associated protein Numb and its cytoplasmic homolog Numblike. Manipulating these factors among others [133–135] by injecting them through indwelling catheters might induce mobilisation of neural stem cells to the injured spinal cord area.

8. Clinical application

8.1. Pre-operative assessment (neurological and radiographic evaluation)

Patients should be evaluated pre-operatively and at monthly intervals. Motor power and sensation should be evaluated using ASIA standards [28]. Confounding factors during motor power evaluation include fake muscle contractions produced by movements of the trunk and cocontractions between abdominal muscles and different muscle groups. Optional elements of ASIA neurologic impairment assessment should be included because the abdominal muscles and medial hamstrings are the first muscles to regain power.

Radiographic evaluation should include plain anteroposterior and lateral radiographs and pre-operative magnetic resonance imaging (MRI). The injury zone on the MRI is determined by the superior and inferior extents of the gliosis; nerve grafts have to be extended beyond the injury zone [136] (**Figure 6**).

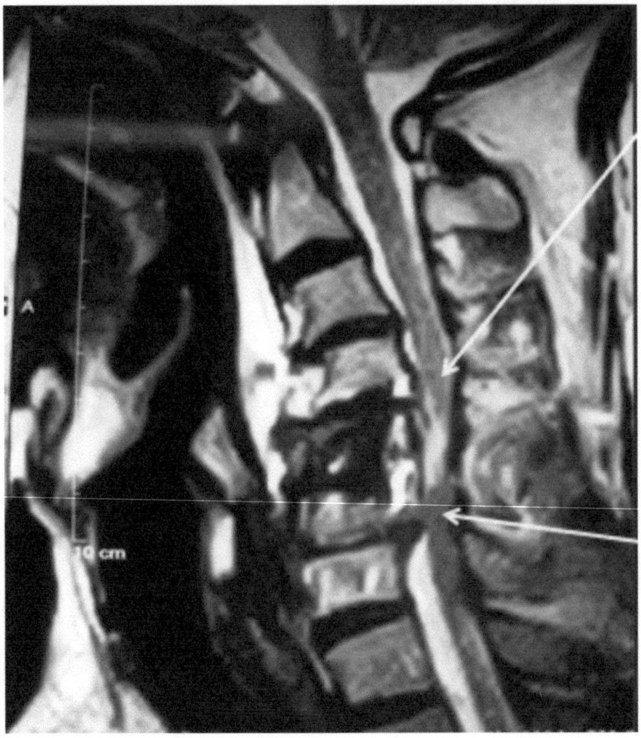

Figure 6. Cervical vertebral C5,6 fracture dislocation in a quadriplegic patient; the gliosis extends from the inferior border of cervical vertebra C4 to the superior border of cervical vertebra C6. The injury zone on the MRI is determined by the superior and inferior extents of the gliosis; nerve grafts have to be extended beyond the injury zone.

8.2. Timing of grafting

Spinal cord injury is considered chronic months to years after injury [6]. At this stage, the primary and secondary injuries have ceased. As the zone of gliosis may extend superiorly or inferiorly during the secondary injury phase, the patient should be operated upon at least 2 months after the injury, i.e., when it has become chronic.

Improvement is also independent of the time delay between the date of injury and the date of definitive surgery. This is supported by the observations made by Li and Raisman [137], who have noted that sprouts from cut corticospinal axons persist despite the presence of astrocytic scarring in long-term lesions of the adult rat spinal cord.

8.3. Operative technique, establishment of CSF circulation and establishment of a continuous drug delivery system (indwelling catheter implantation for post-operative drug and cell administration)

After exploring the injured cord through a posterior spinal laminectomy incision, sural nerves are side-grafted to the cord, especially on its ventral aspect [20, 138] (**Figures 7(a** and **b)** and **8)**. The cord graft construct invariably adheres to the dura preventing CSF circulation. The

http://dx.doi.org/10.5772/64211

latter is important for nutrient, cell and growth factor transport [139, 140]. To prevent the cord adhering to the dura, it has become the author's practice to wrap the cord graft construct with a silicone membrane (**Figure 9**). In fact, silicone chambers or tubes have been used as scaffolds for peripheral nerve regeneration [141–143]. Interest to use them as scaffolds for cellular growth has been rekindled [144, 145]. They have been modified physically to increase porosity or coated to allow for growth of mesenchymal stem cells [146–148] or even to allow neuron-like differentiation of mesenchymal stem cells [149]. They have been modified physically to increase porosity or chemically (with hyaluronic acid and hyaluronic acid--collagen conjugate) to allow for growth of neural cells [150, 151] or to inhibit glial tissue formation [152, 153]. To establish a continuous drug and cell delivery system, an indwelling percutaneous catheter is placed in the interstitium between the membrane and the dura; the dura is finally closed (**Figure 9**). **Figure 10** is a schematic drawing of the hypothetical spinal cord-graft-scaffold-catheter construct.

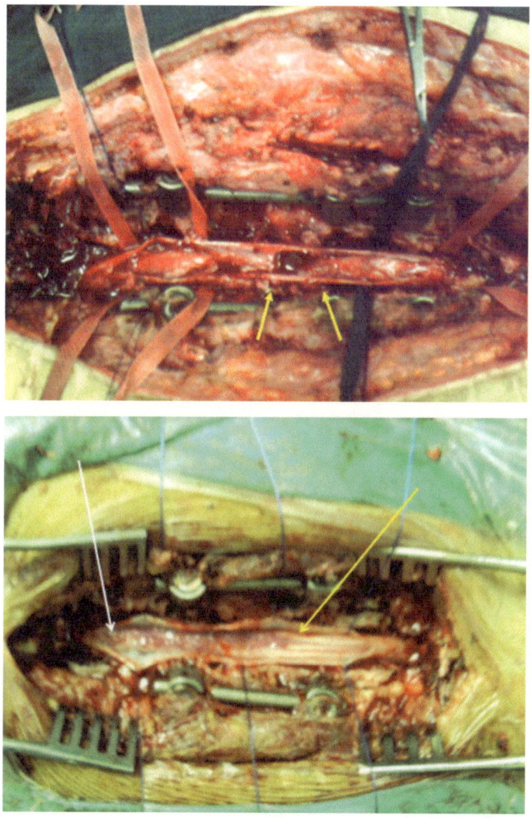

Figure 7. (a) Through a midline dorsal incision, a formal laminectomy is performed preserving the facet joints and pedicles. The dura is exposed. The dura is incised longitudinally and held with stay sutures exposing the cord lesion. The yellow arrows points to the defect in the cord. (b) Spinal cord lesion without defect but with a completely gliotic segment in a paraplegic patient suffering from a dorsolumbar fracture dislocation. The gliotic segment extends from the cord (white arrow) up to the cauda equine (yellow arrow).

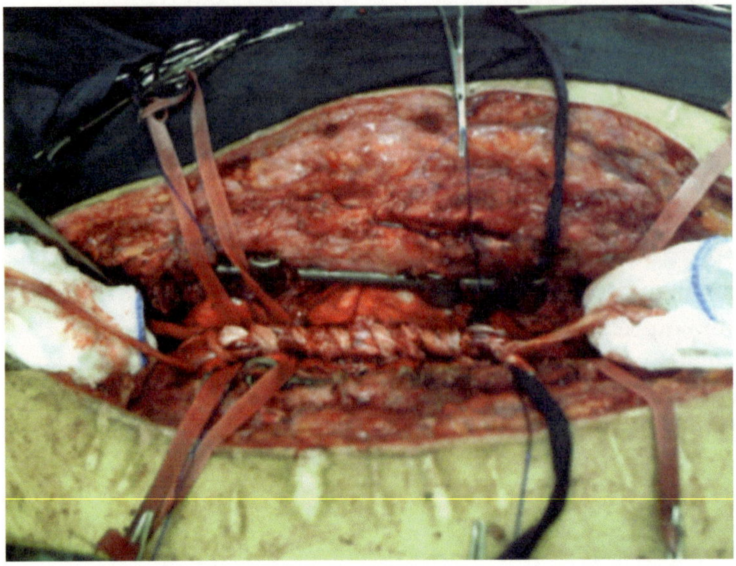

Figure 8. Sural nerve grafts having been side-grafted to the cord.

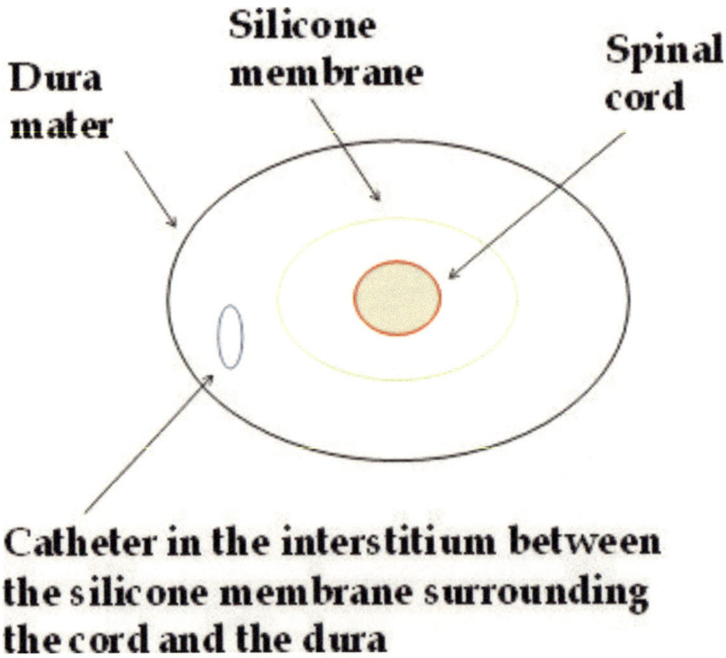

Figure 9. To prevent the cord adhering to the dura, it has become the author's practice to wrap the cord graft construct with a silicone membrane. To establish a continuous drug and cell delivery system, an indwelling catheter is placed in the interstitium between the membrane and the dura; the dura is finally closed.

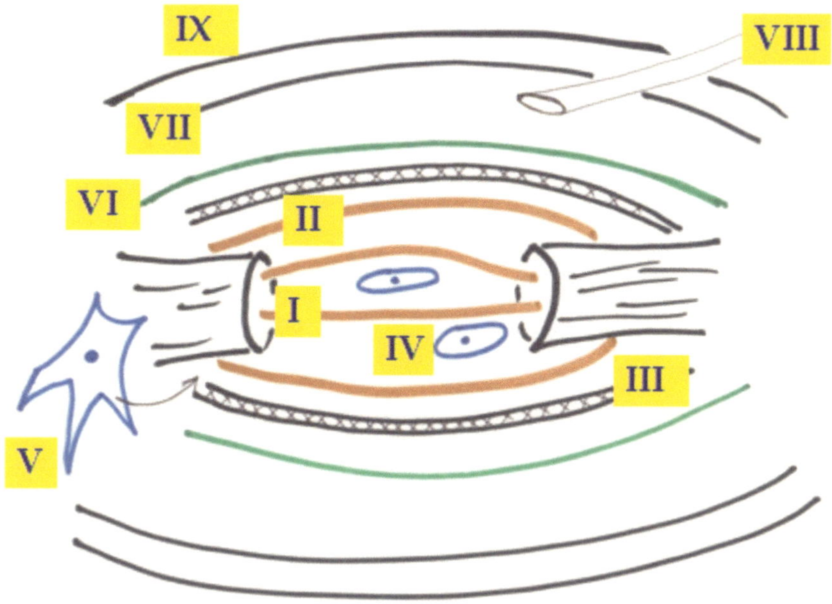

Figure 10. A schematic drawing of the hypothetical spinal cord-graft-scaffold-catheter construct: (I) end-to-end grafts; (II) side grafts; (III) synthetic scaffolds; (IV) cellular transplants; (V) modulated astrocytes; (VI) silicone membrane; (VII) dura mater; (VIII) indwelling catheter for post-operative delivery of neurolyzing agents (chondroitinase ABC, heparin), neurotrophic factors, neurite outgrowth promoting factors, injectable scaffolds and cellular transplants; (IX) skin.

8.4. Post-operative drug and cellular transplant administration through the catheter

The catheter can be used for post-operative administration of growth factors, neurolyzing agents, cellular transplants or even scaffolds. The author's practice has been as follows. Starting from the fifth post-operative day calcium heparin (5000 IU) is injected every second day through the catheter. Chondroitinase ABC (5 IU, Sigma) is dissolved in 2 cc normal saline and injected on a weekly basis.

8.5. Catheter-related complications: keeping the indwelling catheter for 18 months or more around the spinal cord as a means of establishing a continuous spinal drug delivery system

Catheter-related complications include tension headache, meningitis, fibrous track formation, catheter slippage, difficult catheter insertion and catheter blockage. Fibrous track formation is noted by increased pressure on injection through the catheter, associated with increased serosanguinous discharge from the catheter skin exit site due to drug extrusion. Tension headache can be avoided by decreasing the volume of injection; meningitis and early catheter blockage and slippage are avoided by proper catheter care. Complications associated with fibrous track formation, such as difficult catheter insertion, late catheter blockage and slippage (during months 9–18) can only be avoided by inserting the catheter in the interstitium between the silicone membrane and the dura. In this way, the catheter need not be exchanged over 18 months.

8.6. Author's clinical experience with heparin and chondroitinase ABC: its clinical safety and limitations

Delayed wound healing and sinus formation is related to repeated calheparin injection. Its incidence decreases when calheparin is administered every other day.

A vasovagal reaction occurs, when chondroitinase ABC is rapidly injected intrathecally. Its manifestations are cough, hypotension, general irritability and spinal cord irritability manifested by lower limb twitches. A vasovagal reaction does not occur, when the enzyme is injected extradurally or slowly intrathecally.

8.7. Results of surgery

In a clinical study [14], the right and left antero-lateral quadrant of the cord at T7-8 levels have been nerve grafted to homolateral L2-4 lumbar ventral roots. Eight months after surgery, voluntary contractions of bilateral adductors and of the left quadriceps have been observed.

Similar improvements have been observed in another study [15] after nerve side-grafting and augmentation by single-stage mesenchymal cell transplantation. Improvement has been hampered by cocontractions between abdominal muscles and different muscle groups. It has also been hampered by spasticity

In a not yet published study, the author has observed that repeated heparin, chondroitinase ABC and cellular transplant injection through an indwelling catheter placed in the interstitium between the membrane and the dura has led to the disappearance of cocontractions between abdominal muscles and different muscle groups. All patients have had pre-operative bouts of a moderate dull aching pain in the abdomen, back and both legs caused by adherence of the cord to the dura and the bony spinal canal. It has been completely resolved by inserting the silicone barrier membrane in the interstitium between the spinal cord and the dura.

Studies using cellular transplantation alone in spinal cord injuries have reported similar motor and sensory score improvement [154–157]. In all these studies, spontaneous or treatment-induced anatomical neural plasticity as well as the adaptive reorganisation of the neural pathways occurring after injury and acting to restore some of the lost function have to be taken into consideration [4].

8.8. False positive results

On evaluating results of surgery after grafting the cord to the cauda equina in thoracolumbar lesions, it should be noted that false positive results could be obtained from intercostal nerves (peripheral nerves) regenerating into the cauda equina (peripheral nerves) via nerve grafts (**Figure 11**).

http://dx.doi.org/10.5772/64211

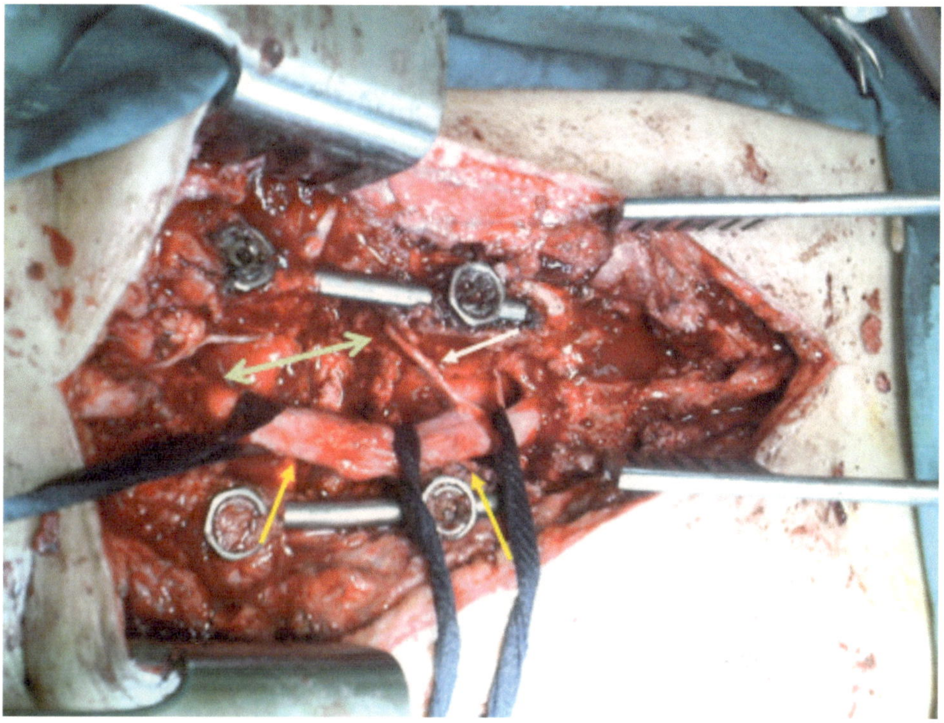

Figure 11. In thoracolumbar lesions, false positive results could be obtained from intercostal nerves (peripheral nerves) at the cranial cord (white arrow) regenerating into to the caua equina (peripheral nerves) (yellow arrow) via nerve grafts.

9. Post-operative target organ derived trophic support

Target organ derived neurotrophic factors, the so-called neurotrophins (nerve growth factor(NGF), brain-derived neurotrophic factor (BDNF), neurotrophin-3(NT-3) and neurotrophin-4/5(NT-4/5)), are transported by retrograde axonal via an endosomal mechanism involving dyneins [158, 159]. Neurotrophins contribute a lot to axonal progression; in the injured spinal cord, this stimulus is lost. After grafting the spinal cord, an important question is whether this stimulus can be restituted by injecting neurotrophins into target organs postoperatively, or whether axonal progression into specific nerves can be restituted by injecting neurotrophins into the specific muscles supplied by them. Experimental evidence points to this [158, 159]. By the same token, it can be questioned whether other neurotrophic factors and neurolyzing agents can be similarly injected into target muscles. Both in vitro and in vivo local infusion of fibroblastic growth factors (FGFs) have been found to rescue motoneuron death induced by spinal cord injury [160]. However, evidence for retrograde axonal transport of heparin-binding growth factors is lacking [161].

10. Conclusions

We have outlined current experimental and clinical experience applying nerve side grafts to the injured spinal cord. Nerve side grafting increases the incidence of nerve regeneration by applying additional grafts extending from the side of the donor end of the cord to the side of the recipient end. A partially regenerated cord cannot be surgically cut and end grafted; nerve side grafting can enhance regeneration through it without incriminating already regained function. Nevertheless, side grafting will fail, unless the gliosis is counteracted or lysed by chondroitinase ABC, sialidase, anti-Nogo, Rho inhibitors and other factors. Side grafting will also fail unless neurons are stimulated to produce neurites. Modulating the function of astrocytes by heparin, aspirin and other factors is one method to stimulate the intrinsic properties of the neurons to produce neurites. Side grafting should be augmented by artificial scaffolds and cellular transplants. Clinically, to prevent the cord adhering to the dura and re-establish CSF circulation, it has become the author's practice to wrap the cord graft construct with a silicone membrane. To establish a continuous drug and cell delivery system, an indwelling catheter is placed in the interstitium between the membrane and the dura; the dura is finally closed. Post-operative injection of paralysed muscles with neurotrophic factors stimulates neurite outgrowth by target-organ-derived neurotrophic support.

Author details

Sherif M. Amr*

Address all correspondence to: sherifamrh@hotmail.com

The Department of Orthopaedics and Traumatology, Cairo University, Cairo, Egypt

References

[1] DeFelipe J, Jones EG: Cajal's degeneration and regeneration of the nervous system (May RM, translator). New York: Oxford University Press, 1991.

[2] Raisman G: A promising therapeutic approach to spinal cord repair. J R Soc Med 2003;96(6):259–261.

[3] Samadikuchaksaraei A: An overview of tissue engineering approaches for management of spinal cord injuries. J Neuroeng Rehabil 2007;4:15.

[4] Bradbury EJ, McMahon SB. Spinal cord repair strategies: why do they work? Nat Rev Neurosci 2006;7:644–653.

[5] Reier PJ: Cellular transplantation strategies for spinal cord injury and translational neurobiology. Neurorx 2004 October;1(4):424–451.

[6] Hyun JK, Kim HW. Clinical and experimental advances in regeneration of spinal cord injury. J Tissue Eng. 2010 Nov 2; Vol. 2010 : 1–20: Article ID 650857. doi: 10.4061/2010/650857. PubMed PMID: 21350645; PubMed Central PMCID: PMC3042682.

[7] David S, Aguayo AJ: Axonal elongation into peripheral nervous system 'bridges' after central nervous system injury in adult rats. Science 1981;214:931–933.

[8] Tuszynski MH, Petersen DA, Ray J, Baird A, Nakahara Y, Gage FH: Fibroblasts genetically modified to produce nerve growth factor induce robust neuritic ingrowth after grafting to the spinal cord. Exp Neurol 1994;126:1–14.

[9] Guenard V, Aebischer P, Bunge RP: The astrocyte inhibition of peripheral nerve regeneration is reversed by Schwann cells. Exp Neurol 1994;126:44–60.

[10] Oudega M, Varon S, Hagg T: Regeneration of adult rat sensory axons into intraspinal nerve grafts: promoting effects of conditioning lesion and graft predegeneration. Exp Neurol 1994;129:194–206.

[11] Liu S, Kadi K, Boisset N, Lacroix C, Said G, Tadie M: Reinnervation of denervated lumbar ventral roots and their target muscle by thoracic spinal motoneurons via an implanted nerve autograft in adult rats after spinal cord injury. J Neurosci Res 1999 Jun 1;56(5):506–517.

[12] Liu S, Aghakhani N, Boisset N, Said G, Tadie M: Innervation of the caudal denervated ventral roots and their target muscles by the rostral spinal motoneurons after implanting a nerve autograft in spinal cord-injured adult marmosets. J Neurosurg 2001 Jan; 94(1 Suppl):82–90.

[13] Dam-Hieu P, Liu S, Choudhri T, Said G, Tadie M: Regeneration of primary sensory axons into the adult rat spinal cord via a peripheral nerve graft bridging the lumbar dorsal roots to the dorsal column. J Neurosci Res 2002 May 1;68(3):293–304.

[14] Tadie M, Liu S, Robert R, Guiheneuc P, Pereon Y, Perrouin-Verbe B, Mathe JF: Partial return of motor function in paralyzed legs after surgical bypass of the lesion site by nerve autografts three years after spinal cord injury. J Neurotrauma 2002 Aug;19(8): 909–916.

[15] Amr SM, Gouda A, Koptan WT, Galal AA, Abdel-Fattah DS, Rashed LA, Atta HM, Abdel-Aziz MT: Bridging defects in chronic spinal cord injury using peripheral nerve grafts combined with a chitosan-laminin scaffold and enhancing regeneration through them by cotransplantation with bone-marrow derived mesenchymal stem cells; a series of 14 patients. J Spinal Cord Medicine 2014;37(1):54–71

[16] Fawcett JW: Bridging spinal cord injuries. J Biol 2008;7:25.

[17] Ray WZ: Mackinnon SE. Management of nerve gaps: autografts, allografts, nerve transfers, and end-to-side neurorrhaphy. Exp Neurol 2010 May ;223(1):77–85. doi: 10.1016/j.expneurol.2009.03.031.

[18] Frostick SP, Yin Q, Kemp G: Schwann cells, neurotrophic factors, and peripheral nerve regeneration. Microsurgery 1998;18:397–405.

[19] Blottner D, Baumgarten HG: Neurotrophy and regeneration in vivo. Acta Anat 1994;150:235–245.

[20] Amr SM, Moharram AN: Repair of brachial plexus lesions by end-to-side side-to-side grafting neurorrhaphy: experience based on 11 cases. Microsurgery 2005, 25(2):126–146.

[21] Rosoff WJ, Urbach JS, Esrick MA, McAllister RG, Richards LJ, Goodhill GJ. A new chemotaxis assay shows the extreme sensitivity of axons to molecular gradients. Nat Neurosci 2004;7(6):678–682. Epub 2004 May 25. Erratum in: Nat Neurosci. 2004;7(7): 785.

[22] Tse TH, Chan BP, Chan CM, Lam J: Mathematical modeling of guided neurite extension in an engineered conduit with multiple concentration gradients of nerve growth factor (NGF). Ann Biomed Eng 2007;35(9):1561–1572. Epub 2007 May 23.

[23] Ciofani G, Sergi PN, Carpaneto J, Micera S. A hybrid approach for the control of axonal outgrowth: preliminary simulation results. Med Biol Eng Comput 2011;49(2):163–170. doi: 10.1007/s11517-010-0687-x. Epub 2010 Oct 6. PubMed PMID: 20924708.

[24] Ciofani G, Raffa V, Menciassi A, Micera S, Dario P: A drug delivery system based on alginate microspheres: mass-transport test and in vitro validation. Biomed Microdevices 2007;9:395–403.

[25] Holmquist B, Kanje M, Kerns JM, Danielsen N. A mathematical model for regeneration rate and initial delay following surgical repair of peripheral nerves. J Neurosci Methods. 1993 Jun;Vol.48(1–2):27–33. PubMed PMID: 8377520.

[26] Cover TM, Thomas JA: Elements of Information Theory, 2nd ed. Hoboken, New Jersey: John Wiley & Sons, Inc., 2006.

[27] Effenberger F. A Primer on Information Theory, with Applications to Neuroscience. In: Rakocevic G., Djukic T., Filipovic N., Milutinović V. (editors) Computational Medicine in Data Mining and Modeling. New York: Springer 2013.

[28] Standards for Neurological Classification of Spinal Injury. American Spinal Injury Association (ASIA) Illinois: Chicago, 1996.

[29] Harel NY, Strittmatter SM: Can regenerating axons recapitulate developmental guidance during recovery from spinal cord injury? Nat Rev Neurosci 2006;7:603–616.

[30] Côté MP, Amin AA, Tom VJ, Houle JD: Peripheral nerve grafts support regeneration after spinal cord injury. Neurotherapeutics 2011;8(2):294–303.

[31] Hill CE, Brodak DM, Bartlett Bunge M: Dissociated predegenerated peripheralnerve transplants for spinal cord injury repair: a comprehensive assessment of their effects on regeneration and functional recovery compared to Schwann cell transplants. J Neurotrauma 2012;29(12):2226–2243. doi: 10.1089/neu.2012.2377. PubMed PMID: 22655857; PubMed Central PMCID: PMC3472680.

[32] Bray GM, Villegas-Perez MP, Vidal-Sanz M, Aguayo AJ: The use of peripheral nerve grafts to enhance neuronal survival, promote growth and permit terminal reconnections in the central nervous system of adult rats. J Exp Biol 1987;132:5–19.

[33] Bunge MB: Bridging areas of injury in the spinal cord. Neuroscientist 2001;7:325–339.

[34] Guzen FP, de Almeida Leme RJ, de Andrade MS, de Luca BA, Chadi G: Glial cell line-derived neurotrophic factor added to a sciatic nerve fragment grafted in a spinal cord gap ameliorates motor impairments in rats and increases local axonal growth. Restor Neurol Neurosci 2009;27(1):1–16.

[35] Cheng H, Cao Y, Olson L: Spinal cord repair in adult paraplegic rats partial restoration of hind limb function. Science 1996;273:510–513.

[36] Lee YS, Hsiao I, Lin VW: Peripheral nerve grafts and aFGF restore partial hindlimb function in adult paraplegic rats. J Neurotrauma 2002;19:1203–1216.

[37] Campos L, Meng Z, Hu G, Chiu DT, Ambron RT, Martin JH: Engineering novel spinal circuits to promote recovery after spinal injury. J Neurosci 2004;24:2090–2101.

[38] Gauthier P, Rega P, Lammari-Barreault N, Polentes J: Functional reconnections established by central respiratory neurons regenerating axons into a nerve graft bridging the respiratory centers to the cervical spinal cord. J Neurosci Res 2002;70:65–81.

[39] Decherchi P, Lammari-Barreault N, Gauthier P: Regeneration of respiratory pathways within spinal peripheral nerve grafts. Exp Neurol 1996;137:1–14.

[40] Aguayo AJ, Bray GM, Rasminsky MM, Zwimpfer T, Carter D, Vidal-Sanz M: Synaptic connections made by axons regenerating in the central nervous system of adult mammals. J Exp Biol 1990;153:199–224.

[41] Plant GW, Bates ML, Bunge MB: Inhibitory proteoglycan immunoreactivity is higher at the caudal than the rostral Schwann cell graft-transected spinal cord interface. Mol Cell Neurosci 2001;17:471–487.

[42] Thuret S, Moon LDF, Gage FH: Therapeutic interventions after spinal cord injury. Nat Rev Neurosci 2006;7:628–643.

[43] Kadoya K, Tsukada S, Lu P, Coppola G, Geschwind D, Filbin MT, Blesch A,Tuszynski MH: Combined intrinsic and extrinsic neuronal mechanisms facilitate bridging axonal regeneration one year after spinal cord injury. Neuron. 2009;64(2):165–172. doi: 10.1016/j.neuron.2009.09.016. PubMed PMID: 19874785; PubMedCentral PMCID: PMC2773653.

[44] Neumann S, Bradke F, Tessier-Lavigne M, Basbaum AI: Regeneration of sensory axons within the injured spinal cord induced by intraganglionic cAMP elevation. Neuron. 2002;34:885–893 [PubMed].

[45] Qiu J, Cai D, Dai H, McAtee M, Hoffman PN, Bregman BS, Filbin MT: Spinal axon regeneration induced by elevation of cyclic AMP. Neuron 2002;34:895–903 [PubMed].

[46] Ferguson TA, Son YJ: Extrinsic and intrinsic determinants of nerve regeneration. J Tissue Eng 2011;2(1):2041731411418392. doi: 10.1177/2041731411418392. Epub 2011 Sep 13. PubMed PMID: 22292105; PubMed Central PMCID: PMC3251917.

[47] Tom VJ, Steinmetz MP, Miller JH, Doller CM, Silver J: Studies on the development and behavior of the dystrophic growth cone, the hallmark of regeneration failure, in an in vitro model of the glial scar and after spinal cord injury. J Neurosci 2004;24(29):6531–6539. PubMed PMID: 15269264.

[48] Blits B, Carlstedt TP, Ruitenberg MJ, de Winter F, Hermens WT, Dijkhuizen PA, Claasens JW, Eggers R, Sluis R van der, Tenenbaum L, Boer GJ, Verhaagen J: Rescue and sprouting of motoneurons following ventral root avulsion and reimplantation combined with intraspinal adeno-associated viral vector-mediated expression of glial cell line-derived neurotrophic factor or brain-derived neurotrophic factor. Exp Neurol 2004;189(2):303–316.

[49] Yiu G, He Z: Glial inhibition of CNS axon regeneration. Nat Rev Neurosci 2006;7:617–627.

[50] McCreedy DA, Sakiyama-Elbert SE: Combination therapies in the CNS: engineering the environment. Neurosci Lett 2012;519(2):115–121. doi: 10.1016/j.neulet.2012.02.025. Epub 2012 Feb 17. Review. PMID: 22343313.

[51] Bradbury EJ, Carter LM: Manipulating the glial scar: chondroitinase ABC as a therapy for spinal cord injury. Brain Res Bull 2011;84:306316 [PubMed: 20620201].

[52] Galtrey CM, Fawcett JW: The role of chondroitin sulfate proteoglycans in regeneration and plasticity in the central nervous system. Brain Res Rev 2007;54:118 [PubMed: 17222456].

[53] Yamagata T, Saito H, Habuchi O, Suzuki S: Purification and properties of bacterial chondroitinases and chondrosulfatases. J Biol Chem 1968;243:15231535 [PubMed: 5647268].

[54] Bradbury EJ, Moon LD, Popat RJ, King VR, Bennett GS, Patel PN, Fawcett JW, McMahon SB: Chondroitinase ABC promotes functional recovery after spinal cord injury. Nature 2002;416:636–640 [PubMed: 11948352].

[55] Houle JD, Tom VJ, Mayes D, Wagoner G, Phillips N, Silver J: Combining an autologous peripheral nervous system "bridge" and matrix modification by chondroitinase allows robust, functional regeneration beyond a hemisection lesion of the adult rat spinal cord. J Neurosci 2006;26(28):7405–7415.

[56] Tom VJ, Sandrow-Feinberg HR, Miller K, Santi L, Connors T, Lemay MA, Houle JD: Combining peripheral nerve grafts and chondroitinase promotes functional axonal regeneration in the chronically injured spinal cord. J Neurosci 2009;29:14881–14890 [PMC free article] [PubMed].

[57] Hwang DH, Kim HM, Kang YM, Joo IS, Cho CS, Yoon BW, Kim SU, Kim BG. Combination of multifaceted strategies to maximize the therapeutic benefits of neural stem cell transplantation for spinal cord repair. Cell Transplant. 2011;20(9):1361–1379. doi: 10.3727/096368910X557155. Epub 2011 Mar 7. PubMed PMID: 21396156.

[58] Kumar P, Choonara YE, Modi G, Naidoo D, Pillay V: Multifunctional therapeutic delivery strategies for effective neuro-regeneration following traumatic spinal cord injury. Curr Pharm Des 2015;21(12):1517–1528 [PubMed PMID: 25594407].

[59] Jain A, Kim YT, McKeon RJ, Bellamkonda RV: In situ gelling hydrogels for conformal repair of spinal cord defects, and local delivery of BDNF after spinal cord injury. Biomaterials 2006;27:497504 [PubMed: 16099038].

[60] Kreider BQ, Messing A, Doan H, Kim SU, Lisak RP, Pleasure DE. Enrichment of Schwann cell cultures from neonatal rat sciatic nerve by differential adhesion. Brain Res 1981;207:433444 [PubMed: 7008901].

[61] Fouad K, Schnell L, Bunge MB, Schwab ME, Liebscher T, Pearse DD. Combining Schwann cell bridges and olfactory-ensheathing glia grafts with chondroitinase promotes locomotor recovery after complete transection of the spinal cord. J Neurosci 2005;25:1169–1178 [PubMed].

[62] Wilems TS, Pardieck J, Iyer N, Sakiyama-Elbert SE: Combination therapy of stem cell derived neural progenitors and drug delivery of anti-inhibitory molecules for spinal cord injury. Acta Biomater 2015. pii: S1742–7061(15)30112–4. doi: 10.1016/j.actbio.2015.09.018. [Epub ahead of print]

[63] Lee H, McKeon RJ, Bellamkonda RV. Sustained delivery of thermostabilized chABC enhances axonal sprouting and functional recovery after spinal cord injury. Proc Natl Acad Sci U S A. 2010 Feb 23;107(8):3340–3345. doi: 10.1073/pnas.0905437106. Epub 2009 Nov 2. PubMed PMID: 19884507; PubMed Central PMCID: PMC2840440.

[64] Tom VJ, Houlé JD: Intraspinal microinjection of chondroitinase ABC following injury promotes axonal regeneration out of a peripheral nerve graft bridge. Exp Neurol 2008;211(1):315–319.

[65] Wilems TS, Sakiyama-Elbert SE: Sustained dual drug delivery of anti-inhibitory molecules for treatment of spinal cord injury. J Control Release 2015;213:103–111. doi: 10.1016/j.jconrel.2015.06.031 [Epub ahead of print] [PubMed PMID: 26122130].

[66] Hyatt AJ, Wang D, Kwok JC, Fawcett JW, Martin KR: Controlled release of chondroitinase ABC from fibrin gel reduces the level of inhibitory glycosaminoglycan chains in

lesioned spinal cord. J Control Release 2010;147(1):24–29. doi: 10.1016/j.jconrel. 2010.06.026.

[67] Hunanyan AS, García-Alías G, Alessi V, Levine JM, Fawcett JW, Mendell LM, Arvanian VL: Role of chondroitin sulfate proteoglycans in axonal conduction in Mammalian spinal cord. J Neurosci 2010;30(23):7761–7769. doi: 10.1523/JNEUROSCI.4659-09.2010.

[68] Cheng CH, Lin CT, Lee MJ, Tsai MJ, Huang WH, Huang MC, Lin YL, Chen CJ, Huang WC, Cheng H: Local delivery of high-dose chondroitinase ABC in the sub-acute stage promotes axonal outgrowth and functional recovery after complete spinal cord transection. PLoS One. 2015;10(9):e0138705. doi:10.1371/journal.pone.0138705. eCollection 2015.

[69] Shields LB, Zhang YP, Burke DA, Gray R, Shields CB: Benefit of chondroitinase ABC on sensory axon regeneration in a laceration model of spinal cord injury in the rat. Surg Neurol 2008;69(6):568–577; discussion 577. doi: 10.1016/j.surneu.2008.02.009.

[70] Iseda T, Okuda T, Kane-Goldsmith N, Mathew M, Ahmed S, Chang YW, Young W, Grumet M: Single, high-dose intraspinal injection of chondroitinase reduces glycosaminoglycans in injured spinal cord and promotes corticospinal axonal regrowth after hemisection but not contusion. J Neurotrauma 2008;25(4):334–349. doi: 10.1089/neu. 2007.0289.

[71] Caggiano AO, Zimber MP, Ganguly A, Blight AR, Gruskin EA: Chondroitinase ABCI improves locomotion and bladder function following contusion injury of the rat spinal cord. J Neurotrauma 2005;22(2):226–239.

[72] Mondello SE, Jefferson SC, Tester NJ, Howland DR: Impact of treatment duration and lesion size on effectiveness of chondroitinase treatment post-SCI. Exp Neurol 2015;267:64–77. doi: 10.1016/j.expneurol.2015.02.028. Epub 2015 Feb 26.

[73] Ma Y, Liu M, Li Y: Secretion of bacterial chondroitinase ABC from bone marrow stromal cells by glycosylation site mutation: a promising approach for axon regeneration. Med Hypotheses 2011;77(5):914–916. doi: 10.1016/j.mehy.2011.08.010. Epub 2011 Aug 31.

[74] Kumar P, Choonara YE, Modi G, Naidoo D, Pillay V(1): Multifunctional therapeutic delivery strategies for effective neuro-regeneration following traumatic spinal cord injury. Curr Pharm Des 2015;21(12):1517–1528.

[75] Steinmetz MP, Horn KP, Tom VJ, Miller JH, Busch SA, Nair D, Silver DJ, Silver J: Chronic enhancement of the intrinsic growth capacity of sensory neurons combined with the degradation of inhibitory proteoglycans allows functional regeneration of sensory axons through the dorsal root entry zone in the mammalian spinal cord. J Neurosci 2005;25(35):8066–8076.

[76] Sarveazad A, Bakhtiari M, Babahajian A, Janzade A, Fallah A, Moradi F, Soleimani M, Younesi M, Goudarzi F, Mohammad Taghi Joghataei: Comparison of human adipose-derived stem cells and chondroitinase ABC transplantation on locomotor recovery in

the contusion model of spinal cord injury in rats. Iran J Basic Med Sci 2014;17(9):685–693. PubMed PMID: 25691946; PubMed Central PMCID:PMC4322153.

[77] Mountney A, Zahner MR, Sturgill ER, Riley CJ, Aston JW, Oudega M, Schramm LP, Hurtado A, Schnaar RL: Sialidase, chondroitinase ABC, and combination therapy after spinal cord contusion injury. J Neurotrauma 2013;30(3):181–190. doi: 10.1089/neu.2012.2353

[78] Lang BT, Cregg JM, DePaul MA, Tran AP, Xu K, Dyck SM, Madalena KM, Brown BP, Weng YL, Li S, Karimi-Abdolrezaee S, Busch SA, Shen Y, Silver J: Modulation of the proteoglycan receptor PTPσ promotes recovery after spinal cord injury. Nature 2015;518(7539):404–408. doi: 10.1038/nature13974. Epub 2014 Dec 3. PubMed PMID: 25470046; PubMed Central PMCID: PMC4336236.

[79] Silver L, Michael JV, Goldfinger LE, Gallo G: Activation of PI3K and R-Ras signaling promotes the extension of sensory axons on inhibitory chondroitin sulfate proteoglycans. Dev Neurobiol 2014;74(9):918–933. doi: 10.1002/dneu.22174. Epub 2014 Mar 27.

[80] Tetzlaff W, Alexander SW, Miller FD, Bisby MA: Response of facial and rubrospinal neurons to axotomy: changes in mRNA expression for cytoskeletal proteins and GAP-43. J Neurosci 1991;11:2528–2544 [PubMed].

[81] Sengottuvel V, Leibinger M, Pfreimer M, Andreadaki A, Fischer D: Taxol facilitates axon regeneration in the mature CNS. J Neurosci 2011;31:2688–2699 [PubMed].

[82] Bates CA, Becker CG, Miotke JA, Meyer RL: Expression of polysialylated NCAM but not L1 or N-cadherin by regenerating adult mouse optic fibers in vitro. Exp Neurol 1999;155:128–139 [PubMed].

[83] Chaisuksunt V, Zhang Y, Anderson PN, et al: Axonal regeneration from CNS neurons in the cerebellum and brainstem of adult rats: correlation with the patterns of expression and distribution of messenger RNAs for L1, CHL1, c-jun and growth-associated protein-43. Neuroscience 2000;100:87–108 [PubMed].

[84] Chen J, Wu J, Apostolova I, et al: Adeno-associated virus-mediated L1 expression promotes functional recovery after spinal cord injury. Brain 2007;130:954–969 [PubMed].

[85] Roonprapunt C, Huang W, Grill R, et al: Soluble cell adhesion molecule L1-Fc promotes locomotor recovery in rats after spinal cord injury. J Neurotrauma 2003;20:871–882 [PubMed].

[86] Chen Y and Swanson RA: Astrocytes and brain injury. Rev Article J Cereb Blood Flow Metab 2003;23(2):137–149.

[87] Mohn TC, Koob AO: Adult astrogenesis and the etiology of cortical neurodegeneration. J Exp Neurosci 2015:9(s) 25–34. doi:10.4137/JEn.s25520.

[88] Hering TM, Beller JA, Calulot CM, Centers A, Snow DM: Proteoglycans of reactive rat cortical astrocyte cultures: abundance of N-unsubstituted glucosamine-enriched heparan sulfate. Matrix Biol 2015;41:8–18. doi: 10.1016/j.matbio.2014.11.006.

[89] Yates D: Synaptogenesis. Asynaptic bridge. Nat Rev Neurosci 2016;17,135. doi:10.1038/nrn.2016.12 Published online 11 February 2016.

[90] Harter K, Levine M, Henderson SO: Anticoagulation drug therapy: a review. West J Emerg Med 2015;16(1):11–17. doi: 10.5811/westjem.2014.12.22933. Epub 2015 Jan 12. Review. PubMed PMID: 25671002; PubMed Central PMCID: PMC4307693.

[91] Kahraman A, Kahveci R: Evaluating the effect of polytetrafluoroethylene and extractum cepae-heparin-allantoin gel in peripheral nerve injuries in a rat model. Plast Surg (Oakv) 2015 Spring;23(1):9–14. PubMed PMID: 25821766; PubMed Central PMCID: PMC4364148.

[92] Akbari H, Rahimi AA, Ghavami Y, Mousavi SJ, Fatemi MJ. Effect of heparin on post-operative adhesion in flexor tendon surgery of the hand. J Hand Microsurg 2015;7(2): 244–249. Epub 2015 Aug 26. PubMed PMID: 26578825; PubMed Central PMCID: PMC4642480.

[93] Aydoseli A, Tahta A, Aras Y, Sabancı A, Keskin M, Balik E, Onder S, Sencer A, Izgi N: Use of antifibrotics to prevent ventriculoperitoneal shunt complications due to intra-abdominal fibrosis: experimental study in a rat model. J Neurol Surg A Cent Eur Neurosurg 2015;76(3):219–223. doi: 10.1055/s-0034-1389369. Epub 2015 Mar 26. PubMed PMID: 25811104.

[94] Alonso Jde M, Rodrigues KA, Yamada AL, Watanabe MJ, Alves AL, Rodrigues CA, Hussni CA: Peritoneal reactivity evaluation in horses subjected to experimental small colon enterotomy and treated with subcutaneous heparin. Vet Med Int 2014;2014:385392. doi: 10.1155/2014/385392. Epub 2014 Nov 11. PubMed PMID: 25436172; PubMed Central PMCID: PMC4243600.

[95] Ho WS, Ying SY, Chan PC, Chan HH: Use of onion extract, heparin, allantoin gel in prevention of scarring in chinese patients having laser removal of tattoos: a prospective randomized controlled trial. Dermatol Surg 2006;32(7):891–896. PubMed PMID: 16875470.

[96] Billings PC, Pacifici M: Interactions of signaling proteins, growth factors and other proteins with heparan sulfate: mechanisms and mysteries. Connect Tissue Res 2015;56(4):272–280. doi: 10.3109/03008207.2015.1045066.

[97] Olczyk P, Mencner Ł, Komosinska-Vassev K: Diverse roles of heparan sulfate and heparin in wound repair. Biomed Res Int 2015;2015:549417. doi: 10.1155/2015/549417. Epub 2015 Jul 7. Review. PubMed PMID: 26236728; PubMed Central PMCID: PMC4508384.

[98] Newman DR, Li CM, Simmons R, Khosla J, Sannes PL: Heparin affects signaling pathways stimulated by fibroblast growth factor-1 and -2 in type II cells. Am J Physiol

Lung Cell Mol Physiol 2004;287(1):L191–L200. Epub 2004 Feb 13. PubMed PMID: 14966081.

[99] Santos-Silva A, Fairless R, Frame MC, Montague P, Smith GM, Toft A, Riddell JS, Barnett SC: FGF/heparin differentially regulates Schwann cell and olfactory ensheathing cell interactions with astrocytes: a role in astrocytosis. J Neurosci 2007;27(27):7154–7167.

[100] Yi-Chao Hsu, Su-Liang Chen, Dan-Yen Wang: Ing-Ming Chiu stem cell-based therapy in neural repair. Biomed J 2013;36:98–105.

[101] Walicke P, Cowan WM, Ueno N, Baird A, Guillemin R: Fibroblast growth factor promotes survival of dissociated hippocampal neurons and enhances neurite extension. Proc Natl Acad Sci U S A 1986;83(9):3012–3016.

[102] Nagayasu T, Miyata S, Hayashi N, Takano R, Kariya Y, Kamei K: Heparin structures in FGF-2-dependent morphological transformation of astrocytes. J Biomed Mater Res A 2005;74(3):374–380. PubMed PMID: 15973728.

[103] Poulsen FR, Lagord C, Courty J, Pedersen EB, Barritault D, Finsen B: Increased synthesis of heparin affin regulatory peptide in the perforant path lesioned mouse hippocampal formation. Exp Brain Res 2000;135(3):319–330. PubMed PMID: 11146810.

[104] Wanaka A, Carroll SL, Milbrandt J: Developmentally regulated expression of pleiotrophin, a novel heparin binding growth factor, in the nervous system of the rat. Brain Res Dev Brain Res 1993;72(1):133–144. PubMed PMID: 8453763.

[105] Hagino S, Iseki K, Mori T, Zhang Y, Sakai N, Yokoya S, Hikake T, Kikuchi S, Wanaka A: Expression pattern of glypican-1 mRNA after brain injury in mice. Neurosci Lett 2003;349(1):29–32. PubMed PMID: 12946579.

[106] Lau E, Margolis RU: Inhibitors of slit protein interactions with the heparin sulphate proteoglycan glypican-1: potential agents for the treatment of spinal cord injury. Clin Exp Pharmacol Physiol 2010;37(4):417–421. doi: 10.1111/j.1440-1681.2009.05318.x.

[107] Modi KK, Sendtner M, Pahan K: Up-regulation of ciliary neurotrophic factor in astrocytes by aspirin: implications for remyelination in multiple sclerosis. J Biol Chem 2013;288(25):18533–18545. doi: 10.1074/jbc.M112.447268.

[108] Khaing ZZ, Milman BD, Vanscoy JE, Seidlits SK, Grill RJ, Schmidt CE: High molecular weight hyaluronic acid limits astrocyte activation and scar formation after spinal cord injury. J Neural Eng 2011;8(4):046033. doi: 10.1088/1741-2560/8/4/046033.

[109] Madigan NN, McMahon S, O'Brien T, Yaszemski MJ, Windebank AJ: Current tissue engineering and novel therapeutic approaches to axonal regeneration following spinal cord injury using polymer scaffolds. Respir Physiol Neurobiol 2009;169(2):183–199. doi: 10.1016/j.resp.2009.08.015. Epub 2009 Sep 6. Review. PubMed PMID: 19737633; PubMed Central PMCID: PMC2981799.

[110] Straley KS, Foo CW, Heilshorn SC: Biomaterial design strategies for the treatment of spinal cord injuries. J Neurotrauma 2010;27(1):1–19. doi: 10.1089/neu.2009.0948. Review. PubMed PMID: 19698073; PubMed Central PMCID: PMC2924783.

[111] Tetzlaff W, Okon EB, Karimi-Abdolrezaee S, Hill CE, Sparling JS, Plemel JR, Plunet WT, Tsai EC, Baptiste D, Smithson LJ, Kawaja MD, Fehlings MG, Kwon BK: A systematic review of cellular transplantation therapies for spinal cord injury. J Neurotrauma 2011;28(8):1611–1682. Epub 2010 Apr 20. Review.

[112] Duncan ID, Milward EA: Glial cell transplants: experimental therapies of myelin diseases. Brain Pathol 1995;5:301–310 [PubMed].

[113] Santos-Silva A, Fairless R, Frame MC, Montague P, Smith GM, Toft A, Riddell JS, Barnett SC: FGF/heparin differentially regulates Schwann cell and olfactory ensheathing cell interactions with astrocytes: a role in astrocytosis. J Neurosci 2007;27(27):7154–7167.

[114] Ramon-Cueto A, Plant GW, Avila J, Bunge MB: Long-distance axonal regeneration in the transected adult rat spinal cord is promoted by olfactory ensheathing glia transplants. J Neurosci 1998;18:3803–3815 [PubMed].

[115] Lu P, Yang H, Culbertson M, Graham L, Roskams AJ, Tuszynski MH: Olfactory ensheathing cells do not exhibit unique migratory or axonal growth-promoting properties after spinal cord injury. J Neurosci 2006;26:11120–11130 [PubMed].

[116] Pearse DD, Sanchez AR, Pereira FC, Andrade CM, Puzis R, Pressman Y, Golden K, Kitay BM, Blits B, Wood PM, Bunge MB: Transplantation of Schwann cells and/or olfactory ensheathing glia into the contused spinal cord: survival, migration, axon association, and functional recovery. Glia 2007;55:976–1000 [PubMed].

[117] Ruitenberg MJ, Plant GW, Hamers FP, Wortel J, Blits B, Dijkhuizen PA, Gispen WH, Boer GJ, Verhaagen J: Ex vivo adenoviral vector-mediated neurotrophin gene transfer to olfactory ensheathing glia: effects on rubrospinal tract regeneration, lesion size, and functional recovery after implantation in the injured rat spinal cord. J Neurosci 2003;23:7045–7058 [PubMed].

[118] Alexanian AR, Crowe MJ, Kurpad SN: Efficient differentiation and integration of lineage-restricted neural precursors in the traumatically injured adult cat spinal cord. J Neurosci Methods 2006;150:41–46 [PubMed].

[119] Cao QL, Zhang YP, Howard RM, Walters WM, Tsoulfas P, Whittemore SR: Pluripotent stem cells engrafted into the normal or lesioned adult rat spinal cord are restricted to a glial lineage. Exp Neurol 2001;167:48–58 [PubMed].

[120] Macias MY, Syring MB, Pizzi MA, Crowe MJ, Alexanian AR, Kurpad SN: Pain with no gain: allodynia following neural stem cell transplantation in spinal cord injury. Exp Neurol 2006;201:335–348 [PubMed].

[121] Jin Y, Bouyer J, Shumsky JS, Haas C, Fischer I: Transplantation of neural progenitor cells in chronic spinal cord injury. Neuroscience 2016;320:69–82. doi: 10.1016/j.neuroscience.2016.01.066. Epub 2016 Feb 4. PubMedPMID: 26852702.

[122] Bambakidis NC, Miller RH: Transplantation of oligodendrocyte precursors and sonic hedgehog results in improved function and white matter sparing in the spinal cords of adult rats after contusion. Spine J 2004;4:16–26 [PubMed].

[123] Cao QL, Howard RM, Dennison JB, Whittemore SR. Differentiation of engrafted neuronal-restricted precursor cells is inhibited in the traumatically injured spinal cord. Exp Neurol 2002;177:349–359 [PubMed].

[124] Ankeny DP, McTigue DM, Jakeman LB: Bone marrow transplants provide tissue protection and directional guidance for axons after contusive spinal cord injury in rats. Exp Neurol 2004;190:17–31 [PubMed].

[125] Yano S, Kuroda S, Lee JB, Shichinohe H, Seki T, Ikeda J, Nishimura G, Hida K, Tamura M, Iwasaki Y: In vivo fluorescence tracking of bone marrow stromal cells transplanted into a pneumatic injury model of rat spinal cord. J Neurotrauma 2005;22:907–918 [PubMed].

[126] Wright KT, Masri WE, Osman A, Roberts S, Trivedi J, Ashton BA, Johnson WE: The cell culture expansion of bone marrow stromal cells from humans with spinal cord injury: implications for future cell transplantation therapy. Spinal Cord 2008;46(12):811–817.

[127] Wright KT, El Masri W, Osman A, Roberts S, Chamberlain G, Ashton BA, Johnson WE: Bone marrow stromal cells stimulate neurite outgrowth over neural proteoglycans (CSPG), myelin associated glycoprotein and Nogo-A. Biochem Biophys Res Commun 2007;354(2):559–566.

[128] Bunge MB: Novel combination strategies to repair the injured mammalian spinal cord. J Spinal Cord Med 2008;31:262–269.

[129] Mackay-Sim A, Feron F, Cochrane J, Bassingthwaighte L, Bayliss C, Davies W, Fronek P, Gray C, Kerr G, Licina P, Nowitzke A, Perry C, Silburn PAS, Urquhart S, Geraghty T: Autologous olfactory ensheathing cell transplantation in human paraplegia: a 3-year clinical trial. Brain 2008;131:2376–2386.

[130] Li H, Wen Y, Luo Y, Lan X, Wang D, Sun Z, Hu L: [Transplantation of bone marrow mesenchymal stem cells into spinal cord injury: a comparison of delivery different times] [Article in Chinese] Zhongguo Xiu Fu Chong Jian Wai Ke Za Zhi 2010;24(2):180–184.

[131] Ichim TE, Solano F, Lara F, Paris E, Ugalde F, Rodriguez JP, Minev B, Bogin V, Ramos F, Woods EJ, Murphy MP, Patel AN, Harman RJ, Riordan NH: Feasibility of combination allogeneic stem celltherapy for spinal cord injury: a case report. Int Archives Med 2010;3:30.

[132] Sullivan R, Duncan K, Dailey T, Kaneko Y, Tajiri N, Borlongan CV: A possible new focus for stroke treatment—migrating stem cells. Expert Opin Biol Ther 2015;15(7):949–958. doi: 10.1517/14712598.2015.1043264.

[133] Klingener M, Chavali M, Aguirre A: N-cadherin promotes recruitment and migration of neural progenitor cells from the SVZ stem cell niche into demyelinated lesions. Int J Dev Neurosci 2015;47(Pt A):107. doi: 10.1016/j.ijdevneu.2015.04.292. PubMed PMID: 26531615.

[134] Kim HJ, Shaker MR, Cho B, Cho HM, Kim H, Kim JY, Sun W: Dynamin-related protein 1 controls the migration and neuronal differentiation of subventricular zone-derived neural progenitor cells. Sci Rep 2015;5:15962. doi: 10.1038/srep15962.

[135] Chen Q, Zhang M, Li Y, Xu D, Wang Y, Song A, Zhu B, Huang Y, Zheng JC: CXCR7 mediates neural progenitor cells migration to CXCL12 independent of CXCR4. Stem Cells 2015;33(8):2574–2585. doi: 10.1002/stem.2022. Epub 2015 May 13. PubMed PMID: 25833331.

[136] Potter K, Saifuddin A: MRI of chronic spinal cord injury. Br J Radiol 2003;76:347–352.

[137] Li Y, Raisman G: Sprouts from cut corticospinal axons persist in the presence of astrocytic scarring in long-term lesions of the adult rat spinal cord. Exp Neurol 1995;134:102–111.

[138] Amr SM, Essam AM, Abdel-Meguid AM, Kholeif AM, Moharram AN, El-Sadek RE: Direct cord implantation in brachial plexus avulsions: revised technique using a single stage combined anterior (first) posterior (second) approach and end-to-side side-to-side grafting neurorrhaphy. J Brachial Plex Peripher Nerve Inj 2009;4:8.

[139] Nakagomi T, Molnár Z, Nakano-Doi A, Taguchi A, Saino O, Kubo S, Clausen M, Yoshikawa H, Nakagomi N, Matsuyama T: Ischemia-induced neural stem/progenitor cells in the pia mater following cortical infarction. Stem Cells Dev 2011 Dec;20(12):2037–2051.

[140] Johanson C, Stopa E, Baird A, Sharma H: Traumatic brain injury and recovery mechanisms: peptide modulation of periventricular neurogenic regions by the choroid plexus-CSF nexus. J Neural Transm 2011;118(1):115–133. Epub 2010 Oct 10.

[141] Francel PC, Francel TJ, Mackinnon SE, Hertl C: Enhancing nerve regeneration across a silicone tube conduit by using interposed short-segment nerve grafts. J Neurosurg 1997;87(6):887–892. PubMed PMID: 9384400.

[142] Spector JG, Lee P, Derby A, Roufa DG: Comparison of rabbit facial nerve regeneration in nerve growth factor-containing silicone tubes to that in autologous neural grafts. Ann Otol Rhinol Laryngol 1995;104(11):875–885.PubMed PMID: 8534028.

[143] Le Beau JM, Powell HC, Ellisman MH: Node of Ranvier formation along fibres regenerating through silicone tube implants: a freeze-fracture and thin-section electron microscopic study. J Neurocytol 1987;16(3):347–358. PubMed PMID: 3612184.

[144] Peláez RJ, Afonso CN, Vega F, Recio-Sánchez G, Torres-Costa V, Manso-Silván M, García-Ruiz JP, Martín-Palma RJ: Laser fabrication of porous silicon-based platforms for cell culturing. J Biomed Mater Res B Appl Biomater 2013;101(8):1463–1468. doi: 10.1002/jbm.b.32966.

[145] Punzón-Quijorna E, Sánchez-Vaquero V, Muñoz-Noval A, Pérez-Roldán MJ, Martín-Palma RJ, Rossi F, Climent-Font A, Manso-Silván M, Ruiz JP, Torres-Costa V: Nanostructured porous silicon micropatterns as a tool forsubstrate-conditioned cell research. Nanoscale Res Lett 2012;7(1):396. PubMed PMID: 22799489; PubMed Central PMCID: PMC3458952.

[146] Collart-Dutilleul PY, Panayotov I, Secret E, Cunin F, Gergely C, Cuisinier F, Martin M: Initial stem cell adhesion on porous silicon surface: molecular architecture of actin cytoskeleton and filopodial growth. Nanoscale Res Lett 2014;9(1):564. doi: 10.1186/1556-276X-9-564. eCollection 2014. PubMed PMID: 25386101; PubMed Central PMCID: PMC4217708.

[147] Pandis C, Trujillo S, Matos J, Madeira S, Ródenas-Rochina J, Kripotou S, Kyritsis A, Mano JF, Gómez Ribelles JL: Porous polylactic acid-silica hybrids: preparation, characterization, and study of mesenchymal stem cell osteogenic differentiation. Macromol Biosci 2015;15(2):262–274. doi: 10.1002/mabi.201400339. Epub 2014 Oct 10. PubMed PMID: 25303745.

[148] Zhou P, Cheng X, Xia Y, Wang P, Zou K, Xu S, Du J: Organic/inorganic composite membranes based on poly(L-lactic-co-glycolic acid) and mesoporous silica for effective bone tissue engineering. ACS Appl Mater Interfaces 2014;6(23):20895–20903. doi: 10.1021/am505493j.

[149] Kim H, Kim I, Choi HJ, Kim SY, Yang EG: Neuron-like differentiation of mesenchymal stem cells on silicon nanowires. Nanoscale 2015;7(40):17131–17138. doi: 10.1039/c5nr05787f. PubMed PMID: 26422757.

[150] Ai H, Lvov YM, Mills DK, Jennings M, Alexander JS, Jones SA: Coating and selective deposition of nanofilm on silicone rubber for cell adhesion and growth. Cell Biochem Biophys 2003;38(2):103–114. PubMed PMID: 12777710.

[151] Yue Z, Liu X, Molino PJ, Wallace GG: Bio-functionalisation of polydimethylsiloxane with hyaluronic acid and hyaluronic acid--collagen conjugate for neural interfacing. Biomaterials 2011;32(21):4714–4724. doi: 10.1016/j.biomaterials.2011.03.032.

[152] Minev IR, Moshayedi P, Fawcett JW, Lacour SP: Interaction of glia with a compliant, microstructured silicone surface. Acta Biomater 2013;9(6):6936–6942. doi: 10.1016/j.actbio.2013.02.048. Epub 2013 Mar 14. PubMed PMID: 23499849.

[153] Patel KR, Tang H, Grever WE, Simon Ng KY, Xiang J, Keep RF, Cao T, McAllister JP II: Evaluation of polymer and self-assembled monolayer-coated silicone surfaces to reduce neural cell growth. Biomaterials 2006;27(8):1519–1526. Epub 2005 Sep 19.

[154] Huang H, Chen L, Wang H, Xiu B, Li B, Wang R, Zhang J, Zhang F, Gu Z, Li Y, Song Y, Hao W, Pang S, Sun J: Influence of patients' age on functional recovery after transplantation of olfactory ensheathing cells into injured spinal cord injury. Chin Med J (Engl) 2003,116:1488–1491.

[155] Lima C, Pratas-Vital J, Escada P, Hasse-Ferreira A, Capucho C, Peduzzi JD: Olfactory mucosa autografts in human spinal cord injury: a pilot clinical study. J Spinal Cord Med 2006;29:191–203; discussion 204–206.

[156] Park HC, Shim YS, Ha Y, Yoon SH, Park SR, Choi BH, Park HS: Treatment of complete spinal cord injury patients by autologous bone marrow cell transplantation and administration of granulocyte-macrophage colony stimulating factor. Tissue Eng 2005;11:913–922.

[157] Yoon SH, Shim YS, Park YH, Chung JK, Nam JH, Kim MO, Park HC, Park SR, Min BH, Kim EY, Choi BH, Park H, Ha Y: Complete spinal cord injury treatment using autologous bone marrow cell transplantation and bone marrow stimulation with granulocyte macrophage-colony stimulating factor: phase I/II clinical trial. Stem Cells 2007;25(8): 2066–2073.

[158] Chowdary PD, Che DL, Cui B: Neurotrophin signaling via long-distance axonal transport. Annu Rev Phys Chem 2012;63:571–594. doi: 10.1146/annurev-physchem-032511-143704. Epub 2012 Jan 30. Review. PubMed PMID: 22404590.

[159] Chowdary PD, Che DL, Kaplan L, Chen O, Pu K, Bawendi M, Cui B: Nanoparticle-assisted optical tethering of endosomes reveals the cooperative function of dyneins in retrograde axonal transport. Sci Rep 2015;5:18059. doi: 10.1038/srep18059. PubMed PMID: 26656461; PubMed Central PMCID: PMC4674899.

[160] Dono R: Fibroblast growth factors as regulators of central nervous system development and function. Am J Physiol Regul Integr Comp Physiol 2003;284(4):R867–R881. Review. PubMed PMID: 12626354.

[161] Hendry IA, Belford DA: Lack of retrograde axonal transport of the heparin-binding growth factors by chick ciliary neurones. Int J Dev Neurosci 1991;9(3):243–250. PubMed PMID: 1718148.

Chapter 9

Stem Cell Therapies for Cervical Spinal Cord Injury

Vanessa M. Doulames, Laura M. Marquardt,
Bhavaani Jayaram, Christine D. Plant and
Giles W. Plant

Additional information is available at the end of the chapter

http://dx.doi.org/10.5772/63580

Abstract

Cervical-level injuries account for the majority of presented spinal cord injuries (SCIs), yet there are few therapies that successfully improve the overall quality of life for patients. Regenerative therapies aimed at ameliorating deficits in respiratory and motor function are urgently needed. Cellular transplantation strategies are a promising therapeutic avenue. These strategies seek to overcome the inhibitory environment of the injury site, increase native regenerative capacities, provide scaffolding to bridge the lesion, or replace injury-lost neurons and glia.

Numerous considerations must be taken into account, however, when designing effective cellular transplantation therapies, most notably of which is cell source. Each cell source offers its own unique attributes—both positive and negative—that directly correspond with functional outcomes and clinical translation. Here we discuss three different cell types currently used in cellular transplantation strategies to treat cervical SCIs: mesenchymal stem cells (MSCs), embryonic stem cells (ESCs), and induced pluripotent stem cells (iPSCs). By illustrating the characteristics of each cell type and outlining the studies and clinical trials in which they have been featured, we hope to provide the reader with a detailed understanding of both their capabilities and also their potential drawbacks in experimental and clinical settings.

Keywords: cervical spinal cord injury, stem cell therapies, cellular transplantation, functional outcomes, regenerative strategies

1. Introduction

1.1. The impact of cervical SCI

Spinal cord injuries (SCIs) create a formidable encumbrance on the US healthcare service with over half of all injuries occurring at the cervical level. While most causes of SCI can be attributed to accidents or violence, the incidence of cervical-specific injuries continues to rise from particularly distinctive causes [1,2]. This is in part due to the ever-increasing spectrum of injury types, such as those sustained in direct military environments or as a result of changes in tactical armor design [3–6]. Others include improvements in emergency medicine leading to better survival rates [7], the growth of the aging population as a result of advances in preventative care [8–10], and lifestyle choices leading to structural degradation of the cervical spine [11,12].

Survivors of cervical SCI are faced with dramatic life changes owing to lengthy and repeated hospitalizations and the need for full- or part-time caretakers, overall resulting in a loss of personal independence. Combined with a frequent inability to maintain employment or contribute to the workforce, patients incur substantial financial expenses—over the course of their lifetime, a 25-year-old SCI patient can expect to accrue up to $4.5 million in direct costs alone. Overall, SCI costs the nation upward of $40.5 billion annually, as per a 2009 report by the Christopher and Dana Reeve Foundation [1,2]. Although recent advances have resulted in increased survival rates, quality of life still remains poor; patients encounter a gradation of sensory deficits, respiratory deficits, motor dysfunction, and paralysis based on their specific injury location. Therapies designed to ameliorate some of these complications, even partially, are drastically needed and would make a radical impact in easing the financial, emotional, and physical burden experienced by cervical SCI patients.

1.2. The pathophysiology of cervical SCI

The cervical spinal cord contains the long tracts connecting the rostral and caudal portions of the central nervous system (CNS), as well as sensory and motor neurons. Cervical SCI in mammals initiates large zones of necrosis at the site of injury, creating gaps in the circuitry and preventing communication within the CNS. Axons within the spinal cord fail to regenerate after injury and retract toward the soma from the lesion border. Overall this culminates in crucial changes to normal upper limb function in mammals and disrupts motor function in humans resulting in paralysis and diaphragm-mediated respiration [13].

SCI is characterized by two distinct phases: primary and secondary injuries. During primary injury, the delicate spinal cord tissue is mechanically compromised due to shearing and compression forces, either by direct contact or inadvertently through manipulation of the vertebrae. This leads to mechanical injury, disruptions in vasculature and respiration, neurogenic shock, inflammation, membrane compromise, and alterations in ion and neurotransmitter levels [14–16]. While the primary injury phase leads to an immediate and often serious impairment of neurological function, it is the secondary injury phase that typically dictates the full magnitude of injury. There are approximately 25 established mechanisms to date by which this occurs, but still much ambiguity as to how these pathways converge upon each other to determine the full manifestation of injury [17,18]. Overall, this biochemical cascade activates the ischemic pathway, inflammation and immune responses, swelling, and neuronal apoptosis and leads to neurotransmitter imbalances that underlie excitotoxicity [19–25].

http://dx.doi.org/10.5772/63580

1.3. Regeneration and plasticity of the CNS

Prior evidence suggested that the adult mammalian CNS did not regenerate, predominantly due to the unlikely event of axonal regeneration through the inhibitory milieu of the spinal lesion [26]. However, some degree of functional recovery is often seen, possibly as a result of reorganization of spared circuitry from innate axonal sprouting of spared and intact fibers [26–28]. Experimental evidence has shown that this process can be influenced and axonal regeneration encouraged via the use of other synergistic therapies. These include the addition of neurotrophic growth factors [29–32], the deletion of inhibitory factors typically associated with the lesion [33–35], and rehabilitation regimens and physical activity [36–38]. Despite this, the innate regenerative capacities of the CNS are often overwhelmed by the extent of injury and functional recovery is limited at best.

Given SCI's multifactorial pathophysiology and the inherent complexity of the CNS, any potentially successful treatment must be effective in positively addressing multiple deficits. Cellular transplantation therapies offer an attractive means of accomplishing this by repopulating SCI-lost neurons and glia, increasing native regenerative capacities through trophic and immunomodulatory factors secreted by transplanted cells, and providing scaffolding to bridge the inhibitory milieu of the lesion site [20,29,30,32,39–43]. Furthermore, the potency of stem cells makes them an ideal candidate by circumventing the impediments of harvesting and transplanting adult neurons. By promoting neurite regeneration and replenishing appropriate cell populations, it may be possible to reconnect rostral and caudal neural circuitry and restore function.

In recent decades, the therapeutic promise of cellular intraspinal transplantation has gained significant interest and has eventuated in preliminary clinical trials. Numerous preclinical experiments have been developed to target SCI using peripheral nerve bridges, Schwann cells,

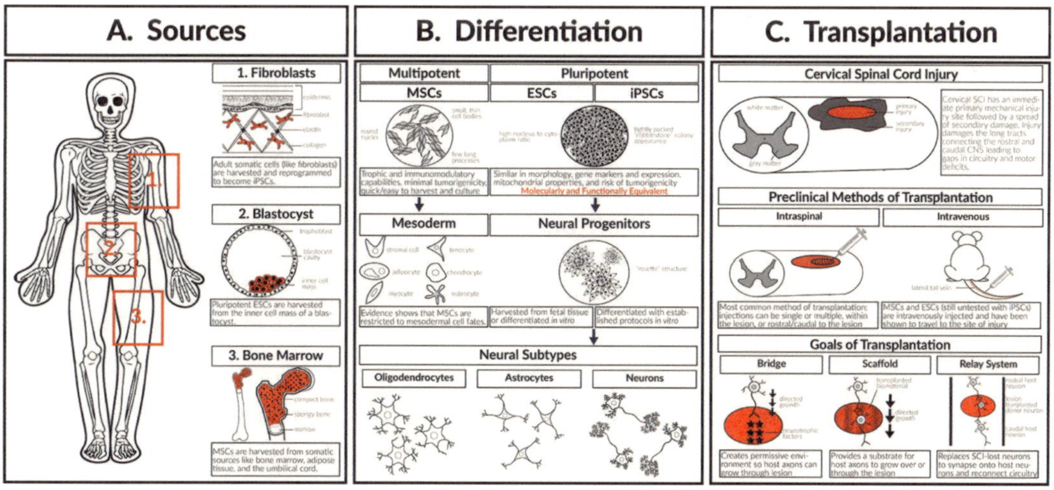

Figure 1. A summary of the different stem cell types. Panel (A) shows the origin and isolation of the cells, (B) shows their differentiation potential, and (C) describes transplantation methods used and their intended goals for treatment of cervical SCI.

olfactory glia, mesenchymal stem cells (MSCs), embryonic-derived stem cells, and induced pluripotent stem cells (iPSCs). However, the vast majority of these do not address cervical-level injury [44–52].

Here, we highlight the current literature on embryonic, mesenchymal, and induced pluripotent stem cell-based cellular transplantation with an emphasis on cervical-level SCI. We discuss the benefits and disadvantages of each cellular source, and consider possible future therapeutic avenues. **Figure 1** provides a summary of these cellular types and their origins, including transplantation methods used and their intended goals for treatment of cervical SCI.

2. Mesenchymal stem cells (MSCs)

2.1. Isolation and purification of MSCs

Transplantation of mesenchymal stem cells (MSCs), also known as bone marrow stromal cells (BMSCs) or mesenchymal progenitor cells, is a strategy currently being investigated to ameliorate the array of deleterious effects following SCI. The terms mesenchymal stromal cells and mesenchymal stem cells have been interchangeably used in the published literature; however there are demonstrable differences between the cells. Mesenchymal stem cells are a subset of stromal cells that maintain the same fibroblast morphology and specific marker expression; however they also have the potential for self-renewal and to differentiate into adipocytes, chondrocytes, and osteoblasts *in vitro* [53–55]. For cultured cells to be defined as MSCs, they should demonstrate the following: (1) adherence to plastic under culture conditions, (2) expression of CD105, CD73, and CD90, (3) lack of expression of CD45, CD34, CD14/CD11b, CD79/CD19, and HLA-DR surface markers, and (4) possession of the transdifferentiation potential to mesodermal lineages *in vitro* [56].

MSCs reside in a wide variety of tissues but are typically extracted from bone marrow and adipose tissue and to a lesser extent the umbilical cord. Their wide distribution and perivascular origin [57] account for their capability to sense and respond to injury by secreting trophic and anti-inflammatory factors [58,59]. The first report of MSCs isolation from bone marrow was by Friedenstein and colleagues. [60]. The spindle-shaped cells isolated were defined as colony-forming units (CFU) with the potential for *in vitro* culture for further transplantation *in vivo* [61]. It was only in 1999 that Pittenger and colleagues established the multi-lineage differentiation potential of MSCs into distinct mesodermal lineages [62]. Originally, Friedenstein and colleagues cultured MSCs by plastic adherence. Since then, many groups have modified this technique by expanding MSCs as a suspension culture [63–65].

Since its origin, bone marrow-derived MSC culture techniques have been continuously validated and improved. While isolation via plastic adherence is effective, the isolation of such cells does not yield a purified population of MSCs leading to varied growth kinetics and differentiation capabilities [66]. The complications of a heterogeneous population can be overcome by the purification of MSCs by using single specific surface markers such as Stro-1, CD271, Stro-3, CD73, and CD2000 [65,67]. Transplantation of MSCs, selected as above, following SCI in a rat model translated to marked improvement in functional recovery and increased tissue sparing [68].

Compared to iPSCs or embryonic stem cells (ESCs), MSCs overcome the ethical concerns of isolation, as MSCs can be extracted from one's own bone marrow or adipose tissue [69]. Recent data has indicated the principal therapeutic advantages of MSCs are their neuroprotective [70,71] and immunomodulatory [71,72] properties.

2.2. Regenerative potential of MSCs

The ubiquitous presence of MSCs around blood vessels makes them more amenable to respond to cues from tissue damage. Recent reports attribute the immunomodulatory function of MSCs as suitable for regenerative therapies and thereby tissue repair. Experimental evidence has shown that the immunomodulatory effect of MSCs is possibly due to their ability to suppress T-cell proliferation by secreting soluble factors such as TGF-beta and hepatocyte growth factor and not via apoptosis [73]. MSCs can also exert their immunomodulatory effect by shifting the balance in favor of regulatory T-cells, known suppressors of the immune system that are triggered by anti-inflammatory cytokines such as IL10. Aggarwal and Pittenger [74] co-cultured populations of immune cells with human MSCS and demonstrated that MSCs altered the secretory cytokine profile, restored balance between helper T-cells and macrophages, reduced pro-inflammatory cytokines, and increased anti-inflammatory molecules, thus favoring the induction of a tolerant anti-inflammatory phenotype [74,75]. Shifting and quenching the inflammatory response then redirects the body's resources toward tissue repair and growth [76,77]. Thus far, preclinical studies have demonstrated the potential for MSCs and their secreted factors to repair damaged tissue through their immunomodulatory and neuroprotective properties.

2.3. Treating cervical SCI with MSCs: toward clinical application

Clinically, the majority of interventions in treating SCI are pharmaceutically based and designed primarily to manage pain and control inflammation. With recent advances in stem cell therapy, there has been an increased interest in clinical studies evaluating the safety and efficacy of stem cells. MSCs are considered a favorable option for transplantation due to a number of factors: ease of isolation, rapid clinical expansion of cultures [78], ability to be cryopreserved and regenerated without loss of potency [79,80], minimal risk of tumorigenicity [81,82], multipotent capabilities, and the clinical possibility for autologous transplantation [83,84]. Furthermore, MSC transplantation has been tested widely in clinical trials and considered safe in a variety of neurological, cardiovascular, and immunological diseases [85]. As such, there is great potential for MSCs as a treatment for SCI, which has been well documented within the literature [53,68,86,87]. There are a number of clinical trials (both ongoing and completed) to test the potential of using MSCs to treat SCI (for the most current information, please refer to www.clinicaltrials.gov). Despite promising results of MSC therapies in animal SCI models and potential for clinical translation, there is yet to be an FDA approved treatment available for SCI patients.

Further investigation is needed to fully understand the basic delivery of MSCs and the mechanistic role in cervical SCI. It has not been established that engraftment and differentiation of MSCs are even needed for a therapeutic effect, and less than 1% of MSCs survive for longer than a week when systemically administered [88–90]. This survival rate would be similar in intraspinal injection. A transplantation study by Paul and colleagues compared the efficacy of hMSC engraftment when delivered either via lumbar puncture (LP), intravenous transfer (IV), or direct injection into the injury site in a rat C5 subtotal hemisection model [91]. Based on their results assessing engraftment volume (direct injection > LP > IV), glial scarring (no difference seen after 21 days of MSC transfer), and host immune response (direct injection had the highest host immune response), it can be concluded that MSC delivery via LP is a viable alternative. LP can overcome some of the difficulties of delivering MSCs in patients at the clinical setting. As a validation, a clinical trial performed by a Japanese group evaluated the effect of MSCs treatment in a single patient with a C5 fracture dislocation [92]. On day 13, he received an autologous MSC transplant via lumbar puncture and showed gradual improvement over the 6-month period in both motor and sensory scores graded according to the American Spinal Injury Association (ASIA) Scoring for International Standards for Neurological Classification of Spinal Cord Injury (ISNCSCI). Though this is a single case reported, it appears to be promising for the future of MSCs as an intervention in cervical SCI.

2.4. Sources of MSCs

2.4.1. From bone marrow stromal cells (BMSCs)

Bone marrow stem/stromal cells (BMSCs) are the most commonly used stem cell source for transplantation in experimental SCI models. These multipotent cells are derived from the heterogeneous stroma of bone marrow, which is also comprised of hematopoietic stem cells (HSC). MSCs are separated from other cells (like HSCs) by the expression of distinctive cell surface markers [53,67]. Though there has been much speculation about the transdifferentiation capacity of MSCs into neuronal and glial lineages [71,93], Hofstetter and colleagues reported that transplanted MSCs could not be induced to differentiate toward a neuronal fate, either *in vitro* or *in vivo,* in spite of the fact the MSCs displayed weak expression of NeuN (a neuronal marker) [94].

As one of the first identified sources of MSCs, BMSCs have been well studied for their anti-inflammatory, neurotrophic, and neuroprotective functions in SCI [95,96]. BMSCs transplanted into the rat spinal cord after a contusion injury demonstrated sensorimotor enhancements, partly due to their anti-inflammatory effects by attenuating activation of microglia and astrocytes [97]. To further support their therapeutic role in SCI, BMSC transplantation has been shown to reduce cavity formation, enhance axonal growth, and also prevent neuronal apoptosis [86]. While the majority of the studies have explored MSCs potential in a thoracic injury model, very few studies demonstrate their effect in a cervical SCI model; here we summarize studies relevant to cervical SCI.

One of the earliest studies to investigate transplantation within the cervical region investigated the use of rat-derived BMSCs in a combinatorial approach with cyclic adenosine monophosphate (cAMP; a neuronal stimulator) and neurotrophin-3 (NT-3; neurotrophic factor) [98]. Using a dorsal column injury as a model system, cAMP and NT-3 were injected 5 days prior to a C4 transection at L4 to precondition the DRG soma. BMSCs were then transplanted 7 days post injury. This combinatorial approach showed successful axon regeneration throughout and beyond the injury site after 12 weeks that was augmented by preconditioning with cAMP and NT-3. Despite this, functional recovery was not supported. The authors attribute the failure to the regenerating axons not reaching their target in the gracile nucleus, a major region that intercepts sensory information.

MSCs can secrete anti-inflammatory molecules and neurotrophic factors, which can lead to immunomodulation and tissue regeneration. In addition, they can also be engineered to secrete factors specific to CNS regeneration. In 2005, Lu and colleagues examined the ability of BMSCs to promote repair in the injured cord by secreting growth factors that overcome the inhibitory environment of the lesion [99]. Native or neurally induced rat-derived BMSCs were modified to either express human brain-derived neurotrophic factor (BDNF) in an acute injury or NT-3 in a chronic injury model [100]. By 1 month post transplantation within a C3 dorsal column lesion, BMSC grafts (both native and neurally induced) supported the growth of host and sensory motor axons, a finding that was augmented by either BDNF or NT-3 transduction. Transduction with neurotrophic factors substantially increased the number of coerulospinal, raphespinal, sensory, and motor axons penetrating the lesion site. Supporting these results, Novikova and colleagues transplanted BMSCs that were pretreated with Schwann-cell differentiating factors into a rat C4 hemisection model and demonstrated that BMSCs prestimulated to secrete neurotrophic factors can also contribute to inhibition of astrogliosis and the post-injury inflammatory response [101].

Another group investigated the combination of BMSCs with rat-derived neural progenitor cells (NPCs) co-transplanted in a rat C3 dorsal hemisection transection model [102]. As demyelination is a significant obstacle following SCI, the strategy was employed with the hypothesis that BMSCs would drive NPCs toward a mature oligodendrocyte lineage. In contrast with their *in vitro* data where BMSCs sufficiently redirected NPC differentiation toward an oligodendrocyte lineage, the group's *in vivo* data failed to demonstrate the same 6 weeks post transplant.

Human-derived BMSCs are a clinically attractive transplantation strategy because they can be reintroduced into patients as autografts or allografts. One preclinical study examined the transplantation of human-derived BMSCs from the iliac crest of four different healthy donors into a rat C3–C4 hemisection model [66]. Regardless of donor source, BMSCs survived and filled the lesion site with minimal migration and substantial axonal growth by 2 weeks post transplantation. By 11 weeks post transplant, no BMSCs were present within the lesion site, having been replaced by host oligodendroglial cells. Axonal infiltration into the lesion site and functional recovery varied by donor; however there was no direct correlation between the amount of axonal growth and forelimb function. One possible explanation for this is that individual donor-based distinctions in the secretory profile of BMSCs contributed to the varied outcome.

As challenging as the pitfalls within previous results may appear, there are currently two active clinical trials (Phase I NCT02574572 and Phase II/III NCT0167644) approved by the FDA to study the safety and efficacy of BMSCs transplanted in patients with chronic SCI. In conjunction with human studies, a clinical study tested the dose-dependent efficacy of autologous human-derived BMSCs in 13 patients with a mix of cervical (five patients) and thoracic (eight patients) chronic SCI. They found no deleterious effect on the patients; however only one of the 13 patients showed improvement [103]. It is possible that the absence of statistical significance can be attributed to the difference in observation of positive outcomes. For example, while one patient showed an improvement in motor power, two other patients had a patchy improvement in sensory outcome below the level of injury. At the chronic stage, the formation of glial scar tissue around the injury lesion is possibly too dense for growing axons to penetrate. While the transplantation of allogenic BMSCs was deemed safe in patients with chronic SCI, there is a need for preclinical studies to establish the mechanism of MSC's contributory role in chronic SCI.

While spinal cord injury models are in the majority represented by a contusion or hemisection injury, damage via herniated discs is also quite a common cause of disability. A herniated disc under traumatic events can lead to spinal cord injury. A discectomy is the surgical removal of the herniated nucleus pulposus of a vertebral disc to reduce pressure on the spinal cord or radiating nerves. Clinically, a discectomy is treated by fusing artificial prostheses to replace the intervertebral disc. In a preliminary proof-of-concept study utilizing an ovine model, one group sought to replicate the intervertebral disc by formulating allogeneic BMSCs with a chondrogenic agent, pentosan polysulfate, to form a cartilaginous matrix when implanted into the animal at the C3–C4 and C4–C5 levels [104]. The implant was devoid of any adverse events, and histological evidence showed predominantly cartilaginous tissue within the interbody cages. This was further confirmed by CT scans at 3 months post transplantation that showed significant bone formation in the cohort receiving BMSCs with pentosan polysulfate when compared to the cohort that received BMSCs alone. Although this particular study had its limitations, it further illustrates the potential for MSCs in preserving spinal function and advancing regenerative medicine.

2.4.2. *From adipose tissue (AMSCs)*

Adipose tissue is equally attractive as a cell therapy source, due to its minimally invasive harvesting procedure. From a clinical standpoint, adipose-derived stem cells (AMSCs) can easily be obtained from the large quantities of fat tissue that are removed by routine and safe procedures such as liposuction and abdominoplasties. Adipose tissue also contains supportive stroma that can be isolated and differentiated toward mesodermal lineages [105].

While a vast majority of the literature indicates that AMSCs support axonal growth, a study utilizing transplanted human-derived AMSCs in a rat C3–C4 hemisection was found to significantly reduce sprouting of the descending serotonergic fibers at the injured site [106]. The authors attributed this to several cumulative factors including enhanced survival of neurons and axons, attenuating the need for excessive sprouting, and reduced astroglial and microglial reactivity favoring the growth of the fibers into and across the transection site. Consistent with other MSC transplantation studies, there was no improvement in functional recovery despite promising microanatomical changes.

Use of AMSCs in humans has been validated for safety and toxicity in both a preclinical testing and a Phase I clinical trial [82]. It is important that every batch of stem cells prepared for transplantation into humans is processed under strict GMP conditions and the cultured cells are verified for absence of toxins and tumorigenic potential in preclinical testing. The purpose of this study was to evaluate any tumorigenic potential for hAMSCs. Twelve weeks post transplantation, the safety of transplanted AMSCs showed no significant difference in adverse events, ECG monitoring, and physical examinations. Though there was no statistical significance in ASIA score, individual patient scores showed improvement at different levels for motor and/or sensory assessment.

2.4.3. From human umbilical cord blood (UMSCs)

Human umbilical cord blood-derived MSCs (UMSCs) offer various therapeutic advantages in SCI treatment with reversal of SCI pathophysiology (downregulation of apoptotic genes and secretion of neurotrophic factors) in as little as 5 days post injury [107]. In an example using a thoracic SCI, transplantation of UMSCs was reported to have been transdifferentiated toward neuronal and oligodendroglial phenotypes. This was viewed as being a successful strategy as evidenced by improved functional motor outcome [86]. These transdifferentiated oligodendrocytes supported the injured spinal cord in remyelination by secreting neurotrophic factors [108]. UMSCs demonstrate a potential application in the treatment of SCI by their reported ability to transdifferentiate into neuronal lineages. For further information on UMSCs in thoracic injury, readers are referred to the review by Park and colleagues [109].

The first clinically based translational study to use UMSCs was in a rat model of radiation myelopathy, in which significant improvement of the microenvironment previously affected by radiation therapy was observed [110]. Radiation myelopathy is a rare, yet serious complication of cancer radiotherapy. Even though radiation myelopathy is not classified as a traditional SCI, there are many similarities in pathophysiology such as vascular damage and demyelination. This particular case study was relevant, as the group studied the efficacy of UMSCs in a radiation myelopathy model restricted to the cervical spine. Administration of the UMSCs clearly improved both microvessel and endothelial cell density, along with functional improvement in blood flow. Concurrent with other studies utilizing MSCs, UMSCs were able to reverse injury induced inflammation by reducing pro-inflammatory and increasing anti-inflammatory cytokines within the spinal cord. **Table 1** shows eight preclinical and clinical trials involving the transplantation of MSCs, describing study design, injury model, observed outcomes, and noted adverse effects.

Study and reference (PMID)	Study designs	Preclinical or clinical trials	Functional Observations	Histological/ imaging datas	Adverse events
Long-term results of spinal cord injury therapy using mesenchymal stem cells derived from bone marrow in humans (22127044)	Cells: autologous MSCs harvested from iliac bone Dosing: MSCs (8×10^6) directly injected into spinal cord and (4×10^7) were injected into intradural space Sample size: *N*=10 patients with ASIA class A or B injury caused by traumatic cervical SCI After 4 and 8 weeks of first injection, 5×10^7 injected via lumbar tapping Measurements: grading of motor power, MRI, electrophysiological recordings	Clinical	At 6-month follow-up: - Six out of 10 patients showed improvement in motor skills - Three out of 10 showed gradual improvement in daily activities	MRI showed a decrease in cavity size and the appearance of fiber-like low-signal intensity streaks	None observed
Intrathecal transplantation of autologous adipose-derived mesenchymal stem cells for treating spinal cord injury: a human trial (26208177)	Cells: autologous ADMSCs isolated from lipoaspirates of patient's subcutaneous fat tissue Dosing: 9×10^7 cells per patient intrathecally through lumbar tapping at day 1, 1 month, and 2 months Sample size: *N*=14 patients with 12 for ASIA A, 1 for B, 1 for D Six patients were injured at cervical, 1 at cervicothoracic, 6 at thoracic, and 1 at lumbar levels Measurements: MRI, hematological	Clinical	At 8-month follow-up: - ASIA motor score was improved in five patients - ASIA sensory score was improved in 10 patients - Voluntary and contraction improvement was seen in two patients - One patient showed median nerve improvement in somatosensory	MRI: no significant interval change for presence of tumorous growth EEG: no significant change after transplantation	Urinary tract infection, headache, nausea, and vomiting were observed in three patients

Study and reference (PMID)	Study designs	Preclinical or clinical trials	Functional Observations	Histological/ imaging datas	Adverse events
	parameters, electrophysiology ASIA motor/sensory scores were assessed before and after transplantation		evoked potential test		
Chronic spinal cord injury treated with transplanted autologous bone marrow-derived mesenchymal stem cells tracked by magnetic resonance imaging: a case report (25885347)	Cells: BM-derived MSCs retrieved from iliac crest were labeled with superparamagnetic iron oxide nanoparticles Dosing: intrathecal transplantation into lumbar spine with 30×10^6 cells (50:50 ratio of both labeled and unlabeled cells) After transplantation, the patient was placed in the Trendelenburg position for 24 hours Sample size: N=1 patient with an incomplete SCI from the atlantoaxial subluxation	Clinical	- ASIA B score did not change over 12 months - At 2 days, 6 months, and 12 months post operative, both upper and lower limbs motor score had not changes from preoperative levels - Light touch and pin prick test also did not change	MRI: showed positive signal from labeled cells in the cervical region after 48 hours No change at the structural level of injured spinal cord at any follow-up	After transplantation, patient experienced fever, headache, and myalgia with increased neurologic pain after 12 months
Transplantation of autologous bone marrow mesenchymal stem cells in the treatment of complete and chronic cervical spinal cord injury (23948102)	Cells: prepared from BM collected from iliac spine Dosing: 8×10^5 cells/μl in 25 μl slowly injected to a depth of 3 mm at multiple sites in the central dorsal area across the junction of injured and uninjured spinal cord Sample size: N=40 patients with complete and chronic cervical SCI divided into control and treatment groups	Clinical	- Ten patients from treatment group showed significant clinical improvement in motor, sensory, and residual urine volume - Nine patients showed changes in AIS scores - Eight out of 20 patients in the treatment group	N/A	One or two patients in the treatment group developed fever and reported headaches

Study and reference (PMID)	Study designs	Preclinical or clinical trials	Functional Observations	Histological/ imaging datas	Adverse events
			showed significant improvement in postoperative EMG		
Localized delivery of brain-derived neurotrophic factor-expressing mesenchymal stem cells enhances functional recovery following cervical spinal cord injury (25093762)	Cells: WT-MSCs or BDNF-MSCs MSCs derived from BM of adult transgenic rats expressing GFP and transduced with murine leukemia virus encoding BDNF MSCs characterized by cell surface expression of CD105 and lack of CD45 Dosing: 2 × 10⁵ cells injected intraspinally at C2 at time of injury Measurements: immunohistochemistry, electromyogram (EMG)	Preclinical: unilateral spinal cord hemisection at C2 in Sprague-Dawley rats; male	N/A	Retrograde labeling with CTB showed localization of MSCs near injection site and primarily in the white matter At day 14 after transplantation, all rats treated with BDNF-MSCs showed functional recovery of diaphragm	N/A
Bone morphogenetic proteins prevent bone marrow stromal cell-mediated oligodendroglial differentiation of transplanted adult neural progenitor cells in the injured spinal cord (23770801)	Cells: NPC isolated from sub-ventricular zone and BMSC isolated from bone marrow Dosing: immediately following the transection, cell suspensions (2 μl) containing either only BMSCs (0.6×10^5 BMSCs/μl; N=5), only NPCs (1.8 × 105 NPCs/μl; N=5), or a mixture of NPCs and BMSCs (1.2×10^5 NPCs/μl mixed with 0.3×10^5 BMSCs/μl; N =6) were administered by a single injection into	Preclinical: C3 complete transection in adult female Fischer 344 rats	None	In vitro assays demonstrate blocking of BMP signaling enables BMSC-induced differentiation of NPCs to oligodendrocytes	

Study and reference (PMID)	Study designs	Preclinical or clinical trials	Functional Observations	Histological/ imaging datas	Adverse events
	the center of the lesion site				
Neuroprotective and growth-promoting effects of bone marrow stromal cells after cervical spinal cord injury in adult rats (21521004)	Cells: harvested from femur and tibia of rats and differentiated to a Schwann-cell phenotype Dosing: 10–12 × 10^6 cells were injected into lateral funiculus at approx. 1 mm from the rostral and caudal site to the lesion Measurements: immunohistochemistry	Preclinical: C4 hemisection in Sprague-Dawley rats; female	N/A	At 6–8 weeks: NF-positive fibers, serotonin-positive raphespinal axons and CGRP sensory axons were seen in the injured cord	N/A
Grafting of human bone marrow stromal cells into spinal cord injury: a comparison of delivery methods (19182705)	Cells: frozen hMSC thawed and transplanted Dosing: animal groups received either 1 × 10^6 cells transplanted via LP or IV or 1.5 × 10^5 cells directly at injury site Measurements: histology, immunohistochemistry	Preclinical: right subtotal hemisection at C4–C5 Sprague-Dawley rats; female	N/A	Cells delivered via LP showed: - Early tissue sparing in immunostaining for GFAP - Reduced host immune response staining for ED1 (macrophage) and CD5 (pan T-cell marker)	N/A

Table 1. Tabulated summary of preclinical and clinical trials involving the transplantation of MSCs; for each trial the study design, injury model, observed outcomes and adverse effects are described.

3. Embryonic-derived stem cells (ESCs)

3.1. Derivation of embryonic stem cells

Embryonic stem cells (ESCs) represent an intriguing avenue to pursue in the race to understand and treat neurodegenerative pathophysiology. Their pluripotency makes them an extremely versatile option when compared to the limitations of MSCs, and the basic cell culture techniques governing them have been established for decades. ESCs are pluripotent cells derived from the inner cell mass harvested at the embryonic blastocyst stage. Unlike multipotent stem cells, such as MSCs, that are limited to mesoderm lineages, ESCs have the ability to give rise to all three germ layer lineages: the ectoderm, endoderm, and mesoderm. The capacity to generate neuronal lineages under directed conditioning makes them an ideal target for cell-based therapies of the nervous system [111–113]. Furthermore, ESCs possess the ability to self-renew, a key characteristic of stem cells that allows for a potentially indefinite source of cells.

ESCs were first harvested and cultured in the early 1980s from murine sources and eventually followed by human sources in the late 1990s [113–116]. Key differences in the *in vitro* culturing of these cells were responsible for the almost 20-year gap between the successful harvesting of murine versus human-derived ESCs. Murine ESCs are capable of surviving without the support of fibroblast feeder layers but require the addition of leukemia inhibitory factor (LIF). This led to earlier xeno-free expansion and characterization than human sources, which were later found to rely on the addition of fibroblast growth factor (FGF) to retain their pluripotency and stem cell characteristics [117].

Despite the positive attributes of ESCs, there are certain shortcomings that cannot be overlooked. Current research utilizing human-derived ESCs is still limited by the lack of chemically defined, *in vitro* culture conditions and is often dependent on the extracellular matrix and growth factor support of Matrigel substrates [118–120]. Additionally, the harvesting and culture of human-derived ESCs raise ethical concerns and extended culturing has been debated to lead to karyotypic stability. *In vivo* use of ESCs often leads to teratoma formation and the need for immunosuppressant drugs, all of which pose a problem for usage in clinical studies [111,121–123]. Current research strategies have centered around developing high-efficiency, high-purity differentiation protocols in order to generate committed or progenitor cell populations that limit their teratogenicity and enhance their therapeutic potential.

3.2. The regenerative potential of ESCs

In treating SCI, groups have looked to generate neural and glial-specific lineages such as oligodendrocytes, astrocytes, and neurons from ESCs. The majority of differentiation protocols lead to high astrocyte and oligodendrocyte populations and relatively few neurons, likely due to the proliferative capacity of the supporting glial cell types compared to neurons [40,111,124–126]. Differentiation methods developed by the McDonald and Keirstead groups have extensively researched the high-efficiency generation of oligodendrocyte progenitor cells (OPCs), which have proven useful in improving myelination and functional outcomes of increased weight support and partial hindlimb gait coordination after thoracic SCI [40,127–131].

Elegantly designed directed differentiation protocols from the Jessell research group using retinoic acid and sonic hedgehog have led to generation of spinal motor neurons from ESCs, which expressed progenitor motor neuron (pMN) marker Olig2 followed by classic motor neuron markers, Isl1, Hb9, and choline acetyltransferase (ChAT) [132]. When grafted into embryonic day 27 chick spinal cords, these cells have shown integration into the ventral spinal cord and acquire appropriate native motor pool identities [132,133], indicating a potential cell source for lost motor neuron pools after SCI. The Keirstead group has also investigated the spontaneous differentiation of human ESC-derived neural progenitor cells (NPCs) into various neuronal phenotypes such as cholinergic, serotonergic, dopaminergic (DA) and/or noradrenergic, and medium spiny striatal neurons [130,134]. Unfortunately, when ES-derived NPCs are transplanted as a heterogenic population, over-proliferation of undifferentiated stem cells can occur and potentially lead to tumor formation [135]. Further research has investigated the ways to mitigate this over-proliferation through antibiotic selection in order to generate high-purity progenitor motor neurons and committed motor neuron populations [136–138].

The first study to demonstrate that stem cells could be induced toward a cortical projection lineage utilized murine ES cells [139]. Appropriate culture conditions and *in vitro* patterning led to the generation of neural precursor cells that initially express forebrain progenitor-specific genes and later features of cortical pyramidal neurons. Most interestingly, transplantation of these cultures into various locations in the mouse brain led to area-specific axonal and dendritic growth, connectivity and integration within the host CNS, and axon extension to developmentally appropriate targets. These results suggest that it is possible to drive stem cells toward committed neural subtypes that can integrate into anatomically relevant circuits *in vivo*.

With all of these various cell populations, numerous cell-based treatment strategies for SCI have been investigated; however the overwhelming majority of these studies have been completed in thoracic injury models. Despite cervical injuries comprising more than 50% of the SCI population, very little preclinical research has been completed to date in this representative model [111].

3.3. Treating cervical SCI with ESCs

The first study to use embryonic-derived stem cells for therapy in a cervical SCI model was from Sharp and colleagues, looking at the use of human ESC-derived OPCs in a severe midline contusion cervical SCI rat model [140]. The hESC-derived OPCs used in this study were derived using the same protocol [130,131,141,142] as those used in earlier thoracic injury models from the Keirstead group [39,142] and in the Geron™-sponsored, clinical trial (first to use human ESCs as a therapeutic) that was halted in 2011 due to financial and safety concerns [143,144]. This study found that transplanting hESC-derived OPCs 7 days post injury led to a decrease in lesion area accompanied by robust white and gray matter sparing 8 weeks post transplant. Transplanted cells remained localized within the lesion epicenter with minimal rostral or caudal migration. Notably, the preservation of endogenous motor neurons was correlated with increased forelimb function. Finally, the use of transplanted hESC-derived OPCs led to differential changes in spinal cord gene expression for neurons, growth factors, apoptosis, and inflammation [140]. As such, injured animals with transplanted cells saw gene expression levels more closely matching their uninjured counterparts when compared to transplant-naïve animals. Since the discontinuation of the Geron™-sponsored thoracic injury clinical trial, Asterias Biotherapeutics, Inc., has undertaken the use of hESC AST-OPC1 cells for clinical use in a new Phase I/IIa efficacy and safety trial for cervical-level injuries (NCT02302157).

While most of the literature utilizes acute injury models to study the intervention of stem cells, one group investigated the use of hESC-derived OPCs in a rat cervical chronic injury model. In the 2013 study by Sun and colleagues, Olig2+ GFP+ OPCs derived from mouse ESCs were transplanted 4 months post rat cervical irradiation injury [145]. The irradiation injury model is a chronic injury commonly caused by radiotherapy for cancer treatment that results in the death of oligodendrocytes, which leads to severe demyelination and increased axon death. By 8 weeks post transplant, there was significantly less demyelination in addition to improved forelimb locomotor function using a clinical degree of weakness scale. Transplanted hESC-OPCs differentiated primarily into mature oligodendrocytes that expressed myelin basic protein. These cells were produced using a retinoic acid/sonic hedgehog differentiation protocol similar to the ones developed by the Jessell and Zhang groups [132,146].

The Keirstead group has also exploited the potential for ESCs to differentiate into neural lineages for use in cervical SCI treatments. They demonstrated successful use of hESC-derived progenitor motor neurons (pMNs) in a cervical SCI contusion model. The pMNs were generated using a retinoic acid differentiation protocol over 28 days and were shown to be Olig1/2+, as well as Tuj1 and Hb9 positive. Electrophysiology of these cells indicated glutamate receptors after 8 weeks in culture and could innervate both human and rodent muscle tissues. *In vivo*, reduced SCI pathology, or lesion size, and greater endogenous neuron survival and growth were observed in hESC-pMN transplanted spinal cords. Furthermore, these outcomes correlated with increased functional recovery on the balance beam task [147]. The authors did note, however, that differentiation of transplanted cells was dependent on location. Cells that were found in the distal ventral horn led to increased differentiation, whereas cells confined to the site of injury reverted to a progenitor state.

Other embryonic or fetal-derived tissues have been used in spinal cord injury therapies, including whole fetal spinal cord transplants (pioneered by Reier and Anderson) and fetal neural progenitor/stem cells taken from brain and spinal tissue [51,111,123,148–157]. In the study by Diener and Bregman, transplantation of fetal spinal cord tissues into cervical hemisections led to supraspinal growth, axon projections, improved skilled forelimb function indicating transplanted cell survival, and potential local circuit formation. Further investigation of fetal spinal cord lineage-restricted NPCs by various groups has indicated differentiation of transplanted cells into all three neural lineages, in both cervical and thoracic level injuries, with long distance cell migration and axon growth leading to functional improvement [123,148–151,158]. Two clinical trials have begun since 2013 investigating the use of fetal-derived tissues for spinal cord injury [144]. StemCells, Inc.® have begun a safety and efficacy study using human-derived CNS-stem cells (proprietary source) in cervical SCI after completing a thoracic injury trial [159]. Neuralstem, Inc., is also investigating the use of fetal stem cells in SCI [160,161] after promising results using such cells in ALS treatment. This trial, however, is determining the efficacy of these cells in a thoracic injury model. While these cells have proven useful in improving functional outcomes after SCI in preclinical trials, they are subject to the same ethical concerns as those for ESCs and have limited differentiation capacity in comparison [162].

In treating SCI, ESCs demonstrate great potential in promoting axon regeneration and functional recovery, but the lack of full characterization of cell safety, efficacy, and phenotype has significantly limited their clinical applications. Furthermore, the use of ESCs in cervical SCI models is limited to less than a handful of peer-reviewed studies. As cervical injuries are becoming more prevalent, future studies must be designed that better replicate clinical injuries in order to more accurately test cell therapeutic strategies.

4. Induced pluripotent stem cells (iPSCs)

4.1. Derivation of iPSCs

Induced pluripotent stem cells (iPSCs) are created by reprogramming adult somatic fibroblasts to revert to a pluripotent stem cell state initially via retroviral delivery of Oct3/4, Sox2, c-Myc, and Klf4 [163–165]. Now iPSCs can be generated via multiple processes, each with its own merits and limitations. Viral transduction is easy to use and reproducible, yields iPSCs efficiently, and is controlled. However there is an increased risk of insertional mutagenesis and transgene reactivation, incomplete splicing, and clone-to-clone variation [166–168]. Reprogramming factors can also be fused to cell-penetrating peptides or introduced through plasmids, which requires no genomic modification but is also a time consuming and potentially inefficient process [169]. Finally iPSCs can be induced via mRNA introduction, which is a highly effective and rapid method; it also requires no genomic modification and is deemed safe due to the transient nature of mRNA. However, repeated transfections are typically required [170,171].

While MSCs are hindered by their limited potency and the harvesting of ESCs is subject to ethical constraints, the pluripotency and source of iPSCs circumvent some of these issues, therefore making them a promising alternative in cellular transplantation therapies. iPSCs share many similarities with ESCs and provide a comparative alternative in that they have the same morphology, gene markers, and potential to form teratomas (ability to differentiate into all three germ layers) [163,165]. Furthermore, the use of iPSCs opens up new possibilities for clinical consideration—ethical concerns are diminished and, in the case of potential transplants, cells can be harvested directly from the patient, therefore avoiding the need for immunosuppression.

4.2. Cell reprogramming technologies for controlled differentiation

There has been a strong motivation to create iPSC differentiation protocols that drive stem cells toward the three main neural lineages *in vitro*. Methods to generate functional neurons have been of particular interest so as to study the differences in neuronal networks in both healthy and impaired states [172–177]. In one report, mature human fibroblasts were directly programmed into synaptically active functional neurons via a cocktail of miR-124, BRN2, and MYT1L [178]. An additional group found that Ascl1 (which has pioneer factor properties) in conjunction with BRN2, and MYT1L, successfully drove murine fibroblasts into neuronal cells with appropriate morphology, expression, and formation of functional synapses [179]. One report demonstrated that the overexpression of neurogenin 2 efficiently transformed iPSCs into functional neurons that were able to spontaneously form excitatory synaptic networks. Furthermore, these networks both synaptically integrate once transplanted into the mouse brain and exhibit plasticity [180]. The majority of research utilizes iPSCs driven toward a neural progenitor state [181,182]; however iPSC differentiation has also been useful in disease modeling. As an example, midbrain dopaminergic (DA) neuron phenotypes have been generated, which has been particularly useful in studying Parkinson's disease (PD), typically characterized by the loss of these DA neurons [183–186]. In one study by the Pera group, a stable iPSC line was derived from a PD patient that carried the most common PD-associated genetic mutation and differentiated into midbrain DA neurons. These iPSC-derived DA neurons exhibited classic hallmarks of PD-related damage including accumulation of α-synuclein and oxidative stress, susceptibility to H_2O_2-induced CASP3 activation, and sensitivity to 6-OHDA and proteasome inhibition. Additionally, other groups have shown that iPSCs can be successfully driven toward glutamatergic, GABAergic, motor, and retinal neuron phenotypes [187–199]. While not specific to SCI, these results demonstrate that developing differentiation protocols capable of generating specific neural subtypes can open up new research avenues in understanding and creating therapies for neuropathologies.

There is also interest in reliably driving iPSCs toward functional glial subtypes, as glial cells are heavily affected in the process of neurodegeneration. In a study by Krencik and Zhang, exogenous patterning molecules were used to transform iPSCs into a neuroepithelial phenotype. From there, administration of mitogens allowed for the generation of astroglial progenitors, which could then be further differentiated into functional astrocytes via ciliary neurotrophic factor [200]. Another protocol utilized the forced expression of Sox10, Olig2, and Zfb536 to directly reprogram rodent fibroblasts into oligodendrocyte precursor cells. The resulting population of precursors exhibited typical morphology and gene expression and gave rise to mature oligodendrocytes that could ensheath dorsal root ganglion cells *in vitro* and form myelin *in vivo* [201].

The intended goal behind SCI therapies is to ameliorate damage and restore the circuitry within the CNS. Cellular transplantation offers an innovative means in accomplishing this, but is obviously extremely dependent upon the characteristics and capabilities of the transplanted cell type. Driving human iPSCs toward neuronal lineages via reproducible and robust differentiation protocols represents a practical interface between developmental neurobiology and SCI research; it may be possible to tailor iPSCs toward a more developmentally appropriate, specific neuronal cell type capable of restoring CNS connectivity rather than the uncharacterized progenitor populations previously used with limited functional recovery.

4.3. Treating cervical SCI with iPSCs

Similar to MSC and ESC-focused SCI therapies, there is a scarcity of targeted preclinical therapies for SCI using iPSC transplantation. Therapies do show positive outcomes yet they are limited in number; to date there are only five published studies using either rodent or

http://dx.doi.org/10.5772/63580

simian models of thoracic SCI [202]. In these studies, iPSCs were driven toward neural stem spheres [203], neural stem cells (NSCs) [202,204], and neurospheres [205,206] with all except one study experiencing amelioration of the inhibitory nature of the lesion site, synaptic integration of transplanted cells, and significant functional improvement in transplanted animals.

Therapies targeting cervical SCI are equally as limited. There are four published studies to date that have examined acute, subacute, and chronic iPSC transplantation following cervical SCI. Li and colleagues evaluated respiratory function following transplantation of iPSC-derived astrocytes engineered to overexpress GLT1, an astroglial glutamate transporter [207]. Both rats and mice underwent a C4 contusion injury resulting in chronic diaphragm dysfunction and phrenic motor neuron deterioration. Immediately post injury, subjects received two separate intraspinal injections rostral and caudal to the lesion within the ventral horn. At time points ranging from 2 days to 4 weeks post transplant, it was demonstrated that transplanted grafts survived and differentiated into GFAP-positive astrocytes, were not tumorigenic, and had less than 10% proliferation (evidenced by Ki67 staining). Furthermore, lesion area and volume were reduced within 1 mm rostral and caudal to the lesion epicenter and innervation of the diaphragm neuromuscular junction was preserved in animals that had received iPSC-derived astrocyte transplants that overexpressed GLT1. Through analysis of spontaneous electromyogram (EMG) activity, GLT1-overexpressing astrocyte transplants significantly magnified EMG amplitude in the dorsal region of the hemidiaphragm, further demonstrating preservation of diaphragmatic respiratory function.

Another study by Lu and colleagues examined the effect of human iPSC-derived NSCs harvested from an elderly donor in a C5 lateral hemisection rat model [208]. While the chosen cell population was minimally characterized, *in vitro* analysis demonstrated reduced expression of Tra1-81 and SSEA4 (pluripotency markers) and maintained expression of nestin and Sox2 (NSC-associated markers). Two weeks post injury, NSCs were intraspinally co-transplanted with a fibrin matrix and a raft of growth factors. By 3 months post transplantation, there was evidence that the grafted cells had survived, distributed throughout the lesion, and integrated with host axons. The majority of grafted cells expressed NeuN and mature neuronal markers MAP2 and Tuj1 alongside mature astrocytic marker GFAP, suggesting preferential differentiation into neuronal and astrocytic lineages. There was also evidence of proliferation and spinal motor neuron identity within a small percentage of transplanted cells via the expression of Ki67 and ChAT, respectively. Most notably, a remarkable amount of axonal growth was present extending from the lesion site toward the olfactory bulbs and lumbar spine sections. Despite robust axonal growth, no behavioral recovery was observed.

In consideration of the substantial lack of existing chronic cervical SCI data, Nutt and colleagues investigated an early chronic injury model mimicking the deficits seen in human injury [209]. Four weeks following a cervical contusion injury at C4, iPSC-derived neural progenitor cells and fibroblasts were co-transplanted rostral and caudal to the lesion in a rat model. Immunohistochemical analysis suggested the differentiation of transplanted cells into mature neurons as well as the intermingling of the host CNS with transplanted cells, as evidenced by NeuN/FOX-3 labeling. Despite interactions between host and donor cells, transplanted cells did not express glutamate receptors. Furthermore, transplanted cells were not positive for serotonin but did express GABA and were shown co-localized with host positive choline acetyltransferase. Behavioral recovery was weak; grasping and weight bearing were only slightly improved by transplants.

	MSCs	ESCs	iPSCs
Source	Bone marrow, adipose, umbilical cord	Fetal tissue	Somatic (adult) cells
Lineage differentiation	Mesodermal lineage	All three germ layers—endoderm, mesoderm, and ectoderm	All three germ layers—endoderm, mesoderm, and ectoderm
Derivation	Purified by surface markers from adult tissue	Embryonic (inner cell mass of blastocyst)	Induced or reprogrammed to "stemness"
Ease of isolation	Easily accessible sources	Difficult; isolated from fetal tissue	Easily accessible sources (e.g., skin)
Differentiation potential	Multipotent	Pluripotent	Pluripotent
Ethical issues	Minimal; cells can be isolated from the patient	Strong concerns	Minimal; even skin cells can be induced to be pluripotent
Axonal regrowth	Yes; by tissue sparing and neuroprotection	Yes; by transdifferentiation	Yes; by transdifferentiation
Functional outcome	Mild to moderate	Moderate	Mild to moderate
Immunomodulatory	Yes	Low	Low
Immunogenicity/ autologous	Low; safe for autologous transplantation	High; often requires immunosuppression	Low; safe for autologous transplantation
Tumorigenicity	No tumor formation	Teratoma formation	Teratoma formation
Clinical trial	Advanced to Phase III	Advanced to Phase II	Preclinical only

Table 2. A comparative scheme of the characteristics of MSCs, ESCs and iPSCs described in this chapter.

In contrast, Kobayashi and colleagues examined the safety and efficacy of iPSC-derived NSC transplants in a simian model of cervical SCI [210]. Human iPSCs were cultured and induced to form neurospheres and passaged a secondary and tertiary time prior to transplantation. Adult female marmosets were given a moderate contusion at the C5 level and received an intraspinal injection of cultured iPSC-neurospheres 9 days post injury at the lesion site. By 12 weeks post transplant, hematoxylin-eosin staining revealed that the grafted cells survived and were positive for NeuN, GFAP, and Olig 1 indicating differentiation into all three neural subtypes. Additionally, animals that received transplants had reduced cystic cavity size, no evidence of tumorigenicity, increased angiogenesis, and a higher amount of neurofilaments and descending motor axons at the lesion center. Severe demyelination was evident surrounding the lesion site in both transplanted and control groups; however, the amount was significantly exacerbated in animals that did not receive cellular transplantation. These findings were further supported by MRI and myelin mapping in which myelin sparing was more evident in the transplanted group and an intramedullary high-signal intensity area in the lesion site of the control group. Calcitonin-generated peptide fibers, which are involved in spinal pain mechanisms, did not differ between transplanted and control groups. In nonhuman primates, contusion at the C5 level in a severed central cord injury model leads to tetraplegia with an expected gradual improvement in motor function. By 8 weeks post injury, there were significant differences in the open field test, bar grip strength test, and cage climbing tests between transplanted and control groups, which stayed consistent throughout the study indicating some level of functional recovery due to transplantation. Promising results from the various cell-based therapies have demonstrated varying degrees of axonal regeneration and functional recovery. **Table 2** provides a summary of the characteristics of MSC, ESC, and iPSC types and also notes their functional outcomes, tumorigenicity, and clinical trial stage to date.

5. Summary and conclusions

Great care and consideration must be taken when choosing an optimal stem cell type as a potential cellular transplantation treatment for cervical SCIs. Of the three main stem cell types discussed here, there are distinct advantages and disadvantages to each. The use of MSCs in treating nervous system injuries remains a hotly debated topic due to their limited survival, differentiation potential, and functional recovery outcomes. Nevertheless, their immunomodulatory properties and growth factor secretion make them potentially beneficial for use in combinatorial strategies especially if delivered noninvasively. ESCs offer significantly more differentiation potential for neural applications than adult stem cells and have the added benefit of promoting functional recovery in cervical SCI models. However, the lack of detailed cell characterization, need for immunosuppression, and overall ethical concerns have led to only a single cervical SCI clinical trial. Moreover, the use of ESCs in preclinical cervical SCI studies is limited to only two ESC-derived phenotypes (OPCs and pMNs). Significant research must still be performed to fully explore alternative appropriate cell types that can potentially promote functional regeneration. Finally iPSCs, the newest technology in stem cell sources, propose an interesting alternative to fate-limited MSCs and ethically restricted ESCs in treating cervical SCI. Promising preclinical data has indicated iPSC-based therapies can improve functional outcomes after injury; however, their recent discovery highlights the need for careful characterization and exploration of secure differentiation protocols. Further studies must still be completed before iPSCs can be approved for clinical applications.

While stem cell transplantation therapies have shown promise in promoting post-injury regeneration, both anatomical and functional recovery still remain imperfect; no preclinical or clinical study to date has dramatically restored significant recovery in patients. Experimental evidence has shown that native regeneration and plasticity occur in limited amounts following injury. These innate processes can be enhanced via the addition of neurotrophic and immunomodulatory factors, the removal of lesion-associated inhibitory factors, and injury-appropriate rehabilitation regimens and physical activity. It would be of great interest to determine whether combinatorial approaches utilizing stem cell transplantation in conjunction with the strategies described above provides a synergistic effect within the living system. Furthermore, the vast majority of cell transplantation studies utilize cell populations driven toward immature final phenotypes. The pluripotent capabilities of ESCs and iPSCs provide the freedom to drive these cell types toward numerous definitive lineages or ages. This, however, will be defined by developing appropriate differentiation protocols that can be used in both preclinical and clinical settings. It is possible that transplanting more mature cells results in the establishment and integration of meaningful circuitry within the host nervous system to restore and promote functional recovery.

The broad scope of stem cell therapies offers a myriad of therapeutic potential. However, due to the limited number of preclinical and clinical studies, extensive logistical questions remain regarding how to optimize their usage. Nonetheless, the great strides made in designing and improving effective stem cell therapies for enhancing function promises an exciting future for the field of spinal cord injury repair.

Author details

Vanessa M. Doulames, Laura M. Marquardt, Bhavaani Jayaram, Christine D. Plant and Giles W. Plant*

*Address all correspondence to: gplant@stanford.edu

Department of Neurosurgery, Stanford University School of Medicine, Stanford, CA, USA

References

[1] Cahill, A., et al. *One Degree of Separation: Paralysis and Spinal Cord Injury in the United States*, 2009, Christopher and Dana Reeves Paralysis Resource Center, p. 1–28.

[2] National Spinal Cord Injury Statistical Center. *Facts and Figures at a Glance*, 2015, University of Alabama at Birmingham: Birmingham, AL.

[3] Wagner, C.S. and A.R. Lehman, *Cervical spine and neck injuries*, in *Musculoskeletal Injuries in the Military*, L.K. Cameron and D.B. Owens, Editors, 2016, Springer New York: New York, NY, p. 229–45.

[4] Breeze, J., et al., *Defining combat helmet coverage for protection against explosively propelled fragments*. J R Army Med Corps, 2015. 161(1): p. 9–13.

[5] Inoue, T., et al., *Combined SCI and TBI: recovery of forelimb function after unilateral cervical spinal cord injury (SCI) is retarded by contralateral traumatic brain injury (TBI), and ipsilateral TBI balances the effects of SCI on paw placement*. Exp Neurol, 2013. 248: p. 136–47.

[6] Yoganandan, N., et al., *Cervical spine injury biomechanics: applications for under body blast loadings in military environments*. Clin Biomech (Bristol, Avon), 2013. 28(6): p. 602–9.

[7] Ropper, A.E., M.T. Neal, and N. Theodore, *Acute management of traumatic cervical spinal cord injury*. Pract Neurol, 2015. 15(4): p. 266–72.

[8] Laing, A.C., et al., *The effects of age on the morphometry of the cervical spinal cord and spinal column in adult rats: an MRI-based study*. Anat Rec (Hoboken), 2014. 297(10): p. 1885–95.

[9] Tetreault, L., et al., *Degenerative cervical myelopathy: a spectrum of related disorders affecting the aging spine*. Neurosurgery, 2015. 77(Suppl 4): p. S51–67.

[10] Wang, T.Y., et al., *Risk assessment and characterization of 30-day perioperative myocardial infarction following spine surgery: a retrospective analysis of 1346 consecutive adult patients*. Spine (Phila Pa 1976), 2016. 41(5): p. 438–44.

[11] Satyanand, V., et al., *Effects of yogasanas on cervical spondylosis*. IAIM, 2015. 2(7): p. 6–10.

[12] Smith, H.E., et al., *Spine care: evaluation of the efficacy and cost of emerging technology*. Am J Med Qual, 2009. 24(6 Suppl): p. 25S–31S.

[13] Gensel, J.C., et al., *Behavioral and histological characterization of unilateral cervical spinal cord contusion injury in rats*. J Neurotrauma, 2006. 23(1): p. 36–54.

[14] Peitzman, A.B., *The trauma manual: trauma and acute care surgery*. 4th ed, C.W.S.M. Rhodes, D.M. Yealy, T.C. Fabian, and A.B. Peitzman, Editors, 2012, Lippincott Williams & Wilkins. Philidelphia. 4th Ed. 2012. pgs:1–824

[15] Sabapathy, V., G. Tharion, and S. Kumar, *Cell therapy augments functional recovery subsequent to spinal cord injury under experimental conditions*. Stem Cells Int, 2015. 2015: p. 132172.

[16] Newman, M.F., L.A. Fleisher, and M.P. Fink, *Perioperative Medicine: Managing for Outcome*, 2008, Elsevier Health Sciences. United States. 2007. pgs:1–752

[17] Ramer, L.M., M.S. Ramer, and J.D. Steeves, *Setting the stage for functional repair of spinal cord injuries: a cast of thousands*. Spinal Cord, 2005. 43(3): p. 134–61.

[18] Tator, C.H., *Biology of neurological recovery and functional restoration after spinal cord injury*. Neurosurgery, 1998. 42(4): p. 696–707; discussion 707-8.

[19] Beattie, M.S., A.A. Farooqui, and J.C. Bresnahan, *Review of current evidence for apoptosis after spinal cord injury*. J Neurotrauma, 2000. 17(10): p. 915–25.

[20] Donnelly, D.J. and P.G. Popovich, *Inflammation and its role in neuroprotection, axonal regeneration and functional recovery after spinal cord injury*. Exp Neurol, 2008. 209(2): p. 378–88.

[21] Dumont, R.J., et al., *Acute spinal cord injury, part I: pathophysiologic mechanisms.* Clin Neuropharmacol, 2001. 24(5): p. 254–64.

[22] Hausmann, O.N., *Post-traumatic inflammation following spinal cord injury.* Spinal Cord, 2003. 41(7): p. 369–78.

[23] Lu, J., K.W. Ashwell, and P. Waite, *Advances in secondary spinal cord injury: role of apoptosis.* Spine (Phila Pa 1976), 2000. 25(14): p. 1859–66.

[24] Mautes, A.E., et al., *Vascular events after spinal cord injury: contribution to secondary pathogenesis.* Phys Ther, 2000. 80(7): p. 673–87.

[25] Park, E., A.A. Velumian, and M.G. Fehlings, *The role of excitotoxicity in secondary mechanisms of spinal cord injury: a review with an emphasis on the implications for white matter degeneration.* J Neurotrauma, 2004. 21(6): p. 754–74.

[26] Horner, P.J. and F.H. Gage, *Regenerating the damaged central nervous system.* Nature, 2000. 407(6807): p. 963–70.

[27] Bernstein, J.J. and M.E. Bernstein, *Axonal regeneration and formation of synapses proximal to the site of lesion following hemisection of the rat spinal cord.* Exp Neurol, 1971. 30(2): p. 336–51.

[28] Ramer, M.S., J.V. Priestley, and S.B. McMahon, *Functional regeneration of sensory axons into the adult spinal cord.* Nature, 2000. 403(6767): p. 312–6.

[29] Bregman, B.S., et al., *Neurotrophic factors increase axonal growth after spinal cord injury and transplantation in the adult rat.* Exp Neurol, 1997. 148(2): p. 475–94.

[30] Grill, R., et al., *Cellular delivery of neurotrophin-3 promotes corticospinal axonal growth and partial functional recovery after spinal cord injury.* J Neurosci, 1997. 17(14): p. 5560–72.

[31] McTigue, D.M., et al., *Neurotrophin-3 and brain-derived neurotrophic factor induce oligodendrocyte proliferation and myelination of regenerating axons in the contused adult rat spinal cord.* J Neurosci, 1998. 18(14): p. 5354–65.

[32] Ye, J.H. and J.D. Houle, *Treatment of the chronically injured spinal cord with neurotrophic factors can promote axonal regeneration from supraspinal neurons.* Exp Neurol, 1997. 143(1): p. 70–81.

[33] Kim, G.M., et al., *Tumor necrosis factor receptor deletion reduces nuclear factor-kappaB activation, cellular inhibitor of apoptosis protein 2 expression, and functional recovery after traumatic spinal cord injury.* J Neurosci, 2001. 21(17): p. 6617–25.

[34] Nishio, Y., et al., *Deletion of macrophage migration inhibitory factor attenuates neuronal death and promotes functional recovery after compression-induced spinal cord injury in mice.* Acta Neuropathol, 2009. 117(3): p. 321–8.

[35] Simonen, M., et al., *Systemic deletion of the myelin-associated outgrowth inhibitor Nogo-A improves regenerative and plastic responses after spinal cord injury.* Neuron, 2003. 38(2): p. 201–11.

[36] Engesser-Cesar, C., et al., *Voluntary wheel running improves recovery from a moderate spinal cord injury.* J Neurotrauma, 2005. 22(1): p. 157–71.

[37] Hamid, S. and R. Hayek, *Role of electrical stimulation for rehabilitation and regeneration after spinal cord injury: an overview.* Eur Spine J, 2008. 17(9): p. 1256–69.

[38] Smith, R.R., et al., *Effects of swimming on functional recovery after incomplete spinal cord injury in rats.* J Neurotrauma, 2006. 23(6): p. 908–19.

[39] Keirstead, H.S., et al., *Human embryonic stem cell-derived oligodendrocyte progenitor cell transplants remyelinate and restore locomotion after spinal cord injury.* J Neurosci, 2005. 25(19): p. 4694–705.

[40] McDonald, J.W., et al., *Transplanted embryonic stem cells survive, differentiate and promote recovery in injured rat spinal cord.* Nat Med, 1999. 5(12): p. 1410–2.

[41] Popovich, P.G., et al., *Depletion of hematogenous macrophages promotes partial hindlimb recovery and neuroanatomical repair after experimental spinal cord injury.* Exp Neurol, 1999. 158(2): p. 351–65.

[42] Thuret, S., L.D. Moon, and F.H. Gage, *Therapeutic interventions after spinal cord injury.* Nat Rev Neurosci, 2006. 7(8): p. 628–43.

[43] Chopp, M., et al., *Spinal cord injury in rat: treatment with bone marrow stromal cell transplantation.* Neuroreport, 2000. 11(13): p. 3001–5.

[44] Barry, F.P. and J.M. Murphy, *Mesenchymal stem cells: clinical applications and biological characterization.* Int J Biochem Cell Biol, 2004. 36(4): p. 568–84.

[45] Carpenter, M.K., E. Rosler, and M.S. Rao, *Characterization and differentiation of human embryonic stem cells.* Cloning Stem Cells, 2003. 5(1): p. 79–88.

[46] Cummings, B.J., et al., *Human neural stem cells differentiate and promote locomotor recovery in spinal cord-injured mice.* Proc Natl Acad Sci U S A, 2005. 102(39): p. 14069–74.

[47] Plant, G.W., M.L. Bates, and M.B. Bunge, *Inhibitory proteoglycan immunoreactivity is higher at the caudal than the rostral Schwann cell graft-transected spinal cord interface.* Mol Cell Neurosci, 2001. 17(3): p. 471–87.

[48] Ramer, L.M., et al., *Peripheral olfactory ensheathing cells reduce scar and cavity formation and promote regeneration after spinal cord injury.* J Comp Neurol, 2004. 473(1): p. 1–15.

[49] Ruitenberg, M.J., et al., *Viral vector-mediated gene expression in olfactory ensheathing glia implants in the lesioned rat spinal cord.* Gene Ther, 2002. 9(2): p. 135–46.

[50] Snyder, E.Y. and Y.D. Teng, *Stem cells and spinal cord repair.* N Engl J Med, 2012. 366(20): p. 1940–2.

[51] Reier, P.J., B.S. Bregman, and J.R. Wujek, *Intraspinal transplantation of embryonic spinal cord tissue in neonatal and adult rats.* J Comp Neurol, 1986. 247(3): p. 275–96.

[52] Reubinoff, B.E., et al., *Neural progenitors from human embryonic stem cells.* Nat Biotechnol, 2001. 19(12): p. 1134–40.

[53] Hodgetts, S.I., P.J. Simmons, and G.W. Plant, *Human mesenchymal precursor cells (Stro-1(+)) from spinal cord injury patients improve functional recovery and tissue sparing in an acute spinal cord injury rat model.* Cell Transplant, 2013. 22(3): p. 393–412.

[54] Horwitz, E.M., et al., *Clarification of the nomenclature for MSC: The International Society for Cellular Therapy position statement.* Cytotherapy, 2005. 7(5): p. 393–5.

[55] Bianco, P., et al., *The meaning, the sense and the significance: translating the science of mesenchymal stem cells into medicine.* Nat Med, 2013. 19(1): p. 35–42.

[56] Dominici, M., et al., *Minimal criteria for defining multipotent mesenchymal stromal cells. The International Society for Cellular Therapy position statement.* Cytotherapy, 2006. 8(4): p. 315–7.

[57] Crisan, M., et al., *A perivascular origin for mesenchymal stem cells in multiple human organs.* Cell Stem Cell, 2008. 3(3): p. 301–13.

[58] Bai, L., et al., *Hepatocyte growth factor mediates mesenchymal stem cell-induced recovery in multiple sclerosis models.* Nat Neurosci, 2012. 15(6): p. 862–70.

[59] Honczarenko, M., et al., *Human bone marrow stromal cells express a distinct set of biologically functional chemokine receptors.* Stem Cells, 2006. 24(4): p. 1030–41.

[60] Friedenstein, A.J., R.K. Chailakhjan, and K.S. Lalykina, *The development of fibroblast colonies in monolayer cultures of guinea-pig bone marrow and spleen cells.* Cell Tissue Kinet, 1970. 3(4): p. 393–403.

[61] Friedenstein, A.J., et al., *Stromal cells responsible for transferring the microenvironment of the hemopoietic tissues. Cloning in vitro and retransplantation in vivo.* Transplantation, 1974. 17(4): p. 331–40.

[62] Pittenger, M.F., et al., *Multilineage potential of adult human mesenchymal stem cells.* Science, 1999. 284(5411): p. 143–7.

[63] Castro-Malaspina, H., et al., *Characterization of human bone marrow fibroblast colony-forming cells (CFU-F) and their progeny.* Blood, 1980. 56(2): p. 289–301.

[64] Goshima, J., V.M. Goldberg, and A.I. Caplan, *The osteogenic potential of culture-expanded rat marrow mesenchymal cells assayed in vivo in calcium phosphate ceramic blocks.* Clin Orthop Relat Res, 1991(262): p. 298–311.

[65] Simmons, P.J. and B. Torok-Storb, *Identification of stromal cell precursors in human bone marrow by a novel monoclonal antibody, STRO-1.* Blood, 1991. 78(1): p. 55–62.

[66] Neuhuber, B., et al., *Axon growth and recovery of function supported by human bone marrow stromal cells in the injured spinal cord exhibit donor variations.* Brain Res, 2005. 1035(1): p. 73–85.

[67] Kfoury, Y. and D.T. Scadden, *Mesenchymal cell contributions to the stem cell niche.* Cell Stem Cell, 2015. 16(3): p. 239–53.

[68] Hodgetts, S.I., P.J. Simmons, and G.W. Plant, *A comparison of the behavioral and anatomical outcomes in sub-acute and chronic spinal cord injury models following treatment with human mesenchymal precursor cell transplantation and recombinant decorin.* Exp Neurol, 2013. 248: p. 343–59.

[69] Gronthos, S., et al., *Surface protein characterization of human adipose tissue-derived stromal cells.* J Cell Physiol, 2001. 189(1): p. 54–63.

[70] Torres-Espin, A., et al., *Neuroprotection and axonal regeneration after lumbar ventral root avulsion by re-implantation and mesenchymal stem cells transplant combined therapy.* Neurotherapeutics, 2013. 10(2): p. 354–68.

[71] Uccelli, A., L. Moretta, and V. Pistoia, *Mesenchymal stem cells in health and disease.* Nat Rev Immunol, 2008. 8(9): p. 726–36.

[72] Bai, L., et al., *Human bone marrow-derived mesenchymal stem cells induce Th2-polarized immune response and promote endogenous repair in animal models of multiple sclerosis.* Glia, 2009. 57(11): p. 1192–203.

[73] Di Nicola, M., et al., *Human bone marrow stromal cells suppress T-lymphocyte proliferation induced by cellular or nonspecific mitogenic stimuli.* Blood, 2002. 99(10): p. 3838–43.

[74] Aggarwal, S. and M.F. Pittenger, *Human mesenchymal stem cells modulate allogeneic immune cell responses.* Blood, 2005. 105(4): p. 1815–22.

[75] Kong, Q.F., et al., *Administration of bone marrow stromal cells ameliorates experimental autoimmune myasthenia gravis by altering the balance of Th1/Th2/Th17/Treg cell subsets through the secretion of TGF-beta.* J Neuroimmunol, 2009. 207(1-2): p. 83–91.

[76] Tidball, J.G. and S.A. Villalta, *Regulatory interactions between muscle and the immune system during muscle regeneration.* Am J Physiol Regul Integr Comp Physiol, 2010. 298(5): p. R1173–87.

[77] Tollervey, J.R. and V.V. Lunyak, *Adult stem cells: simply a tool for regenerative medicine or an additional piece in the puzzle of human aging?* Cell Cycle, 2011. 10(24): p. 4173–6.

[78] Sekiya, I., et al., *Expansion of human adult stem cells from bone marrow stroma: conditions that maximize the yields of early progenitors and evaluate their quality.* Stem Cells, 2002. 20(6): p. 530–41.

[79] Kotobuki, N., et al., *Cultured autologous human cells for hard tissue regeneration: preparation and characterization of mesenchymal stem cells from bone marrow.* Artif Organs, 2004. 28(1): p. 33–9.

[80] Lee, M.W., et al., *Isolation of mesenchymal stem cells from cryopreserved human umbilical cord blood.* Int J Hematol, 2005. 81(2): p. 126–30.

[81] Lalu, M.M., et al., *Safety of cell therapy with mesenchymal stromal cells (SafeCell): a systematic review and meta-analysis of clinical trials.* PLoS One, 2012. 7(10): p. e47559.

[82] Ra, J.C., et al., *Safety of intravenous infusion of human adipose tissue-derived mesenchymal stem cells in animals and humans.* Stem Cells Dev, 2011. 20(8): p. 1297–308.

[83] Fouillard, L., et al., *Infusion of allogeneic-related HLA mismatched mesenchymal stem cells for the treatment of incomplete engraftment following autologous haematopoietic stem cell transplantation.* Leukemia, 2007. 21(3): p. 568–70.

[84] Marmont, A.M., et al., *Allogeneic bone marrow transplantation (BMT) for refractory Behcet's disease with severe CNS involvement.* Bone Marrow Transplant, 2006. 37(11): p. 1061–3.

[85] Parekkadan, B. and J.M. Milwid, *Mesenchymal stem cells as therapeutics.* Annu Rev Biomed Eng, 2010. 12: p. 87–117.

[86] Dasari, V.R., K.K. Veeravalli, and D.H. Dinh, *Mesenchymal stem cells in the treatment of spinal cord injuries: A review.* World J Stem Cells, 2014. 6(2): p. 120–33.

[87] Vawda, R. and M.G. Fehlings, *Mesenchymal cells in the treatment of spinal cord injury: current & future perspectives.* Curr Stem Cell Res Ther, 2013. 8(1): p. 25–38.

[88] White, S.V., et al., *Intravenous transplantation of mesenchymal progenitors distribute solely to the lungs and improve outcomes in cervical spinal cord injury.* Stem Cells, 2016. DOI: 10.1002/STEM.2364

[89] Lee, R.H., et al., *Intravenous hMSCs improve myocardial infarction in mice because cells embolized in lung are activated to secrete the anti-inflammatory protein TSG-6.* Cell Stem Cell, 2009. 5(1): p. 54–63.

[90] Zangi, L., et al., *Direct imaging of immune rejection and memory induction by allogeneic mesenchymal stromal cells.* Stem Cells, 2009. 27(11): p. 2865–74.

[91] Paul, C., et al., *Grafting of human bone marrow stromal cells into spinal cord injury: a comparison of delivery methods.* Spine (Phila Pa 1976), 2009. 34(4): p. 328–34.

[92] Saito, F., et al., *Spinal cord injury treatment with intrathecal autologous bone marrow stromal cell transplantation: the first clinical trial case report.* J Trauma, 2008. 64(1): p. 53–9.

[93] Kopen, G.C., D.J. Prockop, and D.G. Phinney, *Marrow stromal cells migrate throughout forebrain and cerebellum, and they differentiate into astrocytes after injection into neonatal mouse brains.* Proc Natl Acad Sci U S A, 1999. 96(19): p. 10711–6.

[94] Hofstetter, C.P., et al., *Marrow stromal cells form guiding strands in the injured spinal cord and promote recovery.* Proc Natl Acad Sci U S A, 2002. 99(4): p. 2199–204.

[95] Martinez, A.M., et al., *Neurotrauma and mesenchymal stem cells treatment: from experimental studies to clinical trials.* World J Stem Cells, 2014. 6(2): p. 179–94.

[96] Uccelli, A., et al., *Neuroprotective features of mesenchymal stem cells.* Best Pract Res Clin Haematol, 2011. 24(1): p. 59–64.

[97] Abrams, M.B., et al., *Multipotent mesenchymal stromal cells attenuate chronic inflammation and injury-induced sensitivity to mechanical stimuli in experimental spinal cord injury.* Restor Neurol Neurosci, 2009. 27(4): p. 307–21.

[98] Lu, P., et al., *Combinatorial therapy with neurotrophins and cAMP promotes axonal regeneration beyond sites of spinal cord injury.* J Neurosci, 2004. 24(28): p. 6402–9.

[99] Lu, P., L.L. Jones, and M.H. Tuszynski, *BDNF-expressing marrow stromal cells support extensive axonal growth at sites of spinal cord injury.* Exp Neurol, 2005. 191(2): p. 344–60.

[100] Lu, P., L.L. Jones, and M.H. Tuszynski, *Axon regeneration through scars and into sites of chronic spinal cord injury.* Exp Neurol, 2007. 203(1): p. 8–21.

[101] Novikova, L.N., et al., *Neuroprotective and growth-promoting effects of bone marrow stromal cells after cervical spinal cord injury in adult rats.* Cytotherapy, 2011. 13(7): p. 873–87.

[102] Sandner, B., et al., *Bone morphogenetic proteins prevent bone marrow stromal cell-mediated oligodendroglial differentiation of transplanted adult neural progenitor cells in the injured spinal cord.* Stem Cell Res, 2013. 11(2): p. 758–71.

[103] Bhanot, Y., et al., *Autologous mesenchymal stem cells in chronic spinal cord injury.* Br J Neurosurg, 2011. 25(4): p. 516–22.

[104] Goldschlager, T., et al., *Cervical motion preservation using mesenchymal progenitor cells and pentosan polysulfate, a novel chondrogenic agent: preliminary study in an ovine model.* Neurosurg Focus, 2010. 28(6): p. E4.

[105] Zuk, P.A., et al., *Multilineage cells from human adipose tissue: implications for cell-based therapies.* Tissue Eng, 2001. 7(2): p. 211–28.

[106] Kolar, M.K., et al., *The therapeutic effects of human adipose-derived stem cells in a rat cervical spinal cord injury model.* Stem Cells Dev, 2014. 23(14): p. 1659–74.

[107] Saporta, S., et al., *Human umbilical cord blood stem cells infusion in spinal cord injury: engraftment and beneficial influence on behavior.* J Hematother Stem Cell Res, 2003. 12(3): p. 271–8.

[108] Dasari, V.R., et al., *Axonal remyelination by cord blood stem cells after spinal cord injury.* J Neurotrauma, 2007. 24(2): p. 391–410.

[109] Park, D.H., et al., *Transplantation of umbilical cord blood stem cells for treating spinal cord injury.* Stem Cell Rev, 2011. 7(1): p. 181–94.

[110] Wei, L., et al., *Multiple injections of human umbilical cord-derived mesenchymal stromal cells through the tail vein improve microcirculation and the microenvironment in a rat model of radiation myelopathy.* J Transl Med, 2014. 12: p. 246.

[111] Tetzlaff, W., et al., *A systematic review of cellular transplantation therapies for spinal cord injury.* J Neurotrauma, 2011. 28(8): p. 1611–82.

[112] Tsuji, O., et al., *Cell therapy for spinal cord injury by neural stem/progenitor cells derived from iPS/ES cells.* Neurotherapeutics, 2011. 8(4): p. 668–76.

[113] Willerth, S.M., *Neural tissue engineering using embryonic and induced pluripotent stem cells.* Stem Cell Res Ther, 2011. 2(2): p. 17.

[114] Evans, M.J. and M.H. Kaufman, *Establishment in culture of pluripotential cells from mouse embryos.* Nature, 1981. 292(5819): p. 154–6.

[115] Martin, G.R., *Isolation of a pluripotent cell line from early mouse embryos cultured in medium conditioned by teratocarcinoma stem cells.* Proc Natl Acad Sci U S A, 1981. 78(12): p. 7634–8.

[116] Thomson, J.A., et al., *Embryonic stem cell lines derived from human blastocysts.* Science, 1998. 282(5391): p. 1145–7.

[117] Pera, M.F. and A.O. Trounson, *Human embryonic stem cells: prospects for development.* Development, 2004. 131(22): p. 5515–25.

[118] Braam, S.R., et al., *Feeder-free culture of human embryonic stem cells in conditioned medium for efficient genetic modification.* Nat Protoc, 2008. 3(9): p. 1435–43.

[119] McElroy, S.L. and R.A. Reijo Pera, *Culturing human embryonic stem cells in feeder-free conditions.* CSH Protoc, 2008. 2008: doi: 10.1101/pdb.prot5044.

[120] Xu, C., et al., *Feeder-free growth of undifferentiated human embryonic stem cells.* Nat Biotech, 2001. 19(10): p. 971–974.

[121] Ko, J.Y., et al., *Human embryonic stem cell-derived neural precursors as a continuous, stable, and on-demand source for human dopamine neurons.* J Neurochem, 2007. 103(4): p. 1417–29.

[122] Richards, M., et al., *Human feeders support prolonged undifferentiated growth of human inner cell masses and embryonic stem cells.* Nat Biotechnol, 2002. 20(9): p. 933–6.

[123] Ruff, C.A., J.T. Wilcox, and M.G. Fehlings, *Cell-based transplantation strategies to promote plasticity following spinal cord injury.* Exp Neurol, 2012. 235(1): p. 78–90.

[124] Bain, G., et al., *Embryonic stem cells express neuronal properties in vitro.* Dev Biol, 1995. 168(2): p. 342–57.

[125] Kumagai, G., et al., *Roles of ES cell-derived gliogenic neural stem/progenitor cells in functional recovery after spinal cord injury.* PLoS One, 2009. 4(11): p. e7706.

[126] Salewski, R.P., et al., *Transplantation of induced pluripotent stem cell-derived neural stem cells mediate functional recovery following thoracic spinal cord injury through remyelination of axons.* Stem Cells Transl Med, 2015. 4(7): p. 743–54.

[127] Cloutier, F., et al., *Transplantation of human embryonic stem cell-derived oligodendrocyte progenitors into rat spinal cord injuries does not cause harm.* Regen Med, 2006. 1(4): p. 469–79.

[128] Faulkner, J. and H.S. Keirstead, *Human embryonic stem cell-derived oligodendrocyte progenitors for the treatment of spinal cord injury.* Transpl Immunol, 2005. 15(2): p. 131–42.

[129] Liu, S., et al., *Embryonic stem cells differentiate into oligodendrocytes and myelinate in culture and after spinal cord transplantation.* Proc Natl Acad Sci U S A, 2000. 97(11): p. 6126–31.

[130] Nistor, G., et al., *Derivation of high purity neuronal progenitors from human embryonic stem cells.* PLoS One, 2011. 6(6): p. e20692.

[131] Sharp, J., et al., *Derivation of oligodendrocyte progenitor cells from human embryonic stem cells.* Methods Mol Biol, 2011. 767: p. 399–409.

[132] Wichterle, H., et al., *Directed differentiation of embryonic stem cells into motor neurons.* Cell, 2002. 110(3): p. 385–97.

[133] Peljto, M., et al., *Functional diversity of ESC-derived motor neuron subtypes revealed through intraspinal transplantation.* Cell Stem Cell, 2010. 7(3): p. 355–66.

[134] Wyatt, T.J., et al., *Human motor neuron progenitor transplantation leads to endogenous neuronal sparing in 3 models of motor neuron loss.* Stem Cells Int, 2011. 2011: p. 207230.

[135] Johnson, P.J., et al., *Tissue-engineered fibrin scaffolds containing neural progenitors enhance functional recovery in a subacute model of SCI.* Soft Matter, 2010. 6(20): p. 5127–5137.

[136] McCreedy, D.A., et al., *A new method for generating high purity motoneurons from mouse embryonic stem cells.* Biotechnol Bioeng, 2014. 111(10): p. 2041–55.

[137] McCreedy, D.A., et al., *Transgenic enrichment of mouse embryonic stem cell-derived progenitor motor neurons.* Stem Cell Res, 2012. 8(3): p. 368–78.

[138] McCreedy, D.A., et al., *Survival, differentiation, and migration of high-purity mouse embryonic stem cell-derived progenitor motor neurons in fibrin scaffolds after sub-acute spinal cord injury.* Biomater Sci, 2014. 2(11): p. 1672–82.

[139] Ideguchi, M., et al., *Murine embryonic stem cell-derived pyramidal neurons integrate into the cerebral cortex and appropriately project axons to subcortical targets.* J Neurosci, 2010. 30(3): p. 894–904.

[140] Sharp, J., et al., *Human embryonic stem cell-derived oligodendrocyte progenitor cell transplants improve recovery after cervical spinal cord injury.* Stem Cells, 2010. 28(1): p. 152–63.

[141] Hatch, M.N., G. Nistor, and H.S. Keirstead, *Derivation of high-purity oligodendroglial progenitors.* Methods Mol Biol, 2009. 549: p. 59–75.

[142] Nistor, G.I., et al., *Human embryonic stem cells differentiate into oligodendrocytes in high purity and myelinate after spinal cord transplantation.* Glia, 2005. 49(3): p. 385–96.

[143] Baker, M., *Stem-cell pioneer bows out.* Nature, 2011. 479(7374): p. 459.

[144] Hayden, E.C., *Funding windfall rescues abandoned stem-cell trial.* Nature, 2014. 510(7503): p. 18.

[145] Sun, Y., et al., *Transplantation of oligodendrocyte precursor cells improves locomotion deficits in rats with spinal cord irradiation injury.* PLoS One, 2013. 8(2): p. e57534.

[146] Du, Z.W., et al., *Induced expression of Olig2 is sufficient for oligodendrocyte specification but not for motoneuron specification and astrocyte repression.* Mol Cell Neurosci, 2006. 33(4): p. 371–80.

[147] Rossi, S.L., et al., *Histological and functional benefit following transplantation of motor neuron progenitors to the injured rat spinal cord.* PLoS One, 2010. 5(7): p. e11852.

[148] Diener, P.S. and B.S. Bregman, *Fetal spinal cord transplants support growth of supraspinal and segmental projections after cervical spinal cord hemisection in the neonatal rat.* J Neurosci, 1998. 18(2): p. 779–93.

[149] Lepore, A.C., et al., *Neural precursor cells can be delivered into the injured cervical spinal cord by intrathecal injection at the lumbar cord.* Brain Res, 2005. 1045(1–2): p. 206–16.

[150] Lepore, A.C. and I. Fischer, *Lineage-restricted neural precursors survive, migrate, and differentiate following transplantation into the injured adult spinal cord.* Exp Neurol, 2005. 194(1): p. 230–42.

[151] Lu, P., et al., *Long-distance growth and connectivity of neural stem cells after severe spinal cord injury.* Cell, 2012. 150(6): p. 1264–73.

[152] Giovanini, M.A., et al., *Characteristics of human fetal spinal cord grafts in the adult rat spinal cord: influences of lesion and grafting conditions.* Exp Neurol, 1997. 148(2): p. 523–43.

[153] Reier, P.J., et al., *Workshop on intraspinal transplantation and clinical application.* J Neurotrauma, 1994. 11(4): p. 369–77.

[154] Reier, P.J., et al., *Fetal cell grafts into resection and contusion/compression injuries of the rat and cat spinal cord.* Exp Neurol, 1992. 115(1): p. 177–88.

[155] Anderson, D.K., D.R. Howland, and P.J. Reier, *Fetal neural grafts and repair of the injured spinal cord.* Brain Pathol, 1995. 5(4): p. 451–57.

[156] Anderson, D.K., et al., *Delayed grafting of fetal CNS tissue into chronic compression lesions of the adult cat spinal cord.* Restor Neurol Neurosci, 1991. 2(4): p. 309–25.

[157] Reier, P.J., *Neural tissue grafts and repair of the injured spinal cord.* Neuropathol Appl Neurobiol, 1985. 11(2): p. 81–104.

[158] Diener, P.S. and B.S. Bregman, *Fetal spinal cord transplants support the development of target reaching and coordinated postural adjustments after neonatal cervical spinal cord injury.* J Neurosci, 1998. 18(2): p. 763–78.

[159] StemCells, Inc., *Study of human central nervous system (CNS) stem cell transplantation in cervical spinal cord injury. In: ClinicalTrials.gov [Internet]*, 2000-2015, National Library of Medicine (US): Bethesda. MD, *Jan 16. Available from: https://clinicaltrials.gov/ct2/show/NCT02163876 NLM Indentifier: NCT02163876.*

[160] Cizkova, D., et al., *Functional recovery in rats with ischemic paraplegia after spinal grafting of human spinal stem cells.* Neuroscience, 2007. 147(2): p. 546–60.

[161] van Gorp, S., et al., *Amelioration of motor/sensory dysfunction and spasticity in a rat model of acute lumbar spinal cord injury by human neural stem cell transplantation.* Stem Cell Res Ther, 2013. 4(3): p. 57.

[162] Salewski, R.P., et al., *Transplantation of neural stem cells clonally derived from embryonic stem cells promotes recovery after murine spinal cord injury.* Stem Cells Dev, 2015. 24(1): p. 36–50.

[163] Miura, K., et al., *Variation in the safety of induced pluripotent stem cell lines.* Nat Biotechnol, 2009. 27(8): p. 743–5.

[164] Takahashi, K., et al., *Induction of pluripotent stem cells from adult human fibroblasts by defined factors.* Cell, 2007. 131(5): p. 861–72.

[165] Takahashi, K. and S. Yamanaka, *Induction of pluripotent stem cells from mouse embryonic and adult fibroblast cultures by defined factors.* Cell, 2006. 126(4): p. 663–76.

[166] Yamanaka, Shinya. "Patient-specific pluripotent stem cells become even more accessible." *Cell Stem Cell* 7.1 (2010): 1–2.

[167] Fusaki, Noemi, et al. "Efficient induction of transgene-free human pluripotent stem cells using a vector based on Sendai virus, an RNA virus that does not integrate into the host genome." *Proceedings of the Japan Academy, Series B* 85.8 (2009): 348–362.

[168] Nori, Satoshi, et al. "Long-term safety issues of iPSC-based cell therapy in a spinal cord injury model: oncogenic transformation with epithelial-mesenchymal transition." *Stem cell reports* 4.3 (2015): 360–373.

[169] Zhou, Hongyan, et al. "Generation of induced pluripotent stem cells using recombinant proteins." *Cell stem cell* 4.5 (2009): 381–384.

[170] Warren, Luigi, et al. "Highly efficient reprogramming to pluripotency and directed differentiation of human cells with synthetic modified mRNA." *Cell stem cell* 7.5 (2010): 618–630.

[171] Rao, Mahendra S., and Nasir Malik. "Assessing iPSC reprogramming methods for their suitability in translational medicine." *Journal of cellular biochemistry* 113.10 (2012): 3061–3068.

[172] Brennand, K.J., et al., *Modeling psychiatric disorders at the cellular and network levels.* Mol Psychiatry, 2012. 17(12): p. 1239–53.

[173] Han, S.S., L.A. Williams, and K.C. Eggan, *Constructing and deconstructing stem cell models of neurological disease.* Neuron, 2011. 70(4): p. 626–44.

[174] Marchetto, M.C. and F.H. Gage, *Modeling brain disease in a dish: really?* Cell Stem Cell, 2012. 10(6): p. 642–5.

[175] Guo, J., et al., *Contribution of mouse embryonic stem cells and induced pluripotent stem cells to chimeras through injection and coculture of embryos.* Stem Cells Int, 2014. 2014: p. 409021.

[176] Parmar, M. and A. Bjorklund, *Generation of transplantable striatal projection neurons from human ESCs.* Cell Stem Cell, 2012. 10(4): p. 349–50.

[177] Barker, R.A., *Developing stem cell therapies for Parkinson's disease: waiting until the time is right.* Cell Stem Cell, 2014. 15(5): p. 539–42.

[178] Ambasudhan, R., et al., *Direct reprogramming of adult human fibroblasts to functional neurons under defined conditions.* Cell Stem Cell, 2011. 9(2): p. 113–8.

[179] Vierbuchen, T., et al., *Direct conversion of fibroblasts to functional neurons by defined factors.* Nature, 2010. 463(7284): p. 1035–41.

[180] Zhang, Y., et al., *Rapid single-step induction of functional neurons from human pluripotent stem cells.* Neuron, 2013. 78(5): p. 785–98.

[181] Molyneaux, B.J., et al., *Neuronal subtype specification in the cerebral cortex.* Nat Rev Neurosci, 2007. 8(6): p. 427–37.

[182] Arlotta, P., et al., *Neuronal subtype-specific genes that control corticospinal motor neuron development in vivo.* Neuron, 2005. 45(2): p. 207–21.

[183] Byers, B., et al., *SNCA triplication Parkinson's patient's iPSC-derived DA neurons accumulate alpha-synuclein and are susceptible to oxidative stress.* PLoS One, 2011. 6(11): p. e26159.

[184] Nguyen, H.N., et al., *LRRK2 mutant iPSC-derived DA neurons demonstrate increased susceptibility to oxidative stress.* Cell Stem Cell, 2011. 8(3): p. 267–80.

[185] Dolmetsch, R. and D.H. Geschwind, *The human brain in a dish: the promise of iPSC-derived neurons.* Cell, 2011. 145(6): p. 831–4.

[186] Pera, M.F., *Stem cells: the dark side of induced pluripotency.* Nature, 2011. 471(7336): p. 46–7.

[187] Boulting, G.L., et al., *A functionally characterized test set of human induced pluripotent stem cells.* Nat Biotechnol, 2011. 29(3): p. 279–86.

[188] Brennand, K.J. and F.H. Gage, *Concise review: the promise of human induced pluripotent stem cell-based studies of schizophrenia.* Stem Cells, 2011. 29(12): p. 1915–22.

[189] Brennand, K.J., et al., *Modelling schizophrenia using human induced pluripotent stem cells.* Nature, 2011. 473(7346): p. 221–5.

[190] Faravelli, I., et al., *iPSC-based models to unravel key pathogenetic processes underlying motor neuron disease development.* J Clin Med, 2014. 3(4): p. 1124–45.

[191] Hirami, Y., et al., *Generation of retinal cells from mouse and human induced pluripotent stem cells.* Neurosci Lett, 2009. 458(3): p. 126–31.

[192] Hodgetts, S.I., M. Edel, and A.R. Harvey, *The state of play with iPSCs and spinal cord injury models.* J Clin Med, 2015. 4(1): p. 193–203.

[193] Hu, B.Y., et al., *Neural differentiation of human induced pluripotent stem cells follows developmental principles but with variable potency.* Proc Natl Acad Sci U S A, 2010. 107(9): p. 4335–40.

[194] Kim, J., et al., *Reprogramming of postnatal neurons into induced pluripotent stem cells by defined factors.* Stem Cells, 2011. 29(6): p. 992–1000.

[195] Kim, J.E., et al., *Investigating synapse formation and function using human pluripotent stem cell-derived neurons.* Proc Natl Acad Sci U S A, 2011. 108(7): p. 3005–10.

[196] Marchetto, M.C., et al., *A model for neural development and treatment of Rett syndrome using human induced pluripotent stem cells.* Cell, 2010. 143(4): p. 527–39.

[197] Zeng, H., et al., *Specification of region-specific neurons including forebrain glutamatergic neurons from human induced pluripotent stem cells.* PLoS One, 2010. 5(7): p. e11853.

[198] Kim, J., et al., *Direct reprogramming of mouse fibroblasts to neural progenitors.* Proc Natl Acad Sci U S A, 2011. 108(19): p. 7838–43.

[199] Marchetto, M.C., B. Winner, and F.H. Gage, *Pluripotent stem cells in neurodegenerative and neurodevelopmental diseases.* Hum Mol Genet, 2010. 19(R1): p. R71–6.

[200] Krencik, R. and S.C. Zhang, *Directed differentiation of functional astroglial subtypes from human pluripotent stem cells.* Nat Protoc, 2011. 6(11): p. 1710–7.

[201] Yang, N., et al., *Generation of oligodendroglial cells by direct lineage conversion.* Nat Biotechnol, 2013. 31(5): p. 434–9.

[202] All, A.H., et al., *Human embryonic stem cell-derived oligodendrocyte progenitors aid in functional recovery of sensory pathways following contusive spinal cord injury.* PLoS One, 2012. 7(10): p. e47645.

[203] Hayashi, K., et al., *Increase of sensitivity to mechanical stimulus after transplantation of murine induced pluripotent stem cell-derived astrocytes in a rat spinal cord injury model.* J Neurosurg Spine, 2011. 15(6): p. 582–93.

[204] Fujimoto, Y., et al., *Treatment of a mouse model of spinal cord injury by transplantation of human induced pluripotent stem cell-derived long-term self-renewing neuroepithelial-like stem cells.* Stem Cells, 2012. 30(6): p. 1163–73.

[205] Nori, S., et al., *Grafted human-induced pluripotent stem-cell-derived neurospheres promote motor functional recovery after spinal cord injury in mice.* Proc Natl Acad Sci U S A, 2011. 108(40): p. 16825–30.

[206] Tsuji, O., et al., *Therapeutic potential of appropriately evaluated safe-induced pluripotent stem cells for spinal cord injury.* Proc Natl Acad Sci U S A, 2010. 107(28): p. 12704–9.

[207] Li, K., et al., *Human iPS cell-derived astrocyte transplants preserve respiratory function after spinal cord injury.* Exp Neurol, 2015. 271: p. 479–92.

[208] Lu, P., et al., *Long-distance axonal growth from human induced pluripotent stem cells after spinal cord injury.* Neuron, 2014. 83(4): p. 789–96.

[209] Nutt, S.E., et al., *Caudalized human iPSC-derived neural progenitor cells produce neurons and glia but fail to restore function in an early chronic spinal cord injury model.* Exp Neurol, 2013. 248: p. 491–503.

[210] Kobayashi, Y., et al., *Pre-evaluated safe human iPSC-derived neural stem cells promote functional recovery after spinal cord injury in common marmoset without tumorigenicity.* PLoS One, 2012. 7(12): p. e52787.

Section 4

Emerging Techniques for the Assessment and Rehabilitation of Motor Recovery

Chapter 10

Orthoses for Spinal Cord Injury Patients

Mokhtar Arazpour, Monireh Ahmadi Bani,
Mohammad Ebrahim Mousavi,
Mahmood Bahramizadeh and
Mohammad Ali Mardani

Additional information is available at the end of the chapter

http://dx.doi.org/10.5772/64092

Abstract

There are some limitations for patients with spinal cord injury (SCI) when walking with assistive devices. Heavy energy expenditure and walking high loads on the upper limb joints are two main reasons of high rejection rate of orthosis by these patients . Many devices have been designed to enable people with paraplegia to ambulate in an upright position as a solution of these limitations such as mechanical orthoses, hybrid orthoses and powered orthoses. All these devices are designed to solve the problem of standing and walking, but there are some other important notes, which should be considered. For example, the size and weight of external orthoses, donning and doffing, cumbersomeness and independency for using are very important.

Keywords: spinal cord injury, orthoses, walking, assistive devices

1. Introduction

Lower limb paralysis resulting from spinal cord injury (SCI) causes inability to walk. Trauma is one of the main causes of SCI that occurs mostly in young people (aged between 16 and 30 years). In 2006, more than 2000 patients with SCI were in the United States and there are more than 10,000 new cases each year [1]. The ability to walk is the ultimate goal of rehabilitation in SCI patients. Ambulation is always influenced in patients with SCI based on the lesion level and the resulting different levels of muscle paralysis, sensory impairment, spasticity and the lack of trunk control. Walking anomalies in patients with SCI included the absence of active sagittal plane motions in the hip and knee joints, increased ankle plantarflexion during swing phase and an inability to positioning the lower extremity for initial foot contact and the existence of the so-called "foot slap" based on paralysis of ankle dorsiflexor muscles. Different types of orthoses are designed to reduce complication of inability to walk.

In this chapter, we introduce different types of orthoses for patients with spinal cord injury and explain important parameters (walking, stability, energy expenditure and independency) for all existent orthoses by current documents.

2. Different types of orthoses

In overall view, there were three mechanisms in orthoses to walking in spinal cord injury patients: mechanical orthoses, hybrid orthoses and power orthoses (exoskeleton).

2.1. Mechanical orthoses

In this category, three types of the mechanical orthoses included were hip-knee-ankle-foot orthoses, reciprocating gait orthoses and medial linkage orthoses.

2.1.1. Hip-knee-ankle-foot orthoses

A simple hip joint with one degree of freedom generally was used in the Hip Knee Ankle Foot Orthosis (HKAFO). Paraplegic patients use a swing through walking pattern during ambulation with this type of orthoses. Walking with this pattern produces a high rate of energy consumption and high rate of loads on the upper limb joints (shoulder joints and wrist) in paraplegic patients [2–5].

2.1.2. Reciprocating gait orthoses

Reciprocating gait orthoses (RGO) were introduced in the late 1960s. The ultimate goal was mobilizing lower limb by trunk extension. Therefore, hip extension in one side created hip flexion in other side. In using this kind of orthosis, patients were able to walk reciprocally, doff and don the orthosis independently, but cannot stand up without assistance [6, 7]. In addition, walking on a ramp and incline is difficult for paraplegic patients when using the original form of RGO [6]. To resolve this problem, the hip joints in this orthosis must have a two condition locking systems: firstly, in a full extension locking position and secondly in 20° flexion from the first position to walking on ramp and incline [6].

A modified version of RGOs is referred to as the Advanced Reciprocating Gait Orthosis (ARGO) with a one pull-push cable within the pelvic section developed to assist walking performance in paraplegic subjects. In comparison, the Hip Guidance Orthosis (HGO), RGO and ARGO demonstrated the same motion in pattern and magnitude, but in using the ARGO the pelvic displayed a jerky movement pattern. A more developed RGO is defined as the Isocentric Reciprocating Gait Orthosis (IRGO) and was introduced by Motlock in 1992 [8].

http://dx.doi.org/10.5772/64092

2.1.3. Medial linkage orthosis (MLO)

Another type of mechanical orthosis is medial linkage orthosis (MLO). There are variations in this type of orthosis, which include the WalkAbout (WA) [9], Moorong [10] and PrimeWalk (PW) [11] and the Hip and Ankle Linked Orthosis (HALO) [12]. These orthosis are based on a medial single hip joint, which provides artificial hip joint movements. Although it is noted that there is no congruency between the anatomical and mechanical hip joints in the Walkabout MLO, this limitation has been resolved in the Primewalk and Moorong MLO [9–11].

Evaluation of the hip joint mechanism when using the IRGO has been reported to demonstrate improved gait parameters, energy consumption compared to other RGOs, HKAFO and MLOs [13]. Therefore, the prescribed option in improvement of walking parameters between mechanical orthoses is the IRGO system. The difference between walking with optimal mechanical orthoses (IRGO) and healthy subjects walking is high. Donning and doffing with this type of orthosis, however, is difficult due to its bulky structure and increased weight. MLOs have less donning and doffing time and light structure compared to IRGOs, but these types of orthoses do not have a reciprocating gait mechanism and pelvic rigid structure. Therefore, the users are forced to use high energy consumption during walking, which in turn can create a poor posture compared to walking with IRGO conditions [13–15].

Walking with a mechanical orthoses is not ideal for SCI patients and is a view based on the associated problems during walking with them that includes high loads on upper limb joints and high rate of energy consumption. Some authors have also stated that walking with mechanical orthoses is boring and exhausted [2, 4, 7, 16]. Recent efforts to improve orthoses for SCI patients have led to systems of orthoses that combine the mechanical orthoses with functional electrical stimulation of selected lower extremity muscles and powered hip orthoses [3, 17–19]. Generally, walking parameters and energy consumption improved with new generation of orthoses [19, 20].

2.2. Hybrid orthoses

Hybrid orthoses are a kind of orthoses, which are activated by functional electrical stimulation (FES). FES is the application of external electrical stimulation to paralyzed muscles to restore their function [6]. The first reported use of FES to facilitate walking for SCI individuals was in 1980, involving the stimulation of quadriceps muscle to enhance stability during stance phase. Two kinds of hybrid orthoses are available: hybrid orthosis based on available mechanical designs (HGO, LSU RGO, ARGO and MLO) and hybrid orthoses based on the new designs (modular hybrid, wrapped spring clutch and spring brake orthoses).

Although some benefits are noted about hybrid orthosis, there are some limitation associated with the use of orthoses, FES or hybrid orthoses, which include premature muscle fatigue, false triggering of nearby muscles and being heavy and orthotics cumbersomeness.

2.3. Power orthoses (exoskeleton)

Powered orthoses (exoskeleton) are kinds of orthoses, which activate with external power. The mechanical orthoses have a simple structure and user-friendly design. This type of orthoses, however, has not progressed in development in recent years with the progression, since technology of the powered orthoses appears to be the main focus of research in rehabilitation and assisted walking and ambulation in SCI patients. There is currently only a limited range of powered orthoses, but there is some evidence of an increase in temporal spatial parameters when walking with powered orthoses [21, 22].

One successful approach used in patient rehabilitation is the use of partial weight bearing when walking on a treadmill using suspension via an overhead harness. This technique, known as body weight support treadmill training (BWSTT), has been used to encourage the regeneration of stepping and walking in incomplete and complete SCI subjects [23, 24]. One of the limitations of BWSTT is that it can only be used in a clinical environment. Provision of hip extension at the end of stance phase, adequate weight bearing through the lower limb during stance phase and the ability to shift weight to the lateral side in the double support phase are essential for BWSTT [25]. However, agreement on the ideal parameters of such gait training does not currently exist [26]. The speed of the treadmill [27], cadence used, and the amount of body unloading are parameters, which can affect gait training in SCI subjects using this system [28]. Therefore, due to these limitations, powered gait orthosis (PGOs) may offer potential in providing an alternative form of gait training for SCI patients.

PGOs can be used as a gait training system to facilitate ambulation in both the clinical situation and in the home via an external power supply using electric motors, pneumatic and/or hydraulic actuators [9]. The first design and construction of PGOs were done in mid-1970s [29]. Belforte [30, 31], and Kang et al. [32], both developed powered orthoses with pneumatic actuators, which demonstrated a positive effect on walking by paraplegic patients, and further developments were subsequently reported by Ruthenberg et al. [33], Ohta et al. [34] and Arazpour et al. [35, 36].

Robert Bogue analyzed some recently developed exoskeletons for military, civil and medical applications and described brain-computer and systems in this review paper [37]. Ferris et al. in another review paper evaluated the recent powered lower limb orthosis for assisting treadmill stepping in disable persons. Practice starting, turning, stopping and avoiding obstacles during overground walking reported main advantage of using powered orthoses as rehabilitation aids in gait rehabilitation after neurological injury. In this study, the powered orthosis that used with bodyweight supported treadmill training for gait rehabilitation in clinical environment analyzed [38]. In the review paper, Dollar and Herr reported the history of the lower limb active orthoses. They reported a design overview of hardware, actuation, sensory and control systems for most of the powered orthosis that have been fabricated until 2007 [39]. Powered orthosis in this literature included full lower limb exoskeletons, modular active orthoses, single joint active orthoses and other orthotic devices. They conducted that the research directions in the future will focus more on the development of light weight exoskeletons and active orthotic devices. All powered orthoses that fabricated for disable

http://dx.doi.org/10.5772/64092

persons discussed in the Dollar and Herr review paper, but the effect of advanced powered orthosis on walking in paraplegia patients was not analyzed in their study [39]. Duerinck et al. reported an overview of the influence of the ankle-foot robot-assisted rehabilitation orthoses to the attributes of normal gait in patients with spinal cord injury. They conducted that pneumatic artificial muscles in combination with proportional myoelectric control can restore the attributes of normal gait. In this review, only powered ankle foot orthosis evaluated on walking in SCI patients [40]. Del-Amae et al. reviewed powered gait orthosis that used FES on the muscles as natural actuators to generate gait in persons with spinal cord injury. Their paper explained an overview of hybrid lower limb exoskeletons, related technologies and advances in actuation and control systems, but the efficiency of this type of assistive devices was not evaluated on walking in SCI patients [41].

3. Daily living of spinal cord injury patients

Daily living including independence, orthosis donning and doffing, sitting and standing, walking on slope surfaces and curbs and toileting have been reported in few documents and literatures. Insufficient evidence exists as to the effect of powered and hybrid orthoses on daily living parameters in comparison with mechanical orthosis because these kinds of orthoses have evaluated in laboratory.

About mechanical orthoses, researchers have noted that in comparison to the RGOs, wearing the WO and HGOs has been reported to be easier to don and doff [42, 43]. In comparison between WO and IRGO, the WO has also been demonstrated to provide easier sitting and standing [15]. In comparison between HGO and RGO, it was demonstrated that the HGO has been reported to be easier to don and doff [42]. There are only three documents that analyzed mechanical orthosis on sloped surfaces and have demonstrated that the RGO was slightly more effective than the HGO when SCI subjects were negotiating curbs or slopes [10, 15, 42]. In a comparison between a MLOs and RGOs, the IRGO was significantly better than the WO (p value = 0.03) in 1:12 and 1:26 gradients [15]. It has demonstrated that using the Moorong orthoses in negotiating slopes surfaces was more functional than the WO due to the ability to align the orthotic and anatomic joints [44]. There is no evidence of any significant difference between any types of orthosis with regards to toileting.

Mechanical orthoses have different effects in improvement of parameters, which affect the daily living activities of SCI patients. No study was found, which considered these factors comprehensively in a selection of patients. From an independence view, the light and uncomplicated structure of the MLOs with removable hip joints and without a rigid spinal component made them easier for donning and doffing than RGOs [21, 22, 45]. The lumbar portion of IRGOs compared to MLOs limited the pelvis and lumbar joints. Unlocked joints in the IRGO caused more crutch support. Therefore, wearing IRGOs makes it more difficult than the MLO to provide sitting and standing [15], and additional document is required to demonstrate how assistive devices can help to provide activity of daily living more easily in the SCI patients. Therefore, from independence view, the comparison between MLO and RGO will be beneficial in this field.

4. Energy expenditure of spinal cord injury patients

Excessive energy expenditure and increased applied force on upper limb joints are two most important factors that increase rejection rates of orthoses in paraplegia patients. There are different methods of evaluation of energy expenditure including O_2 cost (ml kg^{-1} m^{-1}), O_2 consumption (ml kg^{-1} min^{-1}), the PCI (beat per m), HR (beat per min), O_2 uptake (l min^{-1}) and the respiratory exchange ratio in SCI patients when using orthoses in all of the documents. However, PCI was introduced as a most sensitive indicator for evaluation of energy expenditure in SCI patients [46]. In other hand, there is little evidence regarding the efficacy of powered gait orthoses (PGOs) and hybrid orthoses when directly compared to mechanical orthoses in reducing energy expenditure in SCI subjects. However, documents have demonstrated that PGOs and hybrid orthoses have less energy expenditure in comparison with mechanical orthoses [5, 47, 48].

SCI patients do not use their mechanical orthoses, with abandonment rates of 61–90% for children with myelomeningocele [49, 50] and 46–54% in adults with spinal cord injury [10, 51–53] due to the high level of energy expenditure needed to ambulate.

One of main reasons for the development of PGOs was to potentially reduce energy consumption when walking with an orthosis. A healthy subject walk with 0.176 mL/kg/m energy expenditure [2] and a SCI subject walk with WBCO 5.41 J/kg/s energy expenditure [54]. The difference between healthy normal subject and walking with a powered orthosis is therefore substantial, but is still improved when compared to that noted when paraplegic subjects walk with mechanical orthoses. There is not enough literature on energy cost of walking with powered orthosis. A further understanding of the energy cost of powered orthosis ambulation is therefore required for patients with SCI.

Kawashima et al., in evaluation of the weight bearing control orthoses on energy consumption stated that the energy consumption of walking has been quoted as being 5.41 J/kg/s [54] for SCI persons, while the mean of this parameter was reported 0.176 mL/kg/m in healthy participants [2]. Arazpour et al. in evaluation of the wearing PGOs compared to the mechanical orthoses such as HKAFO and IRGO reported that wearing PGO provided improved speed of walking and distance walked. The value of the PCI reduced in using the PGO compared to other mechanical orthoses. Active hip and knee joints in providing activated sagittal plane motions were announced as responsible for these results [55]. In a comparison between the WPAL and Primewalk orthoses on energy consumption in four people with paraplegia, Tanabe et al. reported that the PCI exhibited was reduced when using the WPAL [56]. The effort of walking has been shown to be reduced when using a powered motorized ARGO compared to mechanical ARGO in SCI patients [34]. Based on limited studies in evaluation of PGOs on energy consumption in paraplegic patients, a further understanding of this parameter is therefore required for patients with SCI when using PGOs.

About hybrid orthoses, Nene and Patrick [57] in evaluation of using hybrid orthoses (combination of Parawalker and electrical stimulation of the gluteal muscles) in three subjects reported that the rate of the energy cost was 11.78 J/kg/m and 10.95 J/kg/m (a 7.1% reduction) in without functional electrical stimulation (FES) and with FES condition, respectively. Using FES announced a considerable responsibility for reduction in the vertical crutch impulse values (mean 21%) [57]. The lowest energy costs (kcal/kg min) were associated with the RGO and FES, followed by the RGO, HGO, LLB and FES for walking speeds below 28 m/s.

Merati et al. [5] compared the energy cost of locomotion demonstrated by 14 SCI patients (lesion level C7 ± T11) during ambulation with different orthoses (the HGO, Parawalker, RGO and RGO + FES). They observed that during locomotion at maximal speed, HR peak values were 160 ± 16, 155 ± 31 and 154 ± 31 bts/min and VO2 1/kg peak values were 18.0 ± 6.1, 18.5 ± 5.4 and 19.1 ± 7.2 for PW, RGO and RGO + FNS, respectively. During orthosis-assisted locomotion at maximal speed, HR peak values were 150 ± 13, 131 ± 21 and 155 ± 23 bts/min, and VO_2 1/kg peak values were 13.4 ± 3.0, 13.8 ± 3.5 and 17.2 ± 4.8 for PW, RGO and RGO + FNS, respectively. They also reported that maximal ventilations at VO2 peak were 63.8 ± 24.0, 68.9 ± 27.1 and 67.6 ± 23.91 1/min during wheelchair ambulation, and 71.8 ± 7.3, 76.5 ± 21.3 and 72.3 ± 12.2 m/kg/min during orthosis locomotion for PW, RGO and RGO + FNS, respectively [5]. The PEDro score for this study was a 4/10, which equals the highest score assigned in this group.

In mechanical orthoses, connector cable ARGO maintains the posture and reduce PCI and IRGO (2.6 beat/m) has been shown to be more effective than an RGO (3.6 beat/m). Participants in this study reported less fatigue when they used the IRGO [46]. In comparison between RGOs and MLOs, RGOs have less energy expenditure, because MLOs do not have flexion-assist system for the SCI patients and have limited trunk stability, which made patients expend additional effort to maintain upright stance [58]. Also in comparison between MLOs, there is no significant difference in PCI.

RGOs produce less energy expenditure than MLOs and KAFOs [58, 59]. This is because RGOs offer more support for pelvis and trunk and possess a reciprocal system [58]. Energy expenditure and endurance have indirect correlation [60]. Muscle dysfunction, locked position of the ankle and knee joints, flexion of the trunk for providing stability and ambulation with assistive devices such as walker and crutch increase energy consumption in paraplegic subjects in wearing and walking with mechanical orthoses. Ankle and knee joints fixed position can increase energy consumption by up to 33% [60, 61]. Development of the ankle and knee joints of mechanical orthoses via powered or movable structures can be announced as the feasible approach to reduce energy expenditure. The energy consumption of using RGOs reported low rate compared to other mechanical orthoses such as MLOs and HKAFOs, based on the reciprocal section of RGOs announced as the responsible for this result. But the effect of the reciprocal link in providing of the reciprocal motion was demonstrated less [62–64]. Using RGOs for SCI patients rather than MLOs is cumbersome due to their bulky structure and using an MLO has high energy consumption compared to RGOs, but MLOs are more user-friendly for people with SCI [15, 65]. As a result, development of the MLOs with additional structure to provide reciprocal motion announced as the better approach in reduction of the energy expenditure in the SCI subjects. Therefore, the comparison of MLOs and IRGOs on the energy cost, energy expenditure and endurance of the ambulation to provide more effective mechanical orthoses in orthotic rehabilitation of ambulation in the SCI subjects will be important and beneficial.

In comparison between IRGO and RGO on energy consumption in four paraplegic SCI subjects with T3–T12 level of injury, the PCI was reduced when wearing the IRGO (2.6 beat/m), compared to condition that the RGO was used (3.6 beat/m). SCI patients announced less rate of the fatigue while walking with the IRGO [46]. Walking with standard ARGOs demonstrated the reduction of the energy consumption compared to an ARGO without a reciprocal connector cable (5.4 beat/m vs. 5.8 beat/m), although this difference was not statistically significant [66]. The standard ARGO provided best trunk posture in the SCI patients. This positioning is critical and important in the subjects with high level of injury. Evaluation of using WO on five SCI patients demonstrated that energy expenditure was 9.61 (ml/kg/min) [67]. The rate of the O_2 consumption and cost were announced as 13.79 (ml/kg/min) and 1.28 (ml/kg/m), respectively, in walking with standard ARGO in six SCI subjects [68].

5. Temporal spatial parameters

The findings of literature show that there is no high level of document to demonstrate that PGOs are better than mechanical orthoses such as RGOs and HGO in improving temporal spatial gait parameters in SCI subjects. From financial view, the PGOs are so expensive, and also the more orthotic gait training time and effort required providing them functionally. Walking with this type of orthosis does not propose any acceptable improvement in temporal spatial parameters compared to mechanical orthoses. Consequently, more additional attempt on structure of the powered orthoses is required to provide more acceptable powered device for SCI patient wearing and using [69]. There shows to be no significant difference in reported speed of walking subjects in walking with different RGOs in the SCI patients. The following text demonstrates the findings resulted by the literature, which analyzed the effect of common mechanical orthoses on temporal spatial parameters in the SCI patients.

5.1. Stride length

In comparison between the RGO and HGO, there was no significant difference in stride length [67]. In comparison of the standard ARGO with RGO without connector cable, 7% increase in stride length (0.89 vs. 0.83) was reported. Improvement in providing vertical positioning of the trunk by the connector cable announced the main responsible in the standard ARGO [62]. The mean of stride length was reported to be 0.56 m in SCI patients when using the WO [70]. In newly developed orthoses, Genda et al. demonstrated that the hip-ankle-linked orthoses (HALO), increased stride length by 3% compared to the WO (1.03 vs. 1.00 m) [12]. Six percent increased stride length was demonstrated when ankle foot orthosis with dorsiflexion-assist ankle joints were used in the ARGO (0.94 vs. 1 m) compared to the ARGO associated with solid ankle-foot orthosis. In this study, it was claimed that the moveable ankle joint in the ankle-foot orthosis section could improve stride length [71]. When comparing two medial linked orthoses (the Primewalk and Walkabout orthosis). Onogi et al. reported that there was significant difference between them in this parameter and the mean of stride length was increased by 19% [72].

5.2. Cadence

In a comparison between the RGO and the HGO, Whittle et al. reported no significant difference between them in this parameter [70]. However, Winchester et al. announced that although cadence was better in the IRGO than the RGO, there was no significant difference between them [46]. Ijzerman et al. in an evaluation of the effect of a connector cable reported that using an ARGO with a connector cable increased cadence compared to without one, but not significantly (31.3 vs. 30.3 steps/min) [66].

Four studies assessed the cadence in walking with orthoses associated with medial single hip joints in SCI patients. The mean of this parameter was reported as being 70.02 steps/min when using the WO [67] and 50.9 steps/min when walking with any type of medial single hip joints orthosis [73]. Significant difference in cadence between the HALO and PW devices (74.1 vs. 58.9) was reported by Genda et al. [12]. In a recently published study, the mean of cadence demonstrated a significant difference in value (40.8 vs. 48 steps/min, respectively) when using the WO and the PW [72].

5.3. Speed of walking

The mean of speed of walking has been reported to be 0.214 m/s when using the Parawalker orthosis during ambulation by SCI patients [45]. When using the ARGO, the mean of this parameter was 0.16 m/s [68]. The mean of speed of walking was reported to be similar between the HGO and the RGO (0.24 m/s) by Whittle et al. [70]. In comparison between RGOs, the IRGO was shown to produce a higher speed of walking (0.22) compared to a cable-type RGO (0.21), but there was no significant difference between them [46]. When comparing the KAFO and the IRGO, there were significant differences noted between them in this parameter ($p = 0.009$) [59]. The effect of a connector cable when using the ARGO has no significant effect on improving walking speed when compared to an ARGO without one (0.24 vs. 0.23 m/s) [62].

The effect of PGOs on walking speed, cadence and step length exhibited by SCI subjects is dependent on which joints are actuated in an orthosis (e.g. the hip or knee actuated separately or by being synchronized). Few studies have directly compared these parameters directly between separately or synchronized movement of the hip and knee joint conditions during walking with PGOs.

Kang et al. [74] in evaluation of the powered IRGO (via using pneumatic actuators in the hip joints) compared to a mechanical IRGO after three months orthotic gait training in three SCI subjects reported that evaluated parameters such as walking speed, pelvic tilt, flexion and extension angles of the knee and hip joints, stance and swing phase times improved. Walking speed was increased by 26% and the percentage swing phase during walking was increased by 25% when walking with the PGO.

Powered lower limb orthoses such as the ReWalk powered orthosis (Argo Medical Technologies), the wearable power-assist locomotor (WPAL) and the eLEGS powered orthosis

(Berkeley Bionics) are all examples of commercially developed powered orthoses designed for walking by paraplegic subjects. The Hybrid Assistive Limb (HAL)—6LB which has six electric motors—bilaterally at the hip, knee and ankle joints, the HAL-5 Type-C, which is previous HAL for paraplegia patients, with only four power units are another examples of power lower limb orthosis. Commercially developed HAL has four power units and uses EMG signals of leg to synchronize the motion support with the wearer's movement, but complete paraplegia patients cannot use this version of HAL.

Speed of walking reported difference between mechanical, hybrid and powered gait orthoses. There was statistically significant difference between orthotic walking and walking in healthy subjects. Since walking with powered orthoses (mechanical orthoses that powered with external actuators in the hip or knee joints) needs to keep balance and other assistive devices such as walker or crutch need to activate the powered joints, therefore, the speed of walking is thought to be adversely affected by these conditions. Commercially developed exoskeletons have shown the potential to significantly improve speed of walking.

Since there were some studies about increased step length and cadence in wearing powered gait orthoses during walking, more research in this field is required. The mechanism of the additional external actuator to mechanical orthosis in the powered gait orthoses in improvement of speed of walking needs more research.

5.3.1. Quiet standing

Mechanical orthosis has been analyzed in a few researches in stability by quite standing. Anterior–posterior (AP) and mediolateral (ML) COP displacement in amplitude and velocity of were measured in SCI patients. Baardman evaluated the effect of connector link in ARGO and reported no difference between ARGO with (35.22 mm in AP and 41.72 mm in ML COP displacement) and without (37.94 mm in AP and 34.53 mm in ML direction) cable in quiet standing in stability [62].

In another study, Middleton et al. compared KAFO with and without a single medial linkage on sway amplitude in SCI patients announced that AP sway amplitude when using a single medial linkage with KAFO was half that when wearing a KAFO without it, but in ML direction amplitude there was no significant difference [75]. In a research Abe et al. compared stability with KAFO, RGO and WO and reported significant difference between KAFO with two other orthoses [75].

5.3.2. Performance

Such as other parameters in PGOs there is no document in relation to performance and powered orthoses. About mechanical orthoses, there are three studies in relation to amplitude and velocity of COP displacement. The first study was reported by Baardman et al., which done on cable connector in the ARGO on performance. These researchers reported no effect of connector cable on performance (COP displacement in quite standing) but demonstrated this cable in ARGO can reduce upper limb load [62].

Middleton et al. compared KAFO with and without single medial linkage and announced no significant difference in sway path and amplitude in the A-P direction between them in SCI patients, but use of KAFO with a medial linkage decreased sway amplitude (p = 0.008) and increased M-L direction of sway path (p = 0.021). Therefore, this research proved using a single medial linkage can increase stability and balance in the mediolateral direction [75]. In the third study, Abe et al. demonstrated that sway amplitude was not significantly different between the WO and the RGO but the KAFO had significantly less stability [76].

6. Future research topics in this field

The following topics can be performed in orthotics rehabilitation of the SCI subjects:

- Based on lack of commercial powered and hybrid orthoses, development of these types of assistive orthoses will be beneficial in this field.
- Analysis of the developed commercial powered and hybrid orthoses on energy cost and energy consumption is essential in this field.
- Finding the solution to reduce energy expenditure during ambulation in SCI patients will be beneficial in rehabilitation of orthotic walking in SCI subjects.
- Analysis of energy expenditure between mechanical orthoses, commercial powered and hybrid orthoses is essential before and after the orthotic gait training in SCI subjects.

7. Summary remarks

- Using the powered gait, orthoses reduced the needed effort during ambulation in SCI subjects. Using external actuators in the hip or knee joints with provided active motions in specific joints announced the main reason for these results.
- Powered gait orthoses can be used in the clinical environment for orthotic gait training purposes. Although the positive effect of the orthotic gait training with WBCO on muscle activity in SCI patients was reported, more research is needed to approve any beneficial influence.
- Based on literature, it is concluded that the powered and hybrid orthoses could be announced as effective devices for orthotic rehabilitation of walking in SCI patients to assist to provide their best ambulation.
- Speed of walking reported difference between mechanical, hybrid and powered gait orthoses. There was statistically significant difference between orthotic walking and waling in healthy subjects.
- Since walking with powered orthoses needs to keep balance and other assistive devices such as walker or crutch need to activate the powered joints, therefore, the speed of walking is

thought to be adversely affected by these conditions. Commercially developed exoskeletons have shown the potential to significantly improve speed of walking.

Author details

Mokhtar Arazpour*, Monireh Ahmadi Bani, Mohammad Ebrahim Mousavi, Mahmood Bahramizadeh and Mohammad Ali Mardani

*Address all correspondence to: M.Arazpour@yahoo.com

Department of Orthotics and Prosthetics, University of Social Welfare and Rehabilitation Sciences, Tehran, Iran

References

[1] Varma AK, Das A, Wallace IV G, Barry J, Vertegel AA, Ray SK, et al. Spinal cord injury: a review of current therapy, future treatments, and basic science frontiers. Neurochemical Research 2013;38(5):895–905.

[2] Bernardi M, Macaluso A, Sproviero E, Castellano V, Coratella D, Felici F, et al. Cost of walking and locomotor impairment. Journal of Electromyography and Kinesiology 1999;9(2):149–57.

[3] Hirokawa S, Grimm M, Solomonow M, Baratta R, Shoji H, D'ambrosia R. Energy consumption in paraplegic ambulation using the reciprocating gait orthosis and electric stimulation of the thigh muscles. Archives of Physical Medicine and Rehabilitation 1990;71(9):687–94.

[4] Johnson W, Fatone S, Gard S. Walking mechanics of persons who use reciprocating gait orthoses. Journal of Rehabilitation Research and Development 2009;46(3):435.

[5] Merati G, Sarchi P, Ferrarin M, Pedotti A, Veicsteinas A. Paraplegic adaptation to assisted-walking: energy expenditure during wheelchair versus orthosis use. Spinal Cord 2000;38(1):37–44.

[6] Nene A, Hermens H, Zilvold G. Paraplegic locomotion: a review. Spinal Cord 1996;34(9):507–24.

[7] Solomonow M, Baratta R, Shoji H, et al., eds. FES powered locomotion of paraplegics fitted with the LSU reciprocating gait orthoses (RGO). Proceeding of Annual International Conferance on IEEE Engineering. Med Biol Soc 1988;10:1672.

[8] Motlock WM. principles of orthotic management for child and adult paraplegia and clinical experience with the isocentric RGO. Proceeding of 7th world congress of the international society in prosthetic and orthotics 1992; Chicago, p 28.

[9] Kirtley C, McKay SK, editors. Total design of the "Walkabout": A new paraplegic walking orthosis. In: ISPO Proceedings 7th World Congress, Chicago, Illinois, 1992, June 28-July 3. ISPO p39.

[10] Middleton J, Fisher W, Davis G, Smith R. A medial linkage orthosis to assist ambulation after spinal cord injury. Prosthetics and Orthotics International 1998;22(3):258–64.

[11] Saitoh E, Baba M, Sonoda S, Tomita Y, Suzuki M, Hayashi M. A new medial single hip joint for paraplegic walkers. In: Ueda S, Nakamura R, Ishigami S (eds). The Eighth World Congress of International Rehabilitation Medicine Association. Monduzzi Editore: Bologna, Italy 1997, pp 1299–1305.

[12] Genda E, Oota K, Suzuki Y, Koyama K, Kasahara T. A new walking orthosis for paraplegics: hip and ankle linkage system. Prosthetics and Orthotics International 2004;28(1):69–74.

[13] Ahmadi Bani M, Arazpour M, Farahmand F, Mousavi ME, Hutchins SW. The efficiency of mechanical orthoses in affecting parameters associated with daily living in spinal cord injury patients: a literature review. Disability and Rehabilitation: Assistive Technology 2014(0):1–8.

[14] Harvey L, Davis G, Smith M, Engel S. Energy expenditure during gait using the walkabout and isocentric reciprocal gait orthoses in persons with paraplegia. Archives of Physical Medicine and Rehabilitation 1998;79(8):945–9.

[15] Harvey LA, Smith MB, Davis GM, Engel S. Functional outcomes attained by T9-12 paraplegic patients with the walkabout and the isocentric reciprocal gait orthoses. Archives of Physical Medicine and Rehabilitation 1997;78(7):706–11.

[16] Bernardi M, Canale I, Castellano V, Di Filippo L, Felici F, Marchetti M. The efficiency of walking of paraplegic patients using a reciprocating gait orthosis. Paraplegia 1995;33(7):409–15.

[17] Karimi MT. Functional walking ability of paraplegic patients: comparison of functional electrical stimulation versus mechanical orthoses. European Journal of Orthopaedic Surgery & Traumatology 2013;23(6):631–8.

[18] Shimada Y, Hatakeyama K, Minato T, Matsunaga T, Sato M, Chida S, et al. Hybrid functional electrical stimulation with medial linkage knee-ankle-foot orthoses in complete paraplegics. The Tohoku Journal of Experimental Medicine 2006;209(2):117–23.

[19] Yang L, Condie D, Granat M, Paul J, Rowley D. Effects of joint motion constraints on the gait of normal subjects and their implications on the further development of hybrid FES orthosis for paraplegic persons. Journal of Biomechanics 1996;29(2):217–26.

[20] Petrofsky J, Smith JB. Physiologic costs of computer-controlled walking in persons with paraplegia using a reciprocating-gait orthosis. Archives of Physical Medicine and Rehabilitation 1991;72(11):890–6.

[21] Arazpour M, Chitsazan A, Hutchins SW, Ghomshe FT, Mousavi ME, Takamjani EE, et al. Design and simulation of a new powered gait orthosis for paraplegic patients. Prosthetics and Orthotics International 2012;36(1):125–30.

[22] Audu ML, To CS, Kobetic R, Triolo RJ. Gait evaluation of a novel hip constraint orthosis with implication for walking in paraplegia. Neural Systems and Rehabilitation Engineering, IEEE Transactions on 2010;18(6):610–8.

[23] Hornby TG, Zemon DH, Campbell D. Robotic-assisted, body-weight-supported treadmill training in individuals following motor incomplete spinal cord injury. Physical Therapy 2005;85(1):52–66.

[24] Colombo G, Joerg M, Schreier R, Dietz V. Treadmill training of paraplegic patients using a robotic orthosis. Journal of Rehabilitation Research and Development 2000;37(6):693–700.

[25] Van Der Salm A, Nene AV, Maxwell DJ, Veltink PH, Hermens HJ, IJzerman MJ. Gait impairments in a group of patients with incomplete spinal cord injury and their relevance regarding therapeutic approaches using functional electrical stimulation. Artificial Organs 2005;29(1):8–14.

[26] Hidler J. What is next for locomotor-based studies? Journal of Rehabilitation Research and Development 2005;42(1):xi.

[27] Harkema SJ, Hurley SL, Patel UK, Requejo PS, Dobkin BH, Edgerton VR. Human lumbosacral spinal cord interprets loading during stepping. Journal of Neurophysiology 1997;77(2):797–811.

[28] Beres-Jones JA, Harkema SJ. The human spinal cord interprets velocity-dependent afferent input during stepping. Brain 2004;127(10):2232–46.

[29] Vukobratovic M, Hristic D, Stojiljkovic Z. Development of active anthropomorphic exoskeletons. Medical and Biological Engineering and Computing 1974;12(1):66–80.

[30] Belforte G, Gastaldi L, Sorli M. Pneumatic active gait orthosis. Mechatronics 2001;11(3): 301–23.

[31] Belforte G, Eula G, Appendino S, Sirolli S. Pneumatic interactive gait rehabilitation orthosis: design and preliminary testing. Proceedings of the Institution of Mechanical Engineers, Part H: Journal of Engineering in Medicine 2011;225(2):158–69.

[32] Kang S, Ryu J, Moon I, Kim K, Mun M. Walker gait analysis of powered gait orthosis for paraplegic. In: Proceedings of world congress on medical physics and biomedical engineering IFMBE, COEX Seoul, Korea, 27 August –1 September 2006, vol. 14, pp. 2889–2891. Springer, 2007.

[33] Ruthenberg B, Wasylewski N, Beard J. An experimental device for investigating the force and power requirements of a powered gait orthosis. Development 1997;34(2):203–13.

[34] Ohta Y, Yano H, Suzuki R, Yoshida M, Kawashima N, Nakazawa K. A two-degree-of-freedom motor-powered gait orthosis for spinal cord injury patients. Proceedings of the Institution of Mechanical Engineers, Part H: Journal of Engineering in Medicine 2007;221(6):629–39.

[35] Arazpour M, Chitsazan A, Hutchins SW, Ghomshe FT, Mousavi ME, Takamjani EE, et al. Evaluation of a novel powered hip orthosis for walking by a spinal cord injury patient: a single case study. Prosthetics and Orthotics International 2012;36(1):105–12.

[36] Arazpour M, Chitsazan A, Hutchins SW, et al. Evaluation of a novel powered hip orthosis for walking by a spinal cord injury patient: a single case study. Prosthet Orthot Int 2012; 36(1): 105–112.

[37] Bogue R. Robotic exoskeletons: a review of recent progress. Industrial Robot: An International Journal 2015;42(1):5–10.

[38] Ferris DP, Sawicki GS, Domingo A. Powered lower limb orthoses for gait rehabilitation. Topics in Spinal Cord Injury Rehabilitation 2005;11(2):34.

[39] Dollar A, Herr H. Lower extremity exoskeletons and active orthoses: challenges and state-of-the-art. Robotics, IEEE Transactions on 2008;24(1):144–58.

[40] Duerinck S, Swinnen E, Beyl P, Hagman F, Jonkers I, Vaes P, et al. The added value of an actuated ankle-foot orthosis to restore normal gait function in patients with spinal cord injury: a systematic review. Journal of Rehabilitation Medicine 2012;44(4):299–309.

[41] Arazpour M, Hutchins SW, Bani MA. The efficacy of powered orthoses on walking in persons with paraplegia. Prosthetics and Orthotics International 2014:0309364613520031.

[42] Whittle M, Cochrane G, Chase A, Copping A, Jefferson R, Staples D, et al. A comparative trial of two walking systems for paralysed people. Paraplegia 1991;29(2):97.

[43] Saitoh E, Suzuki T, Sonoda S, Fujitani J, Tomita Y, Chino N. Clinical experience with a new hip-knee-ankle-foot orthotic system using a medial single hip joint for paraplegic standing and walking 1. American Journal of Physical Medicine & Rehabilitation 1996;75(3):198.

[44] Middleton J, Yeo J, Blanch L, Vare V, Peterson K, Brigden K. Clinical evaluation of a new orthosis, the 'walkabout', for restoration of functional standing and short distance mobility in spinal paralysed individuals. Spinal Cord 1997;35(9):574–9.

[45] Nenel A, Hermensl H, Zilvold G. Paraplegic locomotion: a review. Spinal Cord 1996;34:507–24.

[46] Winchester P, Carollo J, Parekh R, Lutz L, Aston J. A comparison of paraplegic gait performance using two types of reciprocating gait orthoses. Prosthetics and Orthotics International 1993;17(2):101–6.

[47] Nene A, Patrick J. Energy cost of paraplegic locomotion using the ParaWalker—electrical stimulation ``hybrid" orthosis. Archives of Physical Medicine and Rehabilitation 1990;71(2):116.

[48] Hirokawa S, Grimm M. Energy consumption in paraplegic ambulation using the reciprocating gait orthosis and electric stimulation of the thigh muscles. Archives of Physical Medicine and Rehabilitation 1990;71(9):687.

[49] Katz-Leurer M, Weber C, Smerling-Kerem J, Rottem H, Meyer S. Prescribing the reciprocal gait orthosis for myelomeningocele children: a different approach and clinical outcome. Pediatric Rehabilitation 2004;7(2):105–9.

[50] Sykes L, Edwards J, Powell ES, Ross ERS. The reciprocating gait orthosis: long-term usage patterns. Archives of Physical Medicine and Rehabilitation 1995;76(8):779–83.

[51] Franceschini M, Baratta S, Zampolini M, Loria D, Lotta S. Reciprocating gait orthoses: a multicenter study of their use by spinal cord injured patients. Archives of Physical Medicine and Rehabilitation 1997;78(6):582–6.

[52] Scivoletto G, Petrelli A, Di Lucente L, Giannantoni A, Fuoco U, D'Ambrosio F, et al. One year follow up of spinal cord injury patients using a reciprocating gait orthosis: preliminary report. Spinal Cord 2000;38(9):555–8.

[53] Jaspers P, Peeraer L, Van Petegem W, Van der Perre G. The use of an advanced reciprocating gait orthosis by paraplegic individuals: a follow-up study. Spinal Cord 1997;35(9):585–9.

[54] Kawashima N, Sone Y, Nakazawa K, Akai M, Yano H. Energy expenditure during walking with weight-bearing control (WBC) orthosis in thoracic level of paraplegic patients. Spinal Cord 2003;41(9):506–10.

[55] Arazpour M, Bani M, Hutchins S, Jones R. The physiological cost index of walking with mechanical and powered gait orthosis in patients with spinal cord injury. Spinal Cord 2013;51(5):356–9.

[56] Tanabe S, Saitoh E, Hirano S, Katoh M, Takemitsu T, Uno A, et al. Design of the Wearable Power-Assist Locomotor (WPAL) for paraplegic gait reconstruction. Disability and Rehabilitation: Assistive Technology 2013;8(1):84–91.

[57] Nene A, Patrick J. Energy cost of paraplegic locomotion with the ORLAU ParaWalker. Spinal Cord 1989;27(1):5–18.

[58] Harvey LA, Davis GM, Smith MB, Engel S. Energy expenditure during gait using the walkabout and isocentric reciprocal gait orthoses in persons with paraplegia. Archives of Physical Medicine and Rehabilitation 1998;79(8):945–9.

[59] Leung AK, Wong AF, Wong EC, Hutchins SW. The physiological cost index of walking with an isocentric reciprocating gait orthosis among patients with T12–L1 spinal cord injury. Prosthetics and Orthotics International 2009;33(1):61–8.

[60] Waters RL, Mulroy S. The energy expenditure of normal and pathologic gait. Gait & Posture 1999;9(3):207–31.

[61] Kerrigan DC, Viramontes BE, Corcoran PJ, LaRaia PJ. Measured versus predicted vertical displacement of the sacrum during gait as a tool to measure biomechanical gait performance. American Journal of Physical Medicine & Rehabilitation 1995;74(1):3–8.

[62] Baardman G, Ijzerman M, Hermen H, Veltink P, Boom H, Zilvold G. The influence of the reciprocal hip joint link in the Advanced Reciprocating Gait Orthosis on standing performance in paraplegia. Prosthetics and Orthotics International 1997;21(3):210–21.

[63] Dall P, Müller B, Stallard I, Edwards J, Granat M. The functional use of the reciprocal hip mechanism during gait for paraplegic patients walking in the Louisiana State University reciprocating gait orthosis. Prosthetics and Orthotics International 1999;23(2):152–62.

[64] Johnson WB, Fatone S, Gard SA. Walking mechanics of persons who use reciprocating gait orthoses. Journal of Rehabilitation Research and & Development 2009;46(3): 435–46.

[65] Harvey LA, Newton-John T, Davis GM, Smith MB, Engel S. A comparison of the attitude of paraplegic individuals to the walkabout orthosis and the isocentric reciprocal gait orthosis. Spinal Cord 1997;35(9):580–4.

[66] Ijzerman M, Baardman G, Hermens H, Veltink P, Boom H, Zilvold G. The influence of the reciprocal cable linkage in the advanced reciprocating gait orthosis on paraplegic gait performance. Prosthetics and Orthotics International 1997;21(1):52–61.

[67] Saitoh E, Suzuki T, Sonoda S, Fujitani J, Tomita Y, Chino N. Clinical experience with a new hip-knee-ankle-foot orthotic system using a medial single hip joint for paraplegic standing and walking 1. American Journal of Physical Medicine & Rehabilitation 1996;75(3):198–203.

[68] Massucci M, Brunetti G, Piperno R, Betti L, Franceschini M. Walking with the advanced reciprocating gait orthosis (ARGO) in thoracic paraplegic patients: energy expenditure and cardiorespiratory performance. Spinal Cord 1998;36(4):223–7.

[69] Arazpour M, Bani MA, Hutchins SW. Reciprocal gait orthoses and powered gait orthoses for walking by spinal cord injury patients. Prosthetics and Orthotics International 2013;37(1):14–21.

[70] Whittle M, Cochrane G, Chase A, Copping A, Jefferson R, Staples D, et al. A comparative trial of two walking systems for paralysed people. Spinal Cord 1991;29(2):97–102.

[71] Bani MA, Arazpour M, Ghomshe FT, Mousavi ME, Hutchins SW. Gait evaluation of the advanced reciprocating gait orthosis with solid versus dorsi flexion assist ankle foot

orthoses in paraplegic patients. Prosthetics and Orthotics International 2013;37(2):161–7.

[72] Onogi K, Kondo I, Saitoh E, Kato M, Oyobe T. Comparison of the effects of sliding-type and hinge-type joints of knee-ankle-foot orthoses on temporal gait parameters in patients with paraplegia. Japanese Journal of Comprehensive Rehabilitation Science 2010;1:1–6.

[73] Suzuki T, Sonoda S, Saitoh E, Onogi K, Fujino H, Teranishi T, et al. Prediction of gait outcome with the knee–ankle–foot orthosis with medial hip joint in patients with spinal cord injuries: a study using recursive partitioning analysis. Spinal Cord 2007;45(1):57–63.

[74] Middleton JW, Sinclair PJ, Smith RM, Davis GM. Postural control during stance in paraplegia: effects of medially linked versus unlinked knee-ankle-foot orthoses. Archives of Physical Medicine and Rehabilitation 1999;80(12):1558–65.

[75] Abe K. Comparison of static balance, walking velocity, and energy consumption with knee-ankle-foot orthosis, walkabout orthosis, and reciprocating gait orthosis in thoracic-level paraplegic patients. JPO: Journal of Prosthetics and Orthotics 2006;18(3):87–91.

Chapter 11

Non-invasive Brain Stimulation to Characterize and Alter Motor Function after Spinal Cord Injury

Aaron Z. Bailey, Hunter J. Fassett, Tea Lulic,
Jenin El Sayes and Aimee J. Nelson

Additional information is available at the end of the chapter

http://dx.doi.org/10.5772/63351

Abstract

Advances in transcranial magnetic stimulation (TMS) now permit the precise assessment of circuitry in human motor cortices that contribute to movement. Further, TMS approaches are used to promote neural plasticity within cortical and spinal circuitry in an attempt to create short-term changes in motor control. This review is focused on the application of TMS techniques in the study of characterizing and promoting neural plasticity within individuals presenting with chronic spinal cord injury. We review TMS research performed in individuals with SCI and consider new opportunities for the use of TMS approaches to promote neural plasticity for improving motor recovery.

Keywords: spinal cord injury, motor recovery, noninvasive brain stimulation, transcranial magnetic stimulation, neural plasticity

1. Introduction

Noninvasive brain stimulation (NIBS) approaches are used to both characterize and modify neural activity within the targeted cortices and the spinal cord. These approaches are, therefore, well-suited for understanding and attempting to improve functional recovery following spinal cord injury. There is, however, a gap in our present understanding of how the cortical physiology is altered in individuals with spinal cord injury (SCI). In this review, we focus on the characterization of motor cortical circuitry in individuals with SCI using transcranial magnetic stimulation (TMS). This basic knowledge is essential to developing therapies that aim to induce long-term changes in neural circuits that participate in motor control. NIBS approaches are also capable of inducing short-term plasticity within motor cortical neural circuits and may be combined with other techniques to promote greater functional changes in individuals with SCI. Therefore, the second goal of this review is to survey the literature that has utilized NIBS approaches for promoting neural plasticity within the motor system in individuals with SCI. We subsequently explore new opportunities for the use of NIBS to characterize and promote neural plasticity in SCI for improving motor recovery.

2. Noninvasive brain stimulation to characterize motor function

NIBS provides an opportunity to assess the neural circuitry within motor cortical areas as well as the excitatory and inhibitory influences on neural output to specific muscles. These circuits may originate within the motor cortex (intracortical) and/or operate between cortical areas (intercortical) or hemispheres (interhemispheric). Following SCI, the excitability of the motor cortex and the corresponding cortical circuits may be altered, and these changes may be, in part, related to the functional reorganization of the central nervous system. TMS techniques offer the opportunity to characterize alterations in cortical circuits following SCI and are described following. Importantly, these techniques are ideal for monitoring changes that accompany motor recovery in SCI populations.

2.1. Motor-evoked potentials (MEPs)

TMS delivered over the motor cortex trans-synaptically activates corticospinal neurons that ultimately give rise to a motor-evoked potential (MEP) recorded in the target muscle. The amplitude of the MEP represents the overall corticospinal excitability including contributions from the upper and lower motorneurons and the functional integrity of the corticospinal path [1]. The MEP amplitude may be modulated by factors such as action planning [2, 3], pharmaceuticals [4], or neuromuscular diseases [5–7]. The evaluation of MEP amplitude is a commonly used method to quantify changes in excitability within the descending motor pathways following experimental manipulation [8] or during the process of recovery [9]. The MEP latency provides an additional source of neurophysiological information and represents the conduction time for descending signals originating within the motor cortex to travel to the muscle effector, a measure that serves a diagnostic purpose for a number of disease states [10].

Following SCI, MEP amplitude and latency are often altered. When using TMS to assess muscles caudal to the spinal lesion level, smaller amplitude and longer latency MEPs are reported [11, 12]. This is thought to be due to the structural damage to descending corticospinal fibers including fewer intact axons and significant demyelination surrounding the lesion [13]. In individuals with SCI, such decrements in MEP amplitude may be lessened by introducing low level active contraction in the muscle of interest [14]. However, voluntary control of a muscle is not necessarily indicative of corticospinal connectivity to that particular muscle since MEPs may be elicited in muscles not under volitional control in individuals with SCI [15].

http://dx.doi.org/10.5772/63351

The origin of MEPs is complex, as pyramidal tract neurons are influenced directly and indirectly (trans-synaptically) in response to cortical stimulation. Additionally, MEPs depend on spinal motorneuron excitability and are influenced by cortical areas outside of motor cortex such as the premotor and supplementary motor areas [8]. As such, the ambiguity in the origin of the MEP creates challenges in its interpretation. Nonetheless, MEP characteristics have a value for assessing motor recovery following SCI such that both MEP amplitude and latency, in the acute stage of injury, predict the recovery of ambulation and hand function [10].

2.2. Motor threshold (MT)

MT is defined as the minimal stimulation intensity that elicits a MEP in a target muscle. MT can be assessed in two ways. Resting motor threshold (RMT) is often obtained by finding the lowest stimulation intensity that produces a MEP of at least 50 μV in 5 out of 10 consecutive trials, while the target muscle is relaxed [16, 17]. Furthermore, motor threshold can be determined while the participant maintains low levels of muscle contraction (i.e., active motor threshold or AMT). AMT is commonly defined as the lowest stimulation intensity to elicit MEPs of at least 200 μV in 5 out of 10 consecutive trials, while the participant maintains a contraction corresponding to 10–15% of their maximum [16]. RMT represents the resting membrane excitability throughout the efferent system at both cortical and spinal levels [18]. During this resting state, spinal motorneurons require a number of descending volleys from the cortex to summate in order to produce a MEP. This requirement for greater corticospinal summation at rest has been speculated to be due to glutamatergic synaptic activity [18]. Pharmacological studies have shown that AMT and RMT depend on the axon membrane excitability, specifically on voltage-gated sodium channel activity [19]. Application of various drugs that block the action of these channels such as carbamazepine and lamotrigine increase the required stimulation intensity to elicit RMT and AMT (see Paulus et al. 2008 for review) [18]. Despite the fact that pharmacological studies have not been able to isolate changes in RMT without a simultaneous change in AMT [18], differences in levels of synaptic excitability have been inferred from studies of MT latency, where RMT is seen to have a longer latency than AMT [20]. By maintaining a small contraction, low levels of synaptic firing are sustained and are thought to be more reliant on levels of excitability at the axonal membrane.[18].

Individuals with SCI may demonstrate increases in RMT and AMT. Davey et al. [11] found that RMT and AMT were higher for muscles below the level of injury whereas muscles innervated by fibers rostral to the injury had thresholds similar to the uninjured control group. Other research has shown that alterations following SCI are more prevalent when examining AMT [21, 22]. Bailey et al. [22] demonstrated increased AMT elicited from the flexor carpi radialis muscle of the forearm in participants with chronic cervical SCI. They suggested that this increase in AMT without a corresponding increase in RMT may be due to abnormalities in regulation of membrane excitability via voltage-gated ion channels. Collectively, the published data suggest that RMT may or may not be altered while AMT is increased in SCI participants. However, it has been established that changes in both RMT and AMT are dependent on the location of the target muscle relative to the level of the lesion. Further, changes in MT in chronic SCI are likely to differ depending on the severity and location of injury.

2.3. Motor cortical maps

The motor cortex is somatotopically organized in that cortical representations of the muscles are found in relatively predictable locations in the medial–lateral direction [23]. The extent of cortical territory occupied by a given muscle representation is thought to correspond to the amount of dexterity and fine motor control needed by the corresponding muscle such that larger representations exist for small distal muscles of the hand while smaller representations are present for larger proximal muscles of the arm and shoulder [12]. Most cortical muscle representations correspond to effectors of the contralateral limb although some degrees of ipsilateral projections have been found in proximal upper limb muscles in uninjured individuals [24]. Motor cortical maps can be obtained by delivering TMS pulses at suprathreshold intensities using a spatial grid aligned with the precentral gyrus and recording MEPs from target muscles [25]. Motor cortical maps are typically evaluated by quantifying the area, volume, and center of gravity for the representation of each muscle of interest. Map area and volume scale linearly with increasing TMS intensity and are considered a reliable method to evaluate cortical organization [26].

Studies of motor maps following SCI revealed enlarged representations of the most proximally spared muscles that tended to shift into cortical territory corresponding to the muscles below the level of injury [27, 28]. Takeover of de-innervated territory was supported by findings in which the representation of the extensor digitorum communis muscle was shifted anterolaterally (into the hand region) following incomplete cervical SCI [21, 29]. Brouwer and Hopkins-Fosseel [12] quantified motor maps in SCI participants for a variety of contracted upper arm muscles and found that proximal muscles were represented to a greater extent than distal hand muscles, and there was an extensive overlap of different muscle representations when compared to uninjured participants. This overlap may be beneficial for organization as the neurons projecting to single muscles are not focally distributed and may act to minimize complete functional losses following neurological injury. Cortical reorganization following SCI occurs rapidly as evident by the changes in the shape and location of biceps brachii motor cortical maps only 6–17 days following SCI [29]. More recently, a study using neuroimaging techniques demonstrated that representations of the tongue were significantly shifted in their location within motor cortex in participants with cervical SCI compared to uninjured participants [30]. Collectively, the motor cortical maps indicate that the reorganization of motor cortex somatotopy takes place following SCI, suggesting that plasticity may compensate for the loss of neuronal communication between the cortex and the muscles of the body. Although the mechanisms for such reorganization are unknown in humans, it may be speculated that changes in cortical organization are shaped through GABA mediated lateral inhibitory circuits [31].

A number of practical considerations are important for cortical mapping studies using TMS. Mapping protocols require many grid points with approximately 3–10 pulses delivered to each point to capture cortical organization with appropriate resolution. This may require a number of hours to generate a motor map if a large number of points are used [26]. Furthermore, heightened motor thresholds commonly accompany SCI, requiring higher stimulation intensities to elicit MEPs, and this may impact the comfort of the participant and increase the likelihood of coil heating.

2.4. Short-interval intracortical inhibition (SICI)

SICI is an inhibitory circuit within the motor cortex that is comprised of low-threshold GABAergic interneurons [18] and can be evaluated using paired-pulse TMS. By delivering an initial subthreshold conditioning stimulus (CS) approximately 1–5 ms prior to a suprathreshold test stimulus (TS) to the motor cortex, the resulting MEP is reduced when compared to MEPs produced when the TS is applied alone [32]. The subthreshold CS is typically set at an intensity of 70–90% of AMT, showing that the MEP modulation is of cortical origin as no descending volleys to the muscles are produced at these intensities [32]. The mechanism of inhibition involves presynaptic inhibition as inhibitory postsynaptic potentials are generated on neurons upstream of the corticospinal output neurons [18]. $GABA_A$ receptors are implicated in SICI since The delivery of Lorazepam or Diazepam ($GABA_A$ Receptor agonist) reduces SICI [33, 34].

It is well documented that SICI is reduced in individuals with SCI. One case report examined SICI in the relaxed extensor digitorum communis muscle using various interstimulus intervals and a single CS intensity [35]. This method was also used elsewhere in the relaxed first dorsal interosseous muscle [36]. Both cases demonstrated a reduction in SICI when compared to controls [35, 36]. However, the aforementioned studies used a single CS and TS intensity, making interpretation difficult, as the required stimulator output to produce MEPs in SCI participants is typically greater relative to able-bodied individuals. Roy et al. [37] explored SICI in SCI participants by measuring recruitment curves whereby CS intensities were altered from 60 to 110% AMT. They recorded responses from both tibialis anterior in the lower leg and the first dorsal interosseous muscle of the hand during contraction of each muscle. The results indicated a reduction of SICI responses in SCI participants compared to controls, although both retained a U-shaped recruitment curve. Individuals with SCI were seen to have a smaller range of CS intensities eliciting inhibition of the MEP when compared to the recruitment curves of uninjured individuals [37]. Therefore, recruitment characteristics of SICI appear to be unchanged following SCI while the overall amount of inhibition is reduced. The authors speculate that this may be due to spinal inhibitory mechanisms, or to reductions in GABAergic activity following cortical reorganization that occurs with SCI. Mi et al. [38] examined SICI in chronic cervical SCI. Similar to the results found by Roy et al. [37], the authors identified a smaller range of CS intensities to elicit SICI in the flexor carpi radialis muscle of the forearm compared to controls. In this case, significant inhibition of the TS-evoked response was only seen at 90% AMT in SCI compared to the wider range of 70, 80, and 90% AMT in controls [38]. This may reflect the reduced excitability of corticospinal neurons following SCI as the pattern of recruitment is maintained, while the range of inhibition is reduced. Therefore, impairment in GABAergic circuitry mediating SICI in the motor cortex has been established following lesion to the spinal cord.

2.5. Long-interval intracortical inhibition (LICI)

LICI represents intracortical circuitry that acts to modulate MEPs and can be observed via paired-pulse TMS to the motor cortex. The inhibitory pathways involved in LICI can be probed by delivering a suprathreshold CS before a subsequent suprathreshold TS with an interval between 50 and 200 ms to the motor cortex [39, 40]. This produces two MEPs; however, the amplitude of the second MEP is reduced (i.e., inhibited) compared to the MEP evoked by delivery of the single TS pulse. Similar to SICI, the interneuron interactions leading to MEP inhibition are mediated by GABA as seen in pharmacological studies [41, 42]. The longer interstimulus intervals leading to the inhibition are due to $GABA_B$ receptor activity which has been confirmed in studies using $GABA_B$ receptor agonists such as baclofen to increase the inhibitory response [43].

Limited research has examined alterations in LICI after SCI. Barry et al. [43] compared LICI in SCI versus uninjured controls in the resting and active muscle states to examine the effects of $GABA_B$ agonist Baclofen. They examined the first dorsal interosseous muscle of the hand, which showed a decrease in LICI in the active state in the control group as well as in SCI individuals that were taking Baclofen. However, SCI participants not medicated with Baclofen did not show a reduction in LICI during active contraction. This finding suggests abnormal $GABA_B$ receptor activity following SCI as the MEP responses continue to be further inhibited with increasing tonic efferent activity introduced by sustained muscle contraction. Interestingly, this decrease in LICI associated with muscle contraction appears to be rectified by the application of Baclofen, normalizing the inhibitory response in SCI to that of the control group. Another study examined the recruitment of the LICI circuitry in the active muscle state by applying CS intensities at 10% increments from 90 to 130% AMT to capture the pattern of $GABA_B$ mediated response in SCI [38]. An increase in LICI was observed in SCI participants at higher CS intensities (120 and 130% AMT), while the uninjured group did not show any LICI with increasing CS intensity. The authors attributed the increase in inhibition to Baclofen, which as a $GABA_B$ agonist may return LICI circuitry to its normative state.

2.6. Intracortical facilitation (ICF)

ICF can be observed within motor cortex, demonstrating the presence of excitatory circuits impacting the descending corticospinal output. ICF is elicited by delivering a subthreshold TMS pulse over the motor representation of a muscle followed by a suprathreshold TS after an interval of 7–20 ms [32]. This paired-pulse TMS method elicits a net facilitation of the MEP as seen by increased response amplitudes when compared to MEPs evoked from the single TS [33]. Pharmacological approaches reveal that ICF is the net effect of both inhibitory and excitatory contributions. Application of $GABA_A$ receptor agonists such as Diazepam result in decreased ICF, showing an influence of GABAergic inhibition onto corticospinal output neurons [44]. This demonstrates that although ICF is affected by GABAergic activity [44], there is a large excitatory component resulting in net facilitation. Thus, it is speculated that that NMDA receptors play a role in the facilitation observed in ICF [45]. These receptors respond to glutamate when nearby AMPA receptors are active to excite postsynaptic neurons. The role of NMDA receptor activity in ICF is supported by the finding that the application of NMDA receptor antagonists also causes a decrease in facilitation, implicating their role in the physiology of ICF [45].

A single case study examined ICF in a participant with cervical myelopathy using a CS intensity of 80% RMT and TS intensity of 120% RMT at a number of different interstimulus intervals. ICF was only observed when the interstimulus interval was 10 ms [35]. Further research with larger sample sizes and control groups should examine alterations in ICF in individuals with SCI. Collection of recruitment curves for ICF may provide a more comprehensive view of excitatory mechanisms contributing to corticospinal output following SCI.

2.7. Short and long latency afferent inhibition (SAI/LAI)

SAI demonstrates the influence of a peripherally evoked afferent volley on the MEP and is observed when an electrical stimulus applied to a peripheral nerve is followed by a single suprathreshold TMS pulse to the motor cortex. The temporal interval between the peripheral and cortical stimulation corresponds to the conduction time for the afferent volley to reach the somatosensory cortex. This timing causes the afferent information to arrive shortly before the suprathreshold TMS pulse, which is subsequently inhibited compared to the MEP evoked by the TS pulse delivered alone. This circuit is commonly studied in intrinsic muscles of the hand where the interstimulus interval is roughly 18–21 ms [46, 47]. The exact mechanisms underpinning this pathway remains unclear, although pharmacological intervention using drugs such as Scopolamine (cholinergic antagonist) or Diazepam indicate that SAI is mediated by both cholinergic and GABAergic circuits [48, 49]. LAI is another example of sensory modulation to cortical pathways involved in MEP generation. The method of eliciting LAI is similar to that of SAI with the exception of a longer interstimulus interval of ~100–200 ms [46, 50]. LAI is speculated to modulate corticospinal output by exclusively GABAergic systems, particularly those mediated by $GABA_B$ receptors [49]. The modulation of MEPs induced by sensory input suggests that SAI and LAI provide insight into sensorimotor integration [51].

The literature surrounding afferent regulation of the motor cortex following SCI is minimal. Roy et al. [14] stimulated the common peroneal nerve at the ankle to modify MEPs elicited from tibialis anterior using interstimulus intervals ranging from 30 to 80 ms. Results indicated an inhibition of MEPs from tibialis anterior when the internal between the TS pulse and the peripheral electrical stimulation corresponded to the latency of the afferent volley from the common peroneal nerve. However, this effect was reduced in the SCI group. The decrease in SAI relative to controls is expected in this population, as the transmission of afferent information from the periphery to the cortex is largely dependent on spinal mechanisms that are likely to be affected by damage to the spinal cord. Further, a recent study examined SAI within the flexor carpi radialis muscle in cervical SCI participants and found that, compared to uninjured controls SAI was reduced when the muscle was in the active and resting state [22]. The authors speculated that this impairment in SAI circuitry is due to plasticity effects in the processing and/or transmission of the information within the cortex as well as reductions in afferent transmission to the cortex. Thus, literature regarding sensory modulation of motor output suggests that afferent integration is impaired following SCI.

2.8. Cortical silent period (CSP)

The CSP represents descending inhibitory signals during active contraction of the muscle. When maintaining a constant level of muscle contraction, stimulation of the motor cortex at suprathreshold intensities produces a CSP in the active contralateral muscle. The duration of the CSP may provide some indication of functional ability. For example, the ability to modulate muscle activity following large descending efferent volleys may impact motor tasks involving fine motor control where small, precise movements are required. The CSP is commonly ~200 ms in duration and is impacted by both cortical and spinal factors. Initial inhibition (~50–75 ms) is attributed to the refractory period of efferent fibers within the spinal cord following suprathreshold TMS, while the remaining duration is thought to originate from the cortex [52–54]. This effect is physiologically mediated by multiple GABAergic systems as treatment with pharmaceuticals that reduce synaptic clearance of GABA increase CSP durations [42, 55]. At the receptor level, $GABA_A$ appears to modulate the CSP at lower TMS intensities as benzodiazepines increase the CSP duration [52]. However, at high TMS stimulation intensities, treatment with benzodiazepines shortens the CSP [56]. The latter finding suggests that $GABA_A$ activity suppresses the effects of $GABA_B$ receptors when such inputs are presented to the motor cortex [56].

The CSP duration appears to be altered in SCI. Shimizu et al. [36] investigated the CSP in three individuals with cervical SCI. In all participants, there was no observable CSP in the foot muscle, and in two individuals, the CSP was additionally absent in the hand muscles. The loss of this silent period suggests that there may have been reorganization at the level of the cortex or hyper excitability of the cortex as GABA systems are suppressed [36]. Barry et al. [43] examined the GABA system involved in producing the CSP in intrinsic hand muscles of chronic, incomplete SCI groups that either were or were not taking Baclofen. Baclofen did not alter the CSP in SCI, and all SCI participants displayed a longer CSP duration than age-matched uninjured controls [43]. Another study examined the CSP, while generating motor maps of forearm extensor muscles and reported an inverse relationship between the duration of the CSP and the amount of spinal cord atrophy via inspection of MRI images [21]. Therefore, when increases in the CSP are observed in SCI, it is likely due to intact inhibitory corticospinal projections to the muscle although spinal modulation of inhibitory circuits is impaired.

2.9. Inter-hemispheric inhibition (IHI)

IHI is a circuit that results from the extensive interconnectivity between the two cerebral hemispheres via the corpus callosum. The integrity of this cross-communication can be assessed by paired-pulse TMS over the motor cortices. By providing a suprathreshold CS over the motor representation of a muscle in one hemisphere followed by a suprathreshold TS over the homologous motor representation in the opposite hemisphere, inhibition of the MEP in response to the CS is observed [57, 58]. This suppression occurs at interstimulus intervals of 10 and 40 ms [57]. Modulation of MEP amplitude with IHI is mediated via GABAergic systems as application of $GABA_B$ agonist Baclofen induces an increase in inhibition at both paired-pulse intervals [59].

http://dx.doi.org/10.5772/63351

IHI in SCI has not been studied extensively. One report used an interstimulus interval of 10 ms for probing IHI in cervical SCI and found that there was neither enhancement nor suppression of the MEP when the participants were at rest or maintaining a contraction at a level that corresponded to either 30 or 70% MVC [60]. The authors speculate that the lack of change in IHI may be due to interactions with other circuitry that has been affected by injury such as SICI. One challenge in measuring IHI in the SCI population is that a MEP must be obtained with amplitude that is large enough to observe suppression following modulation from the opposite hemisphere. Decreased muscle responses are well established in SCI, making it difficult to elicit a MEP that is large enough to be modulated by the CS of the opposite hemisphere. Therefore, the IHI protocol may need to be adapted for the SCI population.

2.10. Summary

Please refer to **Table 1** for a summary of the previous findings. Changes in motor cortical excitability and circuitry follow SCI and yield alterations in corticospinal output. The available information regarding changes in cortical circuitry for motor output in SCI is limited, making a comprehensive view of neurophysiological rehabilitation difficult in this population. Thus, further studies should identify and quantify aberrant motor cortical circuits in SCI.

Measure	Source	Classification	Muscle tested	Response
Motor-evoked	Davey et al. [11]	Tetraplegic	Thenar Muscles	↓Amplitude
potentials	Brouwer and Hopkins-	Tetraplegic	(APB)	↓ Amplitude (no MEP response in
	Rosseel [12]	Para/Tetraplegic	Biceps, Triceps,	most SCI subjects)
	Roy et al. [37]	Para/Tetraplegic	Deltoid	↓Amplitude
	Roy et al. [14]	Tetraplegic	TA, FDI	↓Amplitude, ↑ MEP duration
	Edwards et al. [15]		TA, FDI	=No change in amplitude
			Biceps, ECR,	
			FCR, APB	
Motor threshold	Davey et al. [11]	Tetraplegic	Biceps, Thenar	No change in biceps (above injury
	Freund et al. [21]	Tetraplegic	Muscles	level), ↑ AMT in APB (below injury
	Bailey et al. [22]	Tetraplegic	EDC	level)
	Saturno et al. [35]	Tetraplegic	FCR	↑ AMT (associated with amount of
			EDC	spinal cord atrophy)
				No change in RMT, ↑ AMT
				↑ RMT
Motor maps	Levy et al. [27]	Tetraplegic	Biceps, Deltoid	↑ Map area, latency, and amplitude
	Cohen et al. [28]	Paraplegic	TA, External	of response inversely related in SCI
	Freund et al. [21]	Tetraplegic	Oblique	↑ Map area of obliques (above
	Streletz et al. [29]	Acute Tetraplegic	EDC	injury), no responses from TA
	Brouwer and Hopins-	Tetraplegic	Biceps, APB	(below injury)
	Rosseel [12]	Tetraplegic	Biceps, Triceps,	CoG shifted posteriorly
	Mikulis et al. [30]		Deltoid	

Measure	Source	Classification	Muscle tested	Response
			Wrist extensors, Tongue	↑ Map area of Biceps, Bicep map shifted laterally ↓ Map volumes, No change in area No change in activation volume, peak response site shifted medially for tongue*
Short-interval intracortical inhibition	Saturno et al. [35] Shimizu et al. [36] Roy et al. [37] Mi et al. [38]	Ischemic Myelopathy Tetraplegic Para/Tetraplegic Tetraplegic	EDC FDI, FHB TA, FDI FDI	↓ SICI ↓SICI in FDI ↓ magnitude of active SICI, similar recruitment with increasing CS intensity No change in magnitude, reduced range of intensities showing SICI
Long-interval intracortical inhibition	Barry et al. [43] Mi et al. [38]	Tetraplegic Tetraplegic	FDI FDI	no change with baclofen, ↑ active LICI without baclofen ↑ active LICI
Intracortical facilitation	Saturno et al. [35]	Ischemic Myelopathy	EDC	No change
Short-latency afferent inhibition	Roy et al. [14] Bailey et al. [22]	Tetraplegia Tetraplegia	TA FCR	↓ SAI (absent) ↓ active and resting SAI
Cortical silent period	Shimizu et al. [36] Barry et al. [43] Freund et al. [21]	Tetraplegic Tetraplegic Tetraplegic	FDI, FHB FDI EDC	↓ CSP duration ↑ CSP duration, correlated with spinal atrophy ↑ CSP duration
Interhemispheric inhibition	Bunday and Perez [60]	Tetraplegic	FDI	No change

Table 1. Cortical circuitry in spinal cord injury.

3. NIBS to induce plasticity in individuals with SCI

NIBS provide an opportunity to modulate the neural circuits that are altered following SCI and have the potential to improve motor function. There are several NIBS protocols that have been used to promote plasticity with the two main forms including repetitive TMS (rTMS), and transcranial direct current stimulation (tDCS). RTMS and tDCS protocols are each founded in the principle of homosynaptic plasticity, while TMS and tDCS protocols paired with peripheral nerve stimulation have effects based on spike-timing dependent plasticity (STDP). Homosynaptic plasticity refers to plasticity occurring at a single synapse that is undergoing stimulation [61, 62]. STDP refers to plasticity induced by timing two stimuli, typically a cortical and a peripheral stimulus, to activate both the presynaptic and postsynaptic neurons coincidentally. These protocols are able to produce effects that resemble long-term potentiation (LTP) or long-term depression (LTD) of synaptic connectivity. Typically, activation of the presynaptic neuron prior to the postsynaptic neuron lends to the generation of LTP while LTD occurs when the postsynaptic neuron is activated first [61]. STDP can be timed such that the two stimuli coincide at different levels of the central nervous system to create either spinal or cortical plasticity. We provide an overview of the literature that has used NIBS approaches to promote plasticity in the motor system in individuals with SCI.

3.1. Repetitive TMS (rTMS)

RTMS is thought to induce homosynaptic plasticity within the target cortex. RTMS may increase or decrease cortical activity via alterations in the activity of glutamatergic NMDA receptors [63]. The frequency, intensity, and duration of rTMS determine whether the plasticity effect is LTD or LTP-like [63, 64]. Typically, rTMS delivered over motor cortex at a frequency of <1 Hz results in LTD-like effects while frequencies >5 Hz yield LTP-like effects [63]. In SCI, the primary focus of rTMS is to modulate descending projections and strengthen the intact corticospinal connections.

In a study by Belci et al. [65], rTMS was applied over the motor cortex for five consecutive days using a protocol that included doublets of TMS delivered at a frequency of 10 Hz with each doublet being separated by 10 s for a total 720 stimuli. Following real rTMS, measures of CSP were reduced. Further, motor and sensory function, determined by the assessment of motor and sensory function by the American Spinal Injury Association (ASIA), was improved, as was performance in the timed peg-board task. Further, the sensory perceptual threshold to an electrical stimulus was reduced suggesting alterations within the somatosensory cortex. These measures remained improved for 2 weeks post-intervention while sham rTMS revealed no benefit [65]. Ellaway et al. [66] delivered real versus sham rTMS via 2 s trains of 5 Hz stimulation separated by 8 s for a total of 15 min over the motor cortex in individuals with SCI. The real and sham interventions were performed over 5 consecutive days. Measurements of the ASIA score, active research arm test (ARAT) which includes testing grasp, grip, pinch and gross movement, electrical stimulation perceptual threshold, MEPs, AMT, and CSP were assessed before and following intervention. Results revealed that AMT was increased and ARAT improved following rTMS compared to the sham intervention, without changes in other measures. Another study delivered real versus sham high-frequency (20 Hz) rTMS over 15 consecutive days to assess improvement in lower limb function [67]. Measurements included lower extremities motor score (LEMS), modified Ashworth scale (MAS), walking index for SCI, ten-meter walking test, step length, cadence assessment, and a timed up and go (TUG) test. At the cessation of the rTMS intervention, LEMS improved, MAS score was reduced, gait was altered (i.e., increased velocity, cadence, step length) and an improvement was observed in TUG without changes in the walking index. Effects returned to baseline 2 weeks following the last intervention [67]. Finally, an rTMS protocol consisting of 4 pulse trains (quadropulse) delivered at a frequency of 250–500 Hz with an inter-train interval of 5–6 s (250–360/day) for either 1 or 5 consecutive days (i.e., ~1000–1440 pulses per day) was delivered to individuals with SCI [68]. Hand dexterity, MEPs, and spinal excitability were measured. After a single session of rTMS, there was no change in hand dexterity although MEPs increased and spinal excitability decreased. Further, after 5 consecutive days of rTMS there was a 10% increase in hand dexterity. These data indicate that rTMS delivered over consecutive days is more effective than single session at promoting motor improvements [68].

3.2. Transcranial direct current stimulation (TDCS)

TDCS is a neuromodulating technique that utilizes homosynaptic plasticity, similar to rTMS. However, unlike rTMS, tDCS does not produce neuronal action potentials since the static field produced by tDCS does not produce the rapid depolarization of neurons [69]. TDCS modifies spontaneous neuronal excitability by either creating tonic depolarization or hyperpolarization [69]. The direction of current flow appears to determine whether the protocol results in LTD or LTP-like effects; anodal tDCS results in neuron depolarization (LTP) while cathodal tDCS results in neuron hyperpolarization (LTD) [69, 70]. There exists one study that has shown evidence for promoting plasticity in individuals with SCI using tDCS. Murray et al. [71] delivered anodal tDCS for 20 min once per week over 3 weeks at varying intensities; 1, 2 mA and sham. Measurements of MEP amplitude, sensory threshold, and muscle strength were performed before and after intervention. MEP amplitude was significantly increased after delivery of 2 mA anodal tDCS but not 1 mA or sham conditions. Sensory threshold was significantly reduced after both 2 and 1 mA but not sham stimulation. No protocol was effective at changing muscle strength [71]. It is evident that the extent of research in tDCS aimed at altering motor function in individuals with SCI is limited. However, early results show that tDCS may be an effective tool to alter corticospinal excitability and improve motor function.

3.3. Paired associative stimulation (PAS) and spinal associative stimulation (SAS)

PAS is a plasticity inducing protocol that utilizes STDP to alter cortical or spinal function. Traditionally, PAS involves timing peripheral electrical nerve stimulation with a TMS pulse over the motor cortex. When these two stimuli are timed to arrive in the cortex at approximately the same time, the protocol is known as PAS and when they are timed to coincide at the level of the spinal cord, the technique is known as spinal associative stimulation (SAS). PAS delivered at an ISI of 25 ms and targeting motor cortex has been effective at increasing MEP amplitude in uninjured individuals [72], while PAS delivered at an ISI of 20 ms has been effective at altering spinal excitability by increasing the amplitude of the spinal H-reflex [73]. There have been three studies performed in SCI where PAS or variations of PAS have been used to induce cortical and/or spinal plasticity promoting functional recovery.

Roy et al. [14] assessed corticospinal excitability in the lower limb before and following PAS delivered at an interval to promote near coincident activation within the motor cortex (i.e., the N20 latency of somatosensory-evoked potential +6 ms). The protocol included 120 pairs of peripheral afferent stimuli and TMS pulses at a frequency of 0.2 Hz [14]. MEPs were measured during tonic 20% contraction (active MEPs) and at rest (resting MEPs). Results indicated significant increases to resting but no change to active MEPs [14]. Bunday and Perez [74] tested the SAS protocol in individuals with SCI and delivered 100 pairs of stimuli at a frequency of 0.1 Hz and timed the ISI such that the TMS efferent volley and the PNS antidromic efferent volley arrived at the corticospinal-motorneuronal synapse at the C7 spinal level nearly simultaneously. Measurements of MEPs, spinal F-waves, voluntary motor output, and manual dexterity were performed post-intervention. Results showed increases in MEPs, no change in F-waves, and increases to both maximum voluntary EMG/force and a reduction in the time to complete the 9-hole pegboard task [74]. Finally, Yamaguchi et al. [75] paired peripheral nerve stimulation with anodal tDCS. During a 20 min, 1 mA anodal tDCS protocol peripheral electrical stimulation trains consisting of 10 pulses delivered at a frequency of 100 Hz were delivered every 2 s. Measurements of reciprocal inhibition from the tibialis anterior and ankle movement were assessed after stimulation. Results indicate reduced reciprocal inhibition, and increased ankle movements following the combination of peripheral electrical stimulation and anodal tDCS [75].

3.4. Summary

Please refer to **Table 2** for a summary of the previous findings. Collectively these studies reveal promising indications that rTMS, TCDS, and PAS approaches can modulate cortical function leading to short-term improvements in the motor system in individuals with SCI. Although, these results are not always unanimous, (i.e., differential effects on MEPs and CSP), they may relate to the specific protocol parameters as existing studies in SCI have utilized variable stimulation parameters. Further research should determine the most effective protocol at yielding changes to neural physiology and improvements in motor function in individuals with SCI. NIBS combined with other techniques might be a promising new avenue for research for the ultimate goal of creating long-term functional improvements.

Intervention	Source	Parameters	Classification	Response
rTMS	Belci et al. [65] Ellaway et al. [66] Benito et al. [67] Alexeeva et al. [68]	- Doublets of TMS delivered at a frequency of 10 Hz - 10 s between doublets - 360 doublets delivered - 90% RMT intensity - 5 consecutive days - trains of TMS delivered at a frequency of 5 HZ over 2 s - 8 s between trains - 15 min of stimulation - 5 consecutive days - TMS delivered at frequ	Incomplete tetraplegic Incomplete tetraplegic Incomplete para/ tetraplegic Incomplete para /tetraplegic	*Physiological* - improved sensory and motor scores on ASIA *Behavioral* - improved time for pegboard task *Physiological* - improved AMT *Behavioral* - improved active reach arm test *Behavioral* - improved lower

Intervention	Source	Parameters	Classification	Response
		ency of 20 Hz - 15 consecutive days - 4 pulses of TMS delivered in trains at a freq uency of 250–500 Hz - 5–6 s between trains - 250–360 pulses delivered - 1–5 consecutive days		extremities motor score - improved modified ashworth scale - improved gait mechanics - improved time up and go *Physiological* - increased motor-evoked potentials - reduced spinal excitability
tDCS	Murray et al. [71]	- Anodal tDCS at 1 or 2 mA - 20 min protocol - once per week for 3 consecutive weeks	Incomplete tetraplegic	*Physiological* - increased motor-evoked potentials - reduced sensory threshold
PAS/SAS	Roy et al. [37] Bunday and Perez [74] Yamaguchi et al. [75]	- ISI of N20 + 6 ms for stimuli to arrive in M1 - 120 pairs of peripheral stimulation and TMS delivered at a frequency of 0.2 Hz - ISI for stimuli to arrive at the C7 spinal level - 100 pairs of peripheral stimulation and TMS delivered at a frequency of 0.1 Hz - pairing of peripheral nerve stimulation with anodal tDCS - 1 mA tDCS delivered over 20 min - peripheral stimulation was trains of 10 stimuli delivered at a	Incomplete para /tetraplegic Incomplete tetraplegic Incomplete para /tetraplegic	*Physiological* - increased resting motor-evoked potentials *Physiological* - increased motor-evoked potentials - increased maximum voluntary EMG activity *Behavioral* - increased maximum voluntary force production - reduced time to complete 9-hole pegboard task

http://dx.doi.org/10.5772/63351

Intervention	Source	Parameters	Classification	Response
		frequency of 100 Hz with 2 s between trains		*Physiological* - reduced recip rocal inhibition *Behavioral* - increased an kle movements

Table 2. Summary of NIBS to promote plasticity in SCI.

4. Coupling NIBS with movement protocols

A primary goal of motor Training is to improve functional ability by repeated exposure to a particular task, such as treadmill training to improve walking ability. In clinical populations, motor training can promote plastic changes in unaffected motor networks by increasing the efficacy of synaptic transmission [76]. Therefore, there is an opportunity to promote neural plasticity via motor training in intact cortical and spinal motor circuitry in individuals with SCI.

4.1. Pairing NIBS with motor training

Previous studies have shown that motor training can influence corticospinal excitability. In participants with SCI, locomotor resistance training using Lokomat facilitates spinal reflexes at 20 and 80 ms in the soleus muscle and improves gait quality as assessed by LEMS, walking index for SCI and velocity [77], as well as MEP amplitudes in tibialis anterior [78]. Treadmill training in SCI participants for ~2 months (5 sessions per week for 1 h) increases MEP amplitudes in tibialis anterior, increases manual muscle strength in ankle dorsiflexors as measured by 11-point manual muscle strength score, and increases the duration of the CSP [79]. Although motor training alone promotes motor recovery, the functional outcomes are often limited and patients still exhibit substantial motor impairments.

Motor training and NIBS are each, independently effective at promoting plasticity in SCI participants. Therefore, the combination of the two may lead to plasticity effects that exceed their individual components. Few studies have tested the effects of pairing NIBS with motor training to facilitate functional motor recovery. Gomes-Osman et al. [80] evaluated upper limb function in SCI participants. They delivered 10 Hz rTMS (800 pulses at 80% RMT) with repetitive task practice involving 30 s of practice with the 9-hole pegboard task. The results revealed a decrease in the time to complete the Jebsen Taylor test following real and sham rTMS paired with repetitive task practice. However, the effects were larger following real versus sham rTMS paired with repetitive task practice. Measures of RMT and AMT were unchanged [80]. Alexeeva et al. [68] combined rTMS with motor training in SCI participants. Participants experienced 5 consecutive days of each intervention: rTMS, motor training, and rTMS + motor training. A washout period of at least 4 weeks elapsed between each intervention. RTMS consisted of 4-pulse trains with a ~0.2–1.5 Hz train delivery rate at an intensity set to 80–90% RMT (i.e., quadropulse rTMS). Motor training consisted of hand tasks in participants 1 and 2 (10 tasks performed 10 times each: grasp and release, hand pronation and supination, isometric and concentric contractions of the wrist, thumb, and interphalangeal joints) and locomotor training in participant 3 (walking on a treadmill at a self-selected pace for 30 min with belt speed ≥0.05 m/s). In participant 1 and 2, "rTMS" and "motor training" improved 9-hole pegboard task performance and increased MEP amplitudes without changing SICI, ICF, or CSP. The combined intervention led to the greatest improvements in 9-hole pegboard task. In participant 3, the largest improvements in treadmill walking speeds were seen following the combined interventions as well [68]. Collectively, studies pairing NIBS with motor training reveal that larger functional gains may be induced compared to the effects of NIBS or motor training delivered in isolation.

4.2. Pairing NIBS with aerobic exercise

Using aerobic exercise to prime the brain prior to NIBS may also lead to larger changes in corticospinal excitability. Regular physical activity and aerobic exercise promote plasticity by increasing levels of growth factors including brain-derived neurotrophic factor (BDNF) and insulin-like growth factor (IGF-1) [81, 82]. Further, aerobic exercise can modify plasticity [83] via increases in cerebral blood flow [84] and angiogenesis [85]. Rojas Vega et al. [86] investigated the effects of aerobic exercise on BDNF and IGF-1 serum concentrations in SCI participants. The SCI participants completed an aerobic exercise session on a hand-bike that included a 10-min warm-up followed by a timed trial over a distance of 42 km. Blood samples were collected before, after the warm-up, and immediately following aerobic exercise. The warm-up resulted in a 1.5-fold increase in BDNF concentration, although no significant differences were seen between pre- and post-aerobic exercise measures. Additionally, IGF-1 concentrations were increased following both the warm-up and aerobic exercise [86] suggesting that aerobic exercise has the ability to prime the central nervous system for neuroplastic changes. This has been supported by recent evidence that aerobic exercise, such as cycling, is able to prime the brain prior to NIBS in healthy participants [87, 88]. In uninjured individuals, priming the cortex with aerobic exercise prior to PAS enhances the plasticity effect relative to PAS alone as measured by increases in the MEP recruitment curve slope [87]. Additionally, recent evidence suggests that individuals who exercise regularly are more prone to motor cortex plasticity following PAS relative to sedentary/low physically active individuals. Those who exercise regularly had increased MEP amplitudes and steeper input/output recruitment curves after intervention, while no significant changes were seen in sedentary/low physically active individuals [89].

4.3. Summary

There are challenges for future research focused on combining NIBS with aerobic exercise or motor training. For example, one consideration involves timing the delivery of NIBS with respect to aerobic exercise and/or motor training. Thus far, NIBS has been delivered simultaneously [80] or in advance of [68] motor training yet their combined effect may be influ-

http://dx.doi.org/10.5772/63351

enced by their order of delivery [90]. In addition, the outcome of pairing protocols may be dependent on parameters of NIBS, aerobic exercise, or motor training, such as intensity and number of sessions; multiple sessions may be needed to induce any significant changes in motor function [91]. Therefore, pairing NIBS with aerobic exercise and/or motor training has the potential to drive neuroplastic changes in SCI participants that may exceed the functional gains achieved by a singular intervention, but further investigation is required.

5. New opportunities for NIBS to promote motor recovery in SCI

Motor recovery in SCI participants via NIBS and paired protocols are promising. However, other forms of NIBS including theta burst stimulation (TBS), rapid rate paired associative stimulation (rPAS), or transspinal direct current stimulation (ts-CCS) have the potential to induce plasticity and promote motor recovery and have yet to be explored in SCI.

TBS is a form of rTMS at low intensity that delivers continuous (cTBS) or intermittent (iTBS) high-frequency pulses inducing homosynaptic plasticity in the stimulated area. TBS effects depend on corticospinal output depend on the nature of stimulation. iTBS over motor cortex increases the amplitude of MEPs [92, 93], while cTBS over motor cortex decreases the amplitude of MEPs [92, 94], although this pattern is not always observed [95–97]. In participants with stroke, iTBS improves hand function [98] and increases MEP amplitudes [98, 99]. In addition, applying multiple sessions of cTBS in participants with amyotrophic lateral sclerosis decrease MEP amplitudes and increase RMT [100]. Although it has yet to be tested, TBS over motor cortex representation of the affected muscle in SCI may have the potential to modulate intracortical (i.e., SICI, ICF) and corticospinal circuitry (i.e., MEP amplitude). Hence, TBS, like rTMS, may be a suitable tool to influence synaptic interactions by strengthening the residual connections [92] and therefore increase motor output from the affected muscle. Further, by modulating plasticity within the cortex, indirect changes in the spinal circuitry may occur. Hence, TBS may provide an alternate method to induce plasticity in the cortex that may lead to motor recovery in SCI participants.

RPAS is based on the principles of STDP and involves pairing 5 Hz rTMS with peripheral nerve stimulation at a specific interstimulus interval [101]. Unlike PAS, which requires ~30 min to deliver, rPAS provides a particularly fast method (i.e., ~3–4 min for 600 pulses) to induce increases in corticospinal excitability. RPAS over the motor cortex increases MEP amplitudes and reduces SAI [101–104] in uninjured individuals. However, rPAS has yet to be investigated in clinical populations presenting with motor impairments. In rPAS, the pairing of TMS with nerve stimuli activates both, afferent and efferent pathways. Recently, it has been speculated that reorganization in the cortex following afferent stimulation may be crucial in neurorehabilitation of the hand [105]. Since rPAS is highly efficient in increasing corticospinal excitability in healthy adults for prolonged periods of time, it may provide a useful tool to promote sensory-motor coupling [102] in SCI participants.

Another promising NIBS technique involves the delivery of 40 min of constant current stimulation to the spinal cord [106]. Long-lasting transspinal constant current stimulation (ts-

CCS) alters cortical, corticospinal, and spinal plasticity in uninjured participants. Knikou et al. [106] found that both cathodal tsCCS and anodal tsCCS decreased afferent-mediated MEP facilitation, increased MEP amplitudes, and decreased transspinal-evoked potentials (TEPs) of knee flexors. Further, cathodal tsCCS increased TMS-mediated tibialis anterior flexor reflex facilitation, while anodal tsCCS decreased TMS-mediated TA flexor reflex facilitation and decreased post-activation depression of TEPs for the soleus H-reflex. This technique provides a way to directly stimulate the spinal cord, changing the synaptic efficacy between descending motor axons and spinal motorneurons, cortical interneurons and descending motor axons and Ia afferents and motorneurons [106]. While more research is required to determine the efficacy of this tool at modulating changes in the cortex and spinal cord to promote motor recovery in clinical populations, it may have the potential to improve voluntary motor function in SCI participants.

Author details

Aaron Z. Bailey, Hunter J. Fassett, Tea Lulic, Jenin El Sayes and Aimee J. Nelson*

*Address all correspondence to: nelsonaj@mcmaster.ca

Department of Kinesiology, McMaster University, Hamilton, Ontario, Canada

References

[1] Siebner HR, Rothwell J. Transcranial magnetic stimulation: new insights into representational cortical plasticity. Exp Brain Res 2003;148:1–16. doi:10.1007/s00221-002-1234-2

[2] Duque J, Labruna L, Verset S, Olivier E, Ivry RB. Dissociating the role of prefrontal and premotor cortices in controlling inhibitory mechanisms during motor preparation. J Neurosci 2012;32:806–16. doi:10.1523/JNEUROSCI.4299-12.2012

[3] Sinclair C, Hammond GR. Excitatory and inhibitory processes in primary motor cortex during the foreperiod of a warned reaction time task are unrelated to response expectancy. Exp Brain Res 2009;194:103–13. doi:10.1007/s00221-008-1684-2

[4] Ziemann U. TMS and drugs. Clin Neurophysiol 2004;115:1717–29. doi:10.1016/j.clinph.2004.03.006.

[5] Bütefisch CM, Netz J, Wessling M, Seitz RJ, Hömberg V. Remote changes in cortical excitability after stroke. Brain 2003;126:470–81.

[6] Neva JL, Lakhani B, Brown KE, Wadden KP, Mang CS, Ledwell NHM, et al. Multiple measures of corticospinal excitability are associated with clinical features of multiple sclerosis. Behav Brain Res 2016;297:187–95. doi:10.1016/j.bbr.2015.10.015

[7] Vucic S, Ziemann U, Eisen A, Hallett M, Kiernan MC. Transcranial magnetic stimulation and amyotrophic lateral sclerosis: pathophysiological insights. J Neurol Neurosurg Psychiatr 2013;84:1161–70. doi:10.1136/jnnp-2012-304019

[8] Bestmann S, Krakauer JW. The uses and interpretations of the motor-evoked potential for understanding behaviour. Exp Brain Res 2015;233:679–89. doi:10.1007/s00221-014-4183-7

[9] Grover HJ, Thornton R, Lutchman LN, Blake JC. Using transcranial magnetic stimulation to evaluate the motor pathways after an intraoperative spinal cord injury and to predict the recovery of intraoperative transcranial electrical motor evoked potentials: a case report. J Clin Neurophysiol 2015:1. doi:10.1097/WNP.0000000000000200

[10] Curt A, Keck ME, Dietz V. Functional outcome following spinal cord injury: significance of motor-evoked potentials and ASIA scores. Arch Phys Med Rehabil 1998;79:81–6.

[11] Davey NJ, Smith HC, Savic G, Maskill DW, Ellaway PH, Frankel HL. Comparison of input–output patterns in the corticospinal system of normal subjects and incomplete spinal cord injured patients. Exp Brain Res 1999;127:382–90.

[12] Brouwer B, Hopkins-Rosseel DH. Motor cortical mapping of proximal upper extremity muscles following spinal cord injury. Spinal Cord 1997;35:205–12.

[13] Smith HC, Savic G, Frankel HL, Ellaway PH, Maskill DW, Jamous MA, et al. Corticospinal function studied over time following incomplete spinal cord injury. Spinal Cord 2000;38:292–300.

[14] Roy FD, Yang JF, Gorassini MA, Roy FD, Yang JF, Gorassini MA. Afferent regulation of leg motor cortex excitability after incomplete spinal cord injury. J Neurophysiol 2010;103:2222–33. doi:10.1152/jn.00903.2009

[15] Edwards DJ, Cortes M, Thickbroom GW, Rykman A, Pascual-Leone A, Volpe BT. Preserved corticospinal conduction without voluntary movement after spinal cord injury. Spinal Cord 2013;51:765–7. doi:10.1038/sc.2013.74

[16] Rossini PM, Burke D, Chen R, Cohen LG, Daskalakis Z, Di Iorio R, et al. Non-invasive electrical and magnetic stimulation of the brain, spinal cord, roots and peripheral nerves: basic principles and procedures for routine clinical and research application. An updated report from an I.F.C.N. Committee. Clin Neurophysiol 2015;126:1071–107. doi:10.1016/j.clinph.2015.02.001

[17] Rothwell JC, Hallett M, Berardelli A. Magnetic stimulation: motor evoked potentials. Electroencephalogr Clin Neurophysiol Suppl 1999;52:9–103.

[18] Paulus W, Classen J, Cohen LG, Large CH, Di Lazzaro V, Nitsche M, et al. State of the art: pharmacologic effects on cortical excitability measures tested by transcranial magnetic stimulation. Brain Stimul 2008;1:151–63. doi:10.1016/j.brs.2008.06.002

[19] Hodgkin AL, Huxley AF. A quantitative description of membrane current and its application to conduction and excitation in nerve. J Physiol (Lond) 1952;117:500–44. doi:10.1111/(ISSN)1469-7793

[20] Day BL, Dressler D, Maertens de Noordhout A, Marsden CD, Nakashima K, Rothwell JC, et al. Electric and magnetic stimulation of human motor cortex: surface EMG and single motor unit responses. J Physiol (Lond) 1989;412:449–73. doi:10.1111/(ISSN)1469-7793

[21] Freund P, Thompson AJ, Rothwell J, Craggs M, Bestmann S. Corticomotor representation to a human forearm muscle changes following cervical spinal cord injury. Eur J Neurosci 2011;34:1839–46. doi:10.1111/j.1460-9568.2011.07895.x

[22] Bailey AZ, Mi YP, Nelson AJ. Short-latency afferent inhibition in chronic spinal cord injury. Transl Neurosci 2015;6:1–9. doi:10.1515/tnsci-2015-0025

[23] Penfield W, Boldrey E. Somatic motor and sensory representation in the cerebral cortex of man as studied by electrical stimulation. Brain J Neurol 1937;60:389–443. doi:10.1093/brain/60.4.389

[24] Raineteau O, Schwab ME. Plasticity of motor systems after incomplete spinal cord injury. Nat Rev Neurosci 2001;2:263–73. doi:10.1038/35067570

[25] Romero JR, Ramirez DM, Aglio LS, Gugino LD. Brain mapping using transcranial magnetic stimulation. Neurosurg Clin N Am 2011;22:141–52–vii. doi:10.1016/j.nec.2010.11.002

[26] van de Ruit M, Grey MJ. The TMS Map Scales with Increased Stimulation Intensity and Muscle Activation. Brain Topogr 2016;29:56–66. doi:10.1007/s10548-015-0447-1

[27] Levy WJ, Amassian VE, Traad M, Cadwell J. Focal magnetic coil stimulation reveals motor cortical system reorganized in humans after traumatic quadriplegia. Brain Res 1990;510:130–4

[28] Cohen LG, Roth BJ, Wassermann EM, Topka H, Fuhr P, Schultz J, et al. Magnetic stimulation of the human cerebral cortex, an indicator of reorganization in motor pathways in certain pathological conditions. J Clin Neurophysiol 1991;8:56–65.

[29] Streletz LJ, Belevich JK, Jones SM, Bhushan A, Shah SH, Herbison GJ. Transcranial magnetic stimulation: cortical motor maps in acute spinal cord injury. Brain Topogr 1995;7:245–50.

[30] Mikulis DJ, Jurkiewicz MT, McIlroy WE, Staines WR, Rickards L, Kalsi-Ryan S, et al. Adaptation in the motor cortex following cervical spinal cord injury. Neurology 2002;58:794–801.

[31] DeFelipe J, Conley M, Jones EG. Long-range focal collateralization of axons arising from corticocortical cells in monkey sensory-motor cortex. J Neurosci 1986;6:3749–66.

[32] Kujirai T, Caramia MD, Rothwell JC, Day BL, Thompson PD, Ferbert A, et al. Corticocortical inhibition in human motor cortex. J Physiol (Lond) 1993;471:501–19. doi:10.1111/(ISSN)1469-7793

[33] Ziemann U, Lönnecker S, Steinhoff BJ, Paulus W. Effects of antiepileptic drugs on motor cortex excitability in humans: a transcranial magnetic stimulation study. Ann Neurol 1996;40:367–78. doi:10.1002/ana.410400306

[34] Ilić TV, Meintzschel F, Cleff U, Ruge D, Kessler KR, Ziemann U. Short-interval paired-pulse inhibition and facilitation of human motor cortex: the dimension of stimulus intensity. J Physiol (Lond) 2002;545:153–67.

[35] Saturno E, Bonato C, Miniussi C, Lazzaro V, Callea L. Motor cortex changes in spinal cord injury: a TMS study. Neurol Res 2008;30:1084–5. doi:10.1179/174313208X332968

[36] Shimizu T, Hino T, Komori T, Hirai S. Loss of the muscle silent period evoked by transcranial magnetic stimulation of the motor cortex in patients with cervical cord lesions. Neurosci Lett 2000;286:199–202.

[37] Roy FD, Zewdie ET, Gorassini MA. Short-interval intracortical inhibition with incomplete spinal cord injury. Clin Neurophysiol 2011;122:1387–95. doi:10.1016/j.clinph.2010.11.020

[38] Mi YP, Bailey AZ, Nelson AJ. Short- and long-intracortical inhibition in incomplete spinal cord injury. Can J Neurol Sci 2016;43:183–91. doi:10.1017/cjn.2015.310

[39] Valls-Solé J, Pascual-Leone A, Wassermann EM, Hallett M. Human motor evoked responses to paired transcranial magnetic stimuli. Electroencephalogr Clin Neurophysiol 1992;85:355–64.

[40] Wassermann EM, Samii A, Mercuri B, Ikoma K, Oddo D, Grill SE, et al. Responses to paired transcranial magnetic stimuli in resting, active, and recently activated muscles. Exp Brain Res 1996;109:158–63.

[41] McDonnell MN, Orekhov Y, Ziemann U. The role of GABA(B) receptors in intracortical inhibition in the human motor cortex. Exp Brain Res 2006;173:86–93. doi:10.1007/s00221-006-0365-2

[42] Werhahn KJ, Kunesch E, Noachtar S, Benecke R, Classen J. Differential effects on motorcortical inhibition induced by blockade of GABA uptake in humans. J Physiol (Lond) 1999;517 (Pt 2):591–7. doi:10.1111/j.1469-7793.1999.0591t.x

[43] Barry MD, Bunday KL, Chen R, Perez MA. Selective effects of baclofen on use-dependent modulation of GABAB inhibition after tetraplegia. J Neurosci 2013;33:12898–907. doi:10.1523/JNEUROSCI.1552-13.2013

[44] Mohammadi B, Krampfl K, Petri S, Bogdanova D, Kossev A, Bufler J, et al. Selective and nonselective benzodiazepine agonists have different effects on motor cortex excitability. Muscle Nerve 2006;33:778–84. doi:10.1002/mus.20531

[45] Schwenkreis P, Witscher K, Janssen F, Addo A, Dertwinkel R, Zenz M, et al. Influence of the N-methyl-D-aspartate antagonist memantine on human motor cortex excitability. Neurosci Lett 1999;270:137–40.

[46] Chen R, Corwell B, Hallett M. Modulation of motor cortex excitability by median nerve and digit stimulation. Exp Brain Res 1999;129:77–86.

[47] Hirashima F, Yokota T. Influence of peripheral nerve stimulation on human motor cortical excitability in patients with ventrolateral thalamic lesion. Arch Neurol 1997;54:619–24.

[48] Di Lazzaro V, Pilato F, Dileone M, Tonali PA, Ziemann U. Dissociated effects of diazepam and lorazepam on short-latency afferent inhibition. J Physiol (Lond) 2005;569:315–23. doi:10.1113/jphysiol.2005.092155

[49] Di Lazzaro V, Oliviero A, Profice P, Pennisi MA, Di Giovanni S, Zito G, et al. Muscarinic receptor blockade has differential effects on the excitability of intracortical circuits in the human motor cortex. Exp Brain Res 2000;135:455–61.

[50] Sailer A, Molnar GF, Cunic DI, Chen R. Effects of peripheral sensory input on cortical inhibition in humans. J Physiol (Lond) 2002;544:617–29.

[51] Tokimura H, Di Lazzaro V, Tokimura Y, Oliviero A, Profice P, Insola A, Mazzone P, Tonali P, Rothwell JC. Short latency inhibition of human hand motor cortex by somatosensory input from the hand. J Physiol 2000;523:503–13.

[52] Kimiskidis VK, Papagiannopoulos S, Sotirakoglou K, Kazis DA, Kazis A, Mills KR. Silent period to transcranial magnetic stimulation: construction and properties of stimulus-response curves in healthy volunteers. Exp Brain Res 2005;163:21–31. doi: 10.1007/s00221-004-2134-4

[53] Fuhr P, Agostino R, Hallett M. Spinal motor neuron excitability during the silent period after cortical stimulation. Electroencephalogr Clin Neurophysiol 1991;81:257–62.

[54] Ziemann U, Netz J, Szelényi A, Hömberg V. Spinal and supraspinal mechanisms contribute to the silent period in the contracting soleus muscle after transcranial magnetic stimulation of human motor cortex. Neurosci Lett 1993;156:167–71.

[55] Pierantozzi M, Marciani MG, Palmieri MG, Brusa L, Galati S, Caramia MD, et al. Effect of Vigabatrin on motor responses to transcranial magnetic stimulation: an effective tool to investigate in vivo GABAergic cortical inhibition in humans. Brain Res 2004;1028:1–8. doi:10.1016/j.brainres.2004.06.009

[56] Inghilleri M, Berardelli A, Marchetti P, Manfredi M. Effects of diazepam, baclofen and thiopental on the silent period evoked by transcranial magnetic stimulation in humans. Exp Brain Res 1996;109:467–72.

[57] Ferbert A, Priori A, Rothwell JC, Day BL, Colebatch JG, Marsden CD. Interhemispheric inhibition of the human motor cortex. J Physiol (Lond) 1992;453:525–46. doi:10.1111/(ISSN)1469-7793

[58] Daskalakis ZJ, Christensen BK, Fitzgerald PB, Roshan L, Chen R. The mechanisms of interhemispheric inhibition in the human motor cortex. J Physiol (Lond) 2002;543:317–26. doi:10.1113/jphysiol.2002.017673

[59] Kukaswadia S, Wagle-Shukla A, Morgante F, Gunraj C, Chen R. Interactions between long latency afferent inhibition and interhemispheric inhibitions in the human motor cortex. J Physiol (Lond) 2005;563:915–24. doi:10.1113/jphysiol.2004.080010

[60] Bunday KL, Perez MA. Impaired crossed facilitation of the corticospinal pathway after cervical spinal cord injury. J Neurophysiol 2012;107:2901–11. doi:10.1152/jn.00850.2011

[61] Chistiakova M, Bannon NM, Bazhenov M, Volgushev M. Heterosynaptic plasticity: multiple mechanisms and multiple roles. Neuroscientist 2014;20:483–98. doi:10.1177/1073858414529829

[62] Tazoe T, Perez MA. Effects of repetitive transcranial magnetic stimulation on recovery of function after spinal cord injury. Arch Phys Med Rehabil 2015;96:S145–55. doi:10.1016/j.apmr.2014.07.418

[63] Ridding MC, Ziemann U. Determinants of the induction of cortical plasticity by non-invasive brain stimulation in healthy subjects. J Physiol (Lond) 2010;588:2291–304. doi:10.1113/jphysiol.2010.190314

[64] Pell GS, Roth Y, Zangen A. Modulation of cortical excitability induced by repetitive transcranial magnetic stimulation: influence of timing and geometrical parameters and underlying mechanisms. Prog Neurobiol 2011;93:59–98. doi:10.1016/j.pneurobio.2010.10.003

[65] Belci M, Catley M, Husain M, Frankel HL, Davey NJ. Magnetic brain stimulation can improve clinical outcome in incomplete spinal cord injured patients. Spinal Cord 2004;42:417–9. doi:10.1038/sj.sc.3101613

[66] Ellaway PH, Maksimovic R, Craggs MD, Mathias CJ, Gall A, Balasubramaniam AV, et al. Action of 5Hz repetitive transcranial magnetic stimulation on sensory, motor and autonomic function in human spinal cord injury. Clin Neurophysiol 2011;122:2452–61. doi:10.1016/j.clinph.2011.04.022

[67] Benito J, Kumru H, Murillo N, Costa U, Medina J, Tormos JM, et al. Motor and gait improvement in patients with incomplete spinal cord injury induced by high-frequency repetitive transcranial magnetic stimulation. Top Spinal Cord Inj Rehabil 2012;18:106–12. doi:10.1310/sci1802-106

[68] Alexeeva N, Calancie B. Efficacy of QuadroPulse rTMS for improving motor function after spinal cord injury: three case studies. J Spinal Cord Med 2016;39:50–7. doi: 10.1179/2045772314Y.0000000279

[69] Nitsche MA, Cohen LG, Wassermann EM, Priori A, Lang N, Antal A, et al. Transcranial direct current stimulation: state of the art 2008. Brain Stimul 2008;1:206–23. doi: 10.1016/j.brs.2008.06.004

[70] Kuo H-I, Paulus W, Batsikadze G, Jamil A, Kuo M-F, Nitsche MA. Chronic enhancement of serotonin facilitates excitatory transcranial direct current stimulation-induced neuroplasticity. Neuropsychopharmacology 2015. doi:10.1038/npp.2015.270

[71] Murray LM, Edwards DJ, Ruffini G, Labar D, Stampas A, Pascual-leone A, et al. Intensity dependent effects of transcranial direct current stimulation on corticospinal excitability in chronic spinal cord injury. Arch Phys Med Rehabil 2015;96:S114–21. doi:10.1016/j.apmr.2014.11.004

[72] Player MJ, Taylor JL, Alonzo A, Loo CK. Paired associative stimulation increases motor cortex excitability more effectively than theta-burst stimulation. Clin Neurophysiol 2012;123:2220–6. doi:10.1016/j.clinph.2012.03.081

[73] Lamy J-C, Russmann H, Shamim EA, Meunier S, Hallett M. Paired associative stimulation induces change in presynaptic inhibition of Ia terminals in wrist flexors in humans. J Neurophysiol 2010;104:755–64. doi:10.1152/jn.00761.2009

[74] Bunday KL, Perez MA. Motor recovery after spinal cord injury enhanced by strengthening corticospinal synaptic transmission. Curr Biol 2012;22:2355–61. doi:10.1016/j.cub. 2012.10.046

[75] Yamaguchi T, Fujiwara T, Tsai Y-A, Tang S-C, Kawakami M, Mizuno K, et al. The effects of anodal transcranial direct current stimulation and patterned electrical stimulation on spinal inhibitory interneurons and motor function in patients with spinal cord injury. Exp Brain Res 2016:1–10. doi:10.1007/s00221-016-4561-4

[76] Rioult-Pedotti MS, Friedman D, Hess G, Donoghue JP. Strengthening of horizontal cortical connections following skill learning. Nat Neurosci 1998;1:230–4. doi: 10.1038/678

[77] Benito Penalva J, Opisso E, Medina J, Corrons M, Kumru H, Vidal J, et al. H reflex modulation by transcranial magnetic stimulation in spinal cord injury subjects after gait training with electromechanical systems. Spinal Cord 2010;48:400–6. doi: 10.1038/sc.2009.151

[78] Chisholm AE, Peters S, Borich MR, Boyd LA, Lam T. Short-term cortical plasticity associated with feedback-error learning after locomotor training in a patient with incomplete spinal cord injury. Phys Ther 2015;95:257–66. doi:10.2522/ptj.20130522

[79] Thomas SL, Gorassini MA. Increases in corticospinal tract function by treadmill training after incomplete spinal cord injury. J Neurophysiol 2005;94:2844–55. doi: 10.1152/jn.00532.2005

[80] Gomes-Osman J, Field-Fote EC. Improvements in hand function in adults with chronic tetraplegia following a multiday 10-Hz repetitive transcranial magnetic stimulation intervention combined with repetitive task practice. J Neurol Phys Ther 2015;39:23–30. doi:10.1097/NPT.0000000000000062

[81] Cotman CW, Berchtold NC, Christie L-A. Exercise builds brain health: key roles of growth factor cascades and inflammation. Trends Neurosci 2007;30:464–72. doi: 10.1016/j.tins.2007.06.011

[82] Colcombe SJ, Kramer AF, Erickson KI, Scalf P, McAuley E, Cohen NJ, et al. Cardiovascular fitness, cortical plasticity, and aging. Proc Natl Acad Sci USA 2004;101:3316–21. doi:10.1073/pnas.0400266101

[83] Kramer AF, Erickson KI. Capitalizing on cortical plasticity: influence of physical activity on cognition and brain function. Trends Cogn Sci (Regul Ed) 2007;11:342–8. doi:10.1016/j.tics.2007.06.009

[84] Xiong J, Ma L, Wang B, Narayana S, Duff EP, Egan GF, et al. Long-term motor training induced changes in regional cerebral blood flow in both task and resting states. NeuroImage 2009;45:75–82. doi:10.1016/j.neuroimage.2008.11.016

[85] Swain RA, Harris AB, Wiener EC, Dutka MV, Morris HD, Theien BE, et al. Prolonged exercise induces angiogenesis and increases cerebral blood volume in primary motor cortex of the rat. Neuroscience 2003;117:1037–46.

[86] Rojas Vega S, Abel T, Lindschulten R, Hollmann W, Bloch W, Strüder HK. Impact of exercise on neuroplasticity-related proteins in spinal cord injured humans. Neuroscience 2008;153:1064–70. doi:10.1016/j.neuroscience.2008.03.037

[87] Mang CS, Campbell KL, Ross CJD, Boyd LA. Promoting neuroplasticity for motor rehabilitation after stroke: considering the effects of aerobic exercise and genetic variation on brain-derived neurotrophic factor. Phys Ther 2013;93:1707–16. doi: 10.2522/ptj.20130053

[88] McDonnell MN, Buckley JD, Opie GM, Ridding MC, Semmler JG. A single bout of aerobic exercise promotes motor cortical neuroplasticity. J Appl Physiol 2013;114:1174–82. doi:10.1152/japplphysiol.01378.2012

[89] Cirillo J, Lavender AP, Ridding MC, Semmler JG. Motor cortex plasticity induced by paired associative stimulation is enhanced in physically active individuals. J Physiol (Lond) 2009;587:5831–42. doi:10.1113/jphysiol.2009.181834

[90] Bolognini N, Pascual-leone A, Fregni F. Using non-invasive brain stimulation to augment motor training-induced plasticity. J Neuroeng Rehabil 2009;6:8. doi: 10.1186/1743-0003-6-8

[91] Froc DJ, Chapman CA, Trepel C, Racine RJ. Long-term depression and depotentiation in the sensorimotor cortex of the freely moving rat. J Neurosci 2000;20:438–45.

[92] Huang Y-Z, Edwards MJ, Rounis E, Bhatia KP, Rothwell JC. Theta burst stimulation of the human motor cortex. Neuron 2005;45:201–6. doi:10.1016/j.neuron.2004.12.033

[93] Zafar N, Paulus W, Sommer M. Comparative assessment of best conventional with best theta burst repetitive transcranial magnetic stimulation protocols on human motor cortex excitability. Clin Neurophysiol 2008;119:1393–9. doi:10.1016/j.clinph.2008.02.006

[94] Wu SW, Shahana N, Huddleston DA, Gilbert DL. Effects of 30Hz θ burst transcranial magnetic stimulation on the primary motor cortex. J Neurosci Methods 2012;208:161–4. doi:10.1016/j.jneumeth.2012.05.014

[95] Gentner R, Wankerl K, Reinsberger C, Zeller D, Classen J. Depression of human corticospinal excitability induced by magnetic theta-burst stimulation: evidence of rapid polarity-reversing metaplasticity. Cereb Cortex 2008;18:2046–53. doi:10.1093/cercor/bhm239

[96] Hamada M, Murase N, Hasan A, Balaratnam M, Rothwell JC. The role of interneuron networks in driving human motor cortical plasticity. Cereb Cortex 2013;23:1593–605. doi:10.1093/cercor/bhs147

[97] López-Alonso V, Cheeran B, Río-Rodríguez D, Fernández-Del-Olmo M. Inter-individual variability in response to non-invasive brain stimulation paradigms. Brain Stimul 2014;7:372–80. doi:10.1016/j.brs.2014.02.004

[98] Talelli P, Greenwood RJ, Rothwell JC. Exploring Theta Burst Stimulation as an intervention to improve motor recovery in chronic stroke. Clin Neurophysiol 2007;118:333–42. doi:10.1016/j.clinph.2006.10.014

[99] Di Lazzaro V, Pilato F, Dileone M, Profice P, Capone F, Ranieri F, et al. Modulating cortical excitability in acute stroke: a repetitive TMS study. Clin Neurophysiol 2008;119:715–23. doi:10.1016/j.clinph.2007.11.049

[100] Munneke MAM, Rongen JJ, Overeem S, Schelhaas HJ, Zwarts MJ, Stegeman DF. Cumulative effect of 5 daily sessions of θ burst stimulation on corticospinal excitability in amyotrophic lateral sclerosis. Muscle Nerve 2013;48:733–8. doi:10.1002/mus.23818

[101] Quartarone A, Rizzo V, Bagnato S, Morgante F, Sant'Angelo A, Girlanda P, et al. Rapid-rate paired associative stimulation of the median nerve and motor cortex can produce long-lasting changes in motor cortical excitability in humans. J Physiol (Lond) 2006;575:657–70. doi:10.1113/jphysiol.2006.114025

[102] Naro A, Russo M, AbdelKader M, Manganotti P, Genovesi V, Marino M, et al. A local signature of LTP-like plasticity induced by repetitive paired associative stimulation. Brain Topogr 2015;28:238–49. doi:10.1007/s10548-014-0396-0

[103] Tsang P, Bailey AZ, Nelson AJ. Rapid-rate paired associative stimulation over the primary somatosensory cortex. Plos One 2015;10:e0120731. doi:10.1371/journal.pone.0120731

[104] Morgante F, Quartarone A, Ricciardi L, Arena MG, Rizzo V, Sant'Angelo A, et al. Impairment of sensory-motor plasticity in mild Alzheimer's disease. Brain Stimul 2013;6:62–6. doi:10.1016/j.brs.2012.01.010

[105] Conforto AB, Kaelin-Lang A, Cohen LG. Increase in hand muscle strength of stroke patients after somatosensory stimulation. Ann Neurol 2002;51:122–5. doi:10.1002/ana.10070

[106] Knikou M, Dixon L, Santora D, Ibrahim MM. Transspinal constant-current long-lasting stimulation: a new method to induce cortical and corticospinal plasticity. J Neurophysiol 2015;114:1486–99. doi:10.1152/jn.00449.2015

Chapter 12

Emerging Techniques for Assessment of Sensorimotor Impairments after Spinal Cord Injury

Filipe Barroso, Diego Torricelli and Juan C. Moreno

Additional information is available at the end of the chapter

Abstract

Gait function can be altered after incomplete spinal cord (iSCI) lesions. Muscular weakness, co-activation of antagonist muscles, and altered muscle mechanics are likely to provoke abnormal gait and postural movements. Functional scales are available for assessment of functional walking in SCI patients, such as walking index for spinal cord injury (WISCI II), timed up and go (TUG) test, 10-meter walk test (10MWT), and 6-minute walk test (6MWT). Novel metrics for a more detailed comprehension of neuromuscular control in terms of degree of voluntary motor control have been recently proposed. This section describes novel techniques based on muscle synergy and frequency domain analysis of electromyographic signals. Such techniques are illustrated as potential tools for assessment of motor function after SCI with experimental data and a case study describing a diagnostic scenario. This chapter presents a discussion of the current status of the emerging metrics for assessment of sensorimotor impairments. Conclusions are given with respect to the availability of enriched information about neuromuscular behavior between functional tasks (walking and pedalling) and the potential relevance of these new techniques to improve the efficacy of treatment to improve locomotion after iSCI.

Keywords: Rehabilitation, spinal cord injury, walking, functional scales

1. Introduction

Gait function can be altered after incomplete spinal cord (iSCI) lesions. Muscular weakness, co-activation of antagonist muscles, and altered muscle mechanics are likely to provoke abnormal gait and postural movements. Human walking involves the coordination of several muscles and its correct activation. One of the main goals of treatment after SCI is to recover the ability to walk again. The assessment of the neurorehabilitation process has traditionally been done based on the qualitative methods (classic clinical scales) or subjective assessment from physiotherapists (based on clinical gaze) [1]. Traditional techniques are prone to low reliability and, as a consequence, may result in inadequate or costly interventions. More importantly, clinical tests focused on behavioral outcomes provide little information about the underlying differences between healthy and impaired nervous system [1]. It is becoming more and more clear that a more profound understanding of impairments may be crucial not only to prescribe effective treatments to individual patients but also to gather comparative results and evidence that are needed to develop novel therapies. Thus, motor neurorehabilitation should be informed by more reliable and repeatable metrics that allow a quantitative assessment of motor control performance and recovery.

Gait analysis is broadly known as means to adequately assess and follow-up patients and supports a clinical decision on the best treatment [2]. Clinical gait analysis involves a variety of techniques including kinematic or joint motion measurements; kinetic or joint torque assessment, electromyographic (EMG) measurements, and video analysis. Measures derived from gait analysis provide a detailed and quantitative description. This might further be used to extract important information to select a task-oriented approach that might enhance therapeutic response, which cannot be provided by clinical evaluation alone [2]. Instrumented clinical gait analysis, despite its objectivity, is not straightforward in practice. Thus, more concise indexes of gait function are to be developed to assess the changes in gait function over time and evaluate interventions.

Most widely used functional scales for gait rehabilitation in SCI patients are walking index for spinal cord injury (WISCI II), timed up and go (TUG) test, 10-meter walk test (10MWT), and 6-minute walk test (6MWT). As mentioned above, to achieve adequate treatment, it is crucial to investigate not only the functional effect but also the mechanisms underlying the impaired function. Recently, the use of quantitative metrics based on electromyography and biomechanical features is bringing a new insight into the motor recovery mechanisms and performance outcomes after neural damage. EMG features provide useful information concerning brain motor control strategies [3]. Muscle activation patterns and muscle synergies have been proposed as a potential technique to measure motor recovery following therapeutic interventions [4]. Muscle synergies, understood as groups of co-activated muscles that are responsible for task execution in different conditions, can explain the way that central nervous system (CNS) solves control of multiple muscles and degrees of freedom by means of a smaller number of neural parameters [5]. This brings a more comprehensive understanding of the underlying motor strategies responsible for impaired locomotion.

The aim of this chapter is to present the emerging indexes based on EMG and biomechanical data to support therapeutic interventions in SCI patients who are commonly affected with spastic paresis and require targeted relearning and activation of a residual motor function. Novel metrics based on computational methods, such as muscle coherence and muscle synergy analysis, are presented as tools for a more detailed comprehension of neuromuscular control in terms of degree of voluntary motor control. Conclusions are given with respect to the availability of enriched information about neuromuscular behavior between functional tasks

http://dx.doi.org/10.5772/64182

(walking and pedalling) and the potential relevance of these new techniques to improve the efficacy of treatment to improve locomotion after iSCI.

2. Sensorimotor impairments after SCI

The spinal lesion leads to sensorimotor impairments in both upper and lower extremities. Ambulation results limited due to the sensory and proprioceptive impairments and muscle spasticity, commonly found even in subjects that reach a sufficient level of ambulation. The mechanisms involved in muscle spasticity are related to the lesion in the CNS that leads to changes in the excitability of spinal reflexes and loss of supraspinal drive. This results in abnormal muscle function and leads to altered mechanical muscle properties. In addition to this, proprioceptive and sensory impairment lead to altered or loss afferent feedback to the CNS, which in turn progressively affects motor control and leads to unstable, non-physiological gait. In particular, symptoms such as muscular weakness, co-activation of antagonist muscles, and altered muscle mechanics provoke abnormal gait and postural movements.

The relationship between hypertonia and gait function is still not clear controversial [6]. The difficulty to classify iSCI subjects as spastic or not is a well-known problem [7]. Spasticity in SCI patients is mostly associated (clinically) with the presence of flexor and extensor spasms triggered by cutaneous stimulation. In practice, it is important to determine whether an impaired gait is mainly caused by disabling paresis but also altered afferent feedback to the CNS. Novel metrics to assess motor control based on detailed EMG analysis are required to complement and optimize interventions that focus on the clinical signs of spasticity, such as exaggerated reflexes and muscle tone (e.g., medication).

3. Clinical assessment of walking ability after SCI

The main goal of clinical assessments is to quantify the motor recovery by observing and measuring the functional changes that occur in the patient after the injury. This is normally done by scales, which quantify the patient's residual functions under a wide spectrum, and therefore support scientifically the clinical practice in making effective choice on the treatment, studying cost-benefit of the rehabilitation process and quantifying objectively the degree of incapacity or handicap. Nevertheless, the sensitivity and reliability of current scales are still limited. For instance, the score assignment still relies on a strong subjective component, which causes high intra and inter-rater variability, even when the scale is carried out by experienced examiners [8]. In addition, scales often have similar content and purpose, which makes difficult to decide which of the available tests are superior and should be used as outcome measures. Therefore, there is a need to incorporate new and more objective methods to assess of motor recovery into the existing panorama. In the following, we present and briefly describe the main measures used in clinical settings to evaluate the functional recovery after SCI.

3.1. ASIA impairment scale (AIS)

This scale [9] provides a correct assessment of the severity of the SCI and can assess the developmental stage of the lesion. The evaluation is mainly based on motor exploration and includes complementary tests for sensory and muscle assessment. Ten muscles are evaluated (covering upper and lower limbs) to get muscle balance score between 0 and 5. The sensory examination measures superficial and deep sensitivity on a scale of 0–2 in 28 sensitive key points (for example, the big toe to C6 or armpit for L2). The sum of the motor and sensory scores reflects the global degree of impairment. According to international standards established by the American Association of SCI AIS, this can be classified into five levels, ranging between complete lesion (A, sensory but not motor function is preserved below the neurological level and includes the sacral segments S4–S5) and normality (E, the sensorimotor functions are completely preserved).

3.2. Walking index for spinal cord injury (WISCI II)

This index [10] specifically measures the functionality of walking and aims to quantify the secondary physical limitations in SCI. A recent study on functional measures of gait in people with SCI [11] showed how previous scales (e.g., 10 m and timed up and go, TUG) were unable to discriminate the improvement in function of patients who needed assistive devices during walking, such as walker or crutches. These data suggest that the WISCII scale serves as a valid tool for measuring changes in locomotion and effectiveness of treatment after SCI when technical help or the assistance of an external person is required to realize gait function. The scoring method is based on visual observation of the patient's ability during walking over at least 10 m. Walking ability is classified in this index, from the level with the most severe disabilities (0), to less severe disability (20). Within this range, the patient is classified according to the use of devices, braces, and physical assistance of one or two people.

3.3. Timed up and go (TUG) test

Originally developed to study the balance in senior age [12], this test demonstrated its validity as a measure of walking performance in neurologically injured subjects [13]. This tool measures the time (in seconds) that patients take to get up from a chair, walk 3 m, and sit back. Walk 3 m is the traditional test TUG, but there are adaptations in which the patient has to walk 10 or 7 m. The score ranges from one (normal) to five points (very abnormal). Times above 20 s are predictors of falls. This test captures the complex interaction between balance and movement, including planning, initiation, and implementation, and completes a series of linked movements that are common in activities of daily living. The validity of the TUG has been studied in different works and found to have a sensitivity and specificity of 87%.

3.4. 10-meter walk test (10MWT)

This test quantifies the walking speed by measuring the time (in seconds) that the patient takes to travel a distance of 10 m [13]. This scale was firstly proposed to assess gait in patients with stroke and Parkinson's disease, and then transferred as an alternative to evaluate patients with

http://dx.doi.org/10.5772/64182

SCI. A study [14] comparing several clinical scales of motion concluded that 10MWT is a more reliable and easier handling tool than the test of 6-minute walk test (see next section). As a drawback, this test requires additional information on technical aids needed during walking.

3.5. 6-minute walk test (6MWT)

This test calculates the distance (in meters) that patients are able to walk in six minutes [15]. Initially, it was used to measure cardiovascular exercise capacity in elderly patients with heart or lung disease, as a submaximal test of the aerobic capacity of the individual. It is one of the most widely used tests to evaluate gait motor recovery in neurologically injured subjects [16].

3.6. Spinal cord (functional) independence measures (FIM and SCIM)

The functional independence measure (FIM) scale was originally developed to assess disability of individuals with stroke [17]. This tool has been then widely applied for the evaluation of the functionality in the SCI. It is a standard and validated scale studying the state of functional recovery of patients from hospital admission to discharge. It is also used globally to monitor the progress of the functionality of patients throughout the rehabilitation treatment. It measures 18 activities, of which 13 items refer to the motor area and five to the cognitive status. These 18 items are grouped into six blocks: self-care, sphincter control, transfers, locomotion, communication, and awareness of the external world. It includes seven levels ranging from total dependence to full independence [18,19].

The SCIM scale was developed specifically to improve some aspects of the FIM scale [13]. This scale consists of 16 items (score range 0–100) and includes three levels of activity: (1) self-care (feeding, grooming, bathing, and dressing), (2) respiration and sphincter management, and (3) mobility (bed and transfers and indoor/outdoor). Scores are obtained by adding up the individual items. The item scores are weighted related to the assumed clinical relevance.

4. Scales to assess clinical conditions of spasticity

The correct measurement of spasticity is of vital importance in SCI for three main reasons: (i) evaluating the effectiveness of anti-spasticity treatments, (ii) optimizing individually the amount of antispastic medication to patients, and (iii) understanding the pathophysiological mechanisms underlying this disorder [20]. However, although spasticity is usually easy to recognize, its quantification is a much more complex process [21]. A unique scale that can provide a general and objective assessment of spasticity is still not available in the literature; therefore, the various tests and clinical measures are usually combined in order to evaluate different aspects of spasticity. The existing clinical measurements include scales that measure muscle hypertonia (modified Ashworth scale (MAS), EAM) [22], the spasms often suffered by patients (frequency spasms scale Penn) [23], and the reflected hyperexcitability after SCI (scale of severity of spasms (SCATS) [24]. In the following sections, these three methods will be briefly described.

4.1. Modified Ashworth scale (MAS)

This scale measures the resistance of muscle to passive stretching [22]. The resistance value is scored between 0 and 4, being "0" the absence of any increase in tone during movement; "1" slight increase in tone and muscle response at the start of movement or increased resistance at the end of the movement; "1+" slight increase in muscle resistance movement followed by minimal resistance throughout the remainder of the range of motion; "2" significant increase in muscle endurance during most arc joint movement, but the joint moves easily; "3" marked increase in muscle strength or passive movement is difficult in flexion or extension; and "4" the affected joints are rigid in flexion or extension. Two physiotherapists should perform this test independently.

4.2. Penn spasm frequency scale (PSFS)

The PENN scale is a tool to quantify spasm frequency suffered by the patient during the 24 h prior to the test [25]. The scores on this scale are between 0 and 4, where "0" is the total absence of spasms, "1" spasms caused only by stimulation, "2" spasms that occur less than once every hour, "3" spasms occur more than once every hour, and "4" spasms that occur more than 10 times an hour. As for the MAS scale, two physiotherapists should perform this test independently.

4.3. Spinal cord assessment tool for spastic reflexes (SCATS)

This scale is a physiologically based measure for spastic reflexes for use in individuals with SCI. It measures the reflected hyperexcitability, which includes clonus, flexor spasms, and cramps in the extensors. This scale is developed to provide a measure of primary spastic reaction, addressing categories of spasms as follows: (1) clonus, (2) flexor spasms, and (3) extensor spasms. The spasm is triggered and rated with a score ranging from 0 to 3. The SCATS does not provide information on patient perspective, which is an important aspect since spasms are sometimes perceived beneficial to the patient. This tool is simple and quick (<5 s) to administer but despite its simplicity it has not been widely accepted yet. The measure could be conducted during a home visit or at a clinic/hospital. A study [24] evaluated the validity of this scale, demonstrating that it correlated significantly with kinematic and electromyographic measures, and with Ashworth scores.

5. Emerging metrics to assess sensorimotor impairments after spinal cord injury

Despite its ability to assess and provide information about underlying mechanisms and changes in motor control, electromyography (EMG) is still rarely employed in the clinical setting to assess SCI patients [26]. Thus, novel approaches using EMG should be explored, as EMG can be very valuable to understand compensatory strategies and for further rehabilitation processes.

This section describes novel techniques based on muscle synergies and frequency-domain analysis of EMG signals (muscle coherence). Such techniques are illustrated as potential tools for assessment of motor function after SCI with experimental data and a case study describing a diagnostic scenario.

5.1. EMG coherence

Neurophysiological studies demonstrate only limited spontaneous recovery of voluntary motor function after incomplete SCI diagnosed with the American Spinal Injury Association (ASIA) Impairment Scale (AIS) [9,27]. Thus, there is a clinical need to identify new comprehensive outcome measures that may be used to assess sensorimotor impairments after incomplete SCI (iSCI). Effective neurophysiological measures should have clinical relevance, reflecting the recovery of volunteer motor force and gait function, as well as the development of maladaptive motor plasticity, such as the spasticity syndrome, which is known to limit the recovery of voluntary motor strength, gait, and daily life activities following SCI [28–34]. These measures may facilitate clinical diagnosis and guidance of individualized neurorehabilitation programs.

5.1.1. Muscle coherence

Lower limb EMG coherence analysis has been used as an indirect measure of voluntary motor control, gait function [35], and spasticity [27] after iSCI. This is a frequency-domain measure of the similarity between two independent EMG signals, having the potential to assess the descending motor drive [36]. The fact that it just needs EMG recording to be calculated makes it suitable for clinical applications. On the other hand, muscle coherence activity estimation can be obtained from the same muscle (intramuscular coherence) [37,38], as well as between two different muscles (intermuscular coherence) [38–40].

Smith et al. [41] have shown that the synchronization of motoneuron discharges (coherence) was reduced after spinal cord injury and also that it could be better recorded during isometric muscle contractions. The analysis of muscle coherence has been used to diagnose lesions in voluntary motor control mechanisms and functionality of SCI patients, for example, gait control [37,38]. Several studies support the use of muscle coherence analysis as an indirect measure of the common descending tracts during the execution of specific motor tasks. For instance, it has been suggested the existence of an association between the force of a maximum isometric contraction and corticospinal activity, based on the evidence of a reduction of intracortical inhibition modulated by training muscle strength [42–45]. Despite the potential of this technique, few studies have investigated which type of movement would be optimal for the use of muscle coherence calculation as a greater diagnostic measure.

Measuring the residual activity of tibialis anterior may represent an interesting diagnostic measure of functionality after SCI, mainly because this muscle receives increased innervation from the corticospinal system [45]. In fact, ankle dorsiflexion movement has been used as an indirect measure of adaptive neuroplasticity during the rehabilitation phase [46], while the recording of tibialis anterior co-activation during plantarflexion may be also used as indicator of maladaptive mechanisms after SCI, such as spasticity or its associated symptoms [47].

5.1.2. An emerging methodology to assess muscle coherence

This section sums up the methodology and main results presented by [27], who analyzed intramuscular TA coherence within specific frequency bands between 10–60 Hz from subjects who suffered an iSCI, while they performed different movement tasks.

Muscle coherence between two TA EMG signals (intramuscular coherence) was calculated during the periods of activation of this muscle during controlled ankle dorsiflexion movements. Specifically, EMG was recorded during the following ankle dorsiflexion tasks: (I) isometric activation at 50, 75, and 100% of maximal voluntary torque (MVT), (II) isokinetic activation at 60 and 120°/s and III) isotonic dorsiflexion at 50% MVT. Periods of activation were visually determined after processing EMG signals. This analysis of EMGs started with demeaning of raw signals, followed by band-pass filtering (3–700 Hz) and rectification.

Muscle coherence was computed using the function "mscohere" of Matlab (Version 7.11). The output of this function is the magnitude-squared coherence estimate of the input signals (both TA signals), using Welch's averaged modified periodogram method [48]. Finally, four bandwidths were analyzed: 10–16, 15–30, 24–40, and 40–60 Hz. For each band, it was computed the mean magnitude squared coherence estimate. A non-significant higher level of coherence activity was identified within the 10–16 Hz band in the iSCI spasticity group, when comparing the isometric activation at 100% of MVT for subjects diagnosed without or with spasticity. For the other bands of frequency, no differences were identified for TA intramuscular coherence [27].

There was also a negative correlation between the TA muscle coherence measured during isometric activation at 100% of MVT and specific symptoms of SCI spasticity muscle hypertonia, passive resistive torque, and involuntary muscle contractions. The modified Ashworth scores correlated negatively with TA coherence within the 24–60 Hz frequency band. The severity spasms measured with the SCATS scale also presented a negative correlation the 40–60 Hz band. On the other hand, a positive correlation was found between the Penn score and the TA coherence for the 15–30 Hz band. A positive correlation was also identified between the degree of clonus activity and TA coherence within the 10–16 Hz bandwidth [27].

TA coherence calculated as the ratio of 120/60°/s isokinetic activation was higher in the iSCI spastic subgroup, when compared with the non-spastic group [27]. In summary, the results presented by Bravo-Esteban et al. [27] suggest that TA muscle coherence activity estimation during the execution of controlled ankle dorsiflexion movements may be used to assess the level of spasticity in iSCI patients.

5.2. Analysis of muscle synergies during cycling

Given the redundancy of the musculoskeletal system, a long-stand idea is that the central nervous system (CNS) controls muscle activation through the use of a synergistic organization constituted by basic control elements called synergies (or motor modules) [49–51]. In 1967, Nikolai Bernstein [52] proposed the existence of muscle synergies as a simplified strategy of motor control. Muscle synergies are functional sets of muscles, co-activated by varying their timing and/or neural drive. This synergistic control is thought to underlie the execution of different biomechanical tasks [53].

Muscle synergies may offer new insight into the underlying motor strategies responsible for impaired locomotion [1]. Thus, muscle synergies have been proposed as a potential technique to measure motor recovery [4]. Nevertheless, it is still difficult to assess or predict motor performance in those patients who lack the required muscle strength to walk during the early stage of the rehabilitation, even with some body weight supports. Given the similarities in kinematics and muscle control with walking [54], cycling may be explored as a novel framework to assess motor performance in iSCI patients.

5.2.1. Comparison of two iSCI patients

Based on the findings presented in our previous research [3], confirming the hypothesis that similar synergistic features are shared between walking and cycling, we further performed a research testing the hypothesis that muscle synergies outcomes extracted during cycling can be used as indicators of gait performance in iSCI patients. Preliminary results of two patients are presented in this section.

5.2.1.1. Subjects

Two iSCI patients gave their written consent to participate in this study and for data publication, after being informed about the procedures and possible discomfort associated with the experiments, in accordance with the Declaration of Helsinki. The local Toledo Paraplegics Hospital (Spain) Clinical Ethical Committee approved this study (07/05/2013 N°47).

Patient ID	Age (years)	Gender	Time post-SCI (months)	Level of lesion	Most affected side	AIS	WISCI II	TUG (s)	10-meter (s)
01	25	M	5	T4	Left	D	15	29.3	27.7
02	77	M	13	C7	Right	D	19	25.1	10.2

M, male; F, female; Level of lesion: C—Cervical, T—Thoracic; AIS, American Spinal Injury Association (ASIA) Impairment Scale. WISCI II, walking index for spinal cord injury; TUG, timed up and go.

Table 1. Individual iSCI patients' description, as well as the amount of physical assistance needed and gait performance.

Detailed information of the patients is presented in **Table 1**. Both patients received the standard rehabilitation program of the hospital. Inclusion criteria were as follows: aged between 18 and 80 years; motor incomplete spinal lesion (AIS C-D) of traumatic and non-traumatic etiology, with a prognosis of recovery of the walking function; evolution of at least 1.5 months. Exclusion criteria were as follows: supraspinal or peripheral neurological involvement; history of epilepsy; musculoskeletal involvement of lower limbs or spasticity higher than 3 (measured with the Modified Ashworth Scale) for each joint, either for extension or flexion.

5.2.1.2. *Experimental protocol*

Prior to the experiment, a trained physiotherapist performed a set of clinical evaluations in order to inform about the functional status of the patients. The gait performance was evaluated using the timed up and go (TUG) test [55] and the 10-meter test [56]. In order to quantify the amount of assistance required by the subjects (10 m walk), the walking index for spinal cord injury (WISCI II) was applied. This is a 21-point scale that ranges from 0 (patient unable to stand and/or participate in assisted walking) to 20 (patient ambulates 10 m with no devices, no braces and no physical assistance) [10].

On the day of the experiment, patients received their standard rehabilitation therapy in the morning. In the afternoon, each iSCI patient performed four cycling trials (at 30, 42, 50, and 60 rpm, revolutions per minute) of 30 s duration each, with 60 s resting between trials. These trials were performed on an electronically braked cycle ergometer (MOTOmed viva2, Reck, Betzenweiler, Germany) in the passive mode. For each patient, the order of the trials was randomized to avoid biased results. Patients were asked to perform the experiment while sat on a regular chair.

An auditory metronome was used in order to synchronize patients' cycling frequency with the desired cadence. An EMG amplifier (EMG-USB, OT Bioelettronica, Torino, Italy) with recording bandwidth of 10–750 Hz, overall gain of 1000 V/V, and acquisition frequency of 2048 Hz was used to record surface electromyography (sEMG) of 13 muscles of the most affected leg of patients. The recorded muscles were as follows: Gluteus Medius, Adductor Longus, Sartorius, Tibialis Anterior, Rectus Femoris, Tensor Fascia Latae, Vastus Lateralis, Vastus Medialis, Biceps Femoris, Semitendinosus, Soleus, Gastrocnemius Lateralis, and Gastrocnemius Medialis. The most affected side was determined based on the muscle score [57] of quadriceps, hamstrings, TA, and gastrocnemius for both limbs.

Bipolar sEMG electrodes (Ag-AgCl, Ambur Neuroline 720, Ambu, Ballerup, Denmark) were fastened with a 2-cm inter-electrode distance on each recorded muscle, following SENIAM recommendations for sEMG recording procedures [58]. One angular sensor (Vishay, Malvern, PA) was applied to estimate the crank angle at a sampling frequency of 100 Hz. Segmentation of pedaling cycles was then performed based on the bottom dead center (BDC) position of the pedal.

5.2.1.3. *Muscle synergies analysis*

For each patient and trial, 10 continuous pedaling cycles were selected for analysis. The selected raw EMG signals were pre-processed using high-pass filtering at 20 Hz, demeaning, rectification, and low-pass filtering at 5 Hz, resulting in the EMG envelopes [49,59]. Muscle synergies were extracted using a Non-Negative Matrix Factorization (NNMF) algorithm [60]. A detailed explanation of the procedure to extract muscles synergies is presented in [49] and [3]. For each trial, the NNMF algorithm was run four times, considering as input two to five

http://dx.doi.org/10.5772/64182

synergies. In order to avoid local minima, for each run, the NNMF was repeated 40 times and the repetition with the lowest reconstruction error was selected.

To assess whether the recorded EMGs were well described as a combination of the identified synergies, two indicators of the quality of reconstruction of the EMG data were used: the *variability accounted for* (VAF_{total}) [49] and the *coefficient of determination* (r^2) [61]. Both VAF_{total} and r^2 have been adopted in most studies on muscle synergies [49,61]. VAF_{total} has been suggested to be more stringent than r^2, since it is sensitive to both shape and amplitude of the signals, whereas r^2 only addresses similarity in shape.

5.2.1.4. Results

Patient 02 presented better motor performance than patient 01. In the case of WISCI II, patient 01 scored 15 points, whereas patient 02 score 19 points. Patient 01 needed 19.3 s to perform TUG test, whereas patient 02 needed 25.1 s to perform the same test. Patient 01 needed 27.7 to perform the 10-meter test, whereas patient 02 just needed 10.2 s to perform the same test.

As a general trend, patient 02 presented higher values of VAF_{total} and r^2 than patient 01, for all speeds and number of synergies. Also, the higher the number of synergies used to reconstruct EMG data, the better the data were reconstructed (higher VAF_{total} and r^2 values). Both patients reached their minimum values of VAF_{total} at 50 rpm, using two synergies to reconstruct EMG data. VAF_{total} values in such condition were 79% (**Figure 1A**) for patient 01 and 76% (**Figure 1B**) for patient 02. Patient 01 reached 92% as maximum VAF_{total} value. This value was observed when using five synergies at 60 rpm. For patient 02, a maximum VAF_{total} of 95% was reached when using five synergies at 42 rpm.

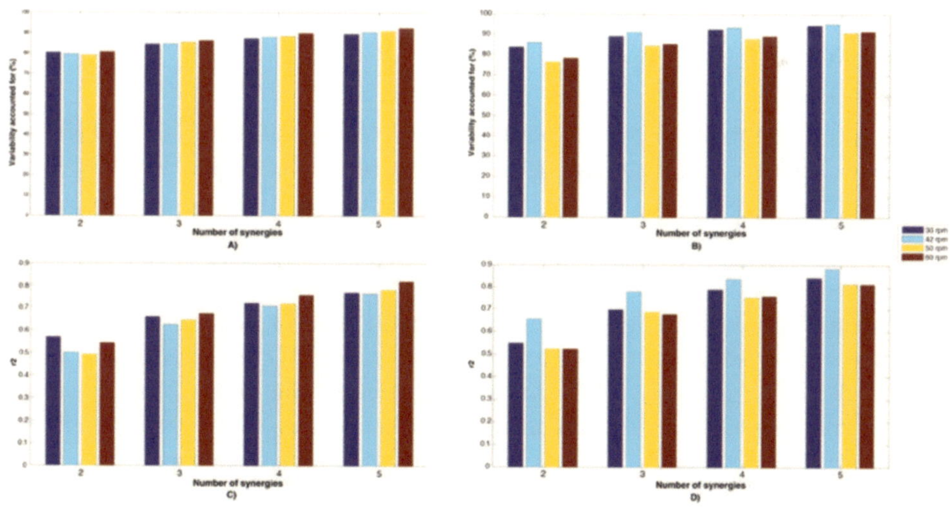

Figure 1. Variability accounted for (VAF_{total}) for patient 01 (A) and patient 02 (B), as well as coefficient of determination (r^2) for patient 01 (C) and patient 02 (D), according to the number of synergies, for each of the four speeds (30, 42, 50, and 60 rpm).

In the case of r^2 values, a minimum of 0.49 (**Figure 1C**) and 0.52 (**Figure 1D**) were obtained for patient 01 (at 50 rpm) and patient 02 (at 60 rpm), respectively. Both values were obtained using two synergies. On the other hand, maximum r^2 values of 0.82 and 0.89 were obtained for patient 01 (at 60 rpm) and patient 02 (at 42 rpm), respectively. Both values were obtained using five synergies. The quality of reconstruction indicators seems to correlate positively with WISCI II scores, that is, patient 02 presented higher values of VAF_{total} and r^2 and also higher values of WISCI II. On the other hand, quality of reconstruction indicators seem to correlate negatively with TUG and 10-meter tests, that is, patient 02 presented higher values of VAF_{total} and r^2 and also needed less time to perform these two gait performance tests.

5.2.1.5. Discussion

Based on the observed common muscle synergies between cycling and walking [3], this preliminary study tested the hypothesis that the analysis of muscle synergies during cycling correlates with gait performance scales in iSCI patients. These preliminary results corroborate this hypothesis.

Results showed positive correlations between WISCI II and EMG reconstruction goodness scores (VAFtotal and r^2) when recording a set of 13 muscles of the most affected leg. In the case of gait speed tests, reconstruction goodness scores correlated negatively with TUG and 10-meter tests. Our results are in agreement with the fact that patients with lower amount of required assistance and good walking performance present higher signal-to-noise ratio in EMG signals than patients with poor walking performance, as severely impaired subjects usually present reduced signal-to-noise ratio in the EMG signals due to reduced signal strength [60]. As a consequence of lower signal-to-noise, lower VAF_{total}, and r^2 values are expected [5].

6. Conclusions

Recovery after SCI is greatly dependent on the severity of the injury as well as the treatment provided in each phase of the lesion, being the subacute phase (up to approximately 6 months) the best phase to promote plastic changes in the CNS. Functional Improvements such as the increase of gait speed increased recovered distance or better WISCI II scores have been observed in acute SCI patients if compared to chronic SCI patients [62].

The application of simple diagnostic measures that might provide comprehensive information regarding the state of adaptive and maladaptive motor control mechanisms after SCI could play a crucial role in guiding rehabilitation strategies in the clinic. Neurophysiological measures should be preferred over qualitative clinical measures, as they are more independent, provide objective data and can be performed in less cooperative patients [63]. However, standardization and clinical validation should be achieved to allow for wide use in the clinical setting.

The analysis of muscle synergies during cycling can be explored as a novel approach for the quantitative assessment of gait performance. This analysis can complement current assessment procedures. On the other hand, the analysis of intramuscular coherence of tibialis anterior can also be explored as a measure of spasticity during the subacute phase of recovery in SCI patients, as it provides information on the mechanisms of maladaptive plasticity (specifically spasticity) [27].

In the future, additional researches are needed in order to validate TA muscle coherence analysis and use it in the clinical setting for the assessment of sensorimotor impairments in SCI patients. Specifically, longitudinal studies have to be performed since the initial stage of recovery, comparing muscle coherence with clinical and functional scales. This will be also useful to provide new information on the neurophysiological mechanisms present during the recovery stage in SCI patients.This work has been partially funded by grant from the European Commission, within the Seventh Framework Programme (IFP7-ICT-2013-10-611695: BioMot - Smart Wearable Robots with Bioinspired Sensory-Motor Skills).

Author details

Filipe Barroso[1,2], Diego Torricelli[2] and Juan C. Moreno[2*]

*Address all correspondence to: jc.moreno@csic.es

1 Department of Physiology, Feinberg School of Medicine – Northwestern University, Chicago, IL, USA

2 Neural Rehabilitation Group, Cajal Institute, Spanish National Research Council (CSIC), Madrid, Spain

References

[1] SAFAVYNIA, S. A.; TORRES-OVIEDO, G.; TING, L. H. Muscle synergies: implications for clinical evaluation and rehabilitation of movement. Top Spinal Cord Inj Rehabil, v. 17, n. 1, p. 16-24, 2011.

[2] NADEAU, S. et al. Guiding task-oriented gait training after stroke or spinal cord injury by means of a biomechanical gait analysis. Progress in Brain Research, v. 192, p. 161-180, 2011.

[3] BARROSO, F. O. et al. Shared muscle synergies in human walking and cycling. Journal of Neurophysiology, v. 112, n. 8, p. 1984-1998, 2014.

[4] ROUTSON, R. L. et al. The influence of locomotor rehabilitation on module quality and post-stroke hemiparetic walking performance. Gait Posture, v. 38, n. 3, p. 511-517, 2013.

[5] STEELE, K. M.; TRESCH, M.; PERREAULT, E. The number and choice of muscles impact the results of muscle synergy analyses. Front Comput Neurosci, v. 7, 2013.

[6] DUFFELL, L. D.; BROWN, G. L.; MIRBAGHERI, M. M. Facilitatory effects of anti-spastic medication on robotic locomotor training in people with chronic incomplete spinal cord injury. J Neuroeng Rehabil, v. 12, n. 29.

[7] REICHENFELSER, W. et al. Monitoring of spasticity and functional ability in individuals with incomplete spinal cord injury with a functional electrical stimulation cycling system. J Rehabil Med, v. 44, n. 5, p. 444-449, 2012.

[8] SAVIC, G. et al. Inter-rater reliability of motor and sensory examinations performed according to American Spinal Injury Association standards. Spinal Cord, v. 45, p. 444-451, 2007.

[9] MAYNARD, F. M. J. et al. International standards for neurological and functional classification of spinal cord injury. American Spinal Injury Association. Spinal Cord, v. 35, n. 5, p. 266-274, 1997.

[10] DITTUNO, P. L.; DITUNNO, J. F. Walking index for spinal cord injury (WISCI II): scale revision. Spinal Cord, v. 39, n. 12, p. 654-656, 2001.

[11] SAENSOOK, W. et al. Discriminative ability of the three functional tests in independent ambulatory patients with spinal cord injury who walked with and without ambulatory assistive devices. J Spinal Cord Med, v. 37, n. 2, p. 212-217, 2014.

[12] PODSIADLO, D.; RICHARDSON, S. The timed "Up & Go": a test of basic functional mobility for frail elderly persons. J Am Geriatr Soc, v. 39, n. 2, p. 142-148, 1991.

[13] FURLAN, J. C. et al. Assessment of disability in patients with acute traumatic spinal cord injury: a systematic review of the literature. J Neurotrauma, v. 28, p. 1413-1430, 2011.

[14] VAN HEDEL, H. J.; WIRZ, M.; DIETZ, V. Assessing walking ability in subjects with spinal cord injury: validity and reliability of 3 walking tests. Arch Phys Med Rehabil., v. 86, n. 2, p. 190-196, 2005.

[15] GUYATT, G. H. et al. The 6-miunte walk: a new measure of exercise capacity in patients with chronic heart failure. Can Med Assoc J, v. 8, n. 919-923, p. 132, 1985.

[16] MAANUM, G. et al. Walking ability and predictors of performance on the 6-minute walk test in adults with spastic cerebral palsy. Dev Med Child Neurol, v. 6, n. e126-e132, p. 52, 2010.

[17] HAMILTON, B. B.; GRANGER, C. V. Disability outcomes following inpatient rehabilitation for stroke. Physical Therapy, v. 74, n. 5, p. 494-503, 1994.

[18] KIRSHBLUM, S. et al. Late neurologic recovery after traumatic spinal cord injury. Arch Phys Med Rehabil, v. 85, p. 1811-1817, 2004.

[19] CATZ, A. et al. A multicenter international study on the spinal cord independence measure, version III: Rasch psychometric validation. Spinal Cord, v. 4, n. 275-291, p. 45, 2007.

[20] BURRIDGE, J. H. et al. Theoretical and methodological considerations in the measurement of spasticity. Disabil Rehabil, v. 27, n. 1-2, p. 69-80, 2005.

[21] BIERING-SORENSEN, F.; NIELSEN, J. B.; KLINGE, K. Spasticity-assessment: a review. Spinal Cord, v. 12, n. 708-722, p. 44, 2006.

[22] BOHANNON, R. W.; SMITH, M. B. Interrater reliability of a modified Ashworth scale of muscle spasticity. Phys Ther, v. 67, n. 2, p. 206-207, 1987.

[23] PENN, R. D. Intrathecal baclofen for severe spasticity. Ann N Y Acad Sci, v. 531, p. 157-166, 1988.

[24] BENZ, E. N.; HORNBY, T. G. A physiologically based clinical measure for spastic reflexes in spinal cord injury. Arch Phys Med Rehabil, v. 86, n. 1, p. 52-59, 2005.

[25] Development and Use of a Knowledge Translation Tool: The Rehabilitation Measures Database Moore, Jennifer L. et al. Archives of Physical Medicine and Rehabilitation, Volume 95, Issue 1, 197–202 January 2014.

[26] WANG, P. et al. Detection of abnormal muscle activations during walking following spinal cord injury (SCI). Res Dev Disabil, v. 34, n. 4, p. 1226-1235, 2013.

[27] BRAVO-ESTEBAN, E. et al. Tibialis anterior muscle coherence during controlled voluntary activation in patients with spinal cord injury: diagnostic potential for muscle strength, gait and spasticity. J Neuroeng Rehabil, v. 11, n. 23, 2014.

[28] BEAUPARLANT, J. et al. Undirected compensatory plasticity contributes to neuronal dysfunction after severe spinal cord injury. Brain, v. 136, n. Pt 11, p. 3347-3361, 2013.

[29] D'Amico, J. M., Condliffe, E. G., Martins, K. J. B., Bennett, D. J., & Gorassini, M. A. (2014). Recovery of neuronal and network excitability after spinal cord injury and implications for spasticity. Frontiers in Integrative Neuroscience, 8, 36. http://doi.org/10.3389/fnint.2014.00036

[30] ZORNER, B. et al. Clinical algorithm for improved prediction of ambulation and patient stratification after incomplete spinal cord injury. J Neurotrauma., v. 27, n. 1, p. 241-252, 2010.

[31] BOAKYE, M. et al. Quantitative testing in spinal cord injury: overview of reliability and predictive validity. J Neurosurg Spine., v. 17, n. 1, p. 141-150, 2012.

[32] PETERSEN, J. A. et al. Spinal cord injury: one-year evolution of motor-evoked potentials and recovery of leg motor function in 255 patients. Neurorehabil Neural Repair, v. 26, n. 8, p. 939-948, 2012.

[33] CURT, A.; KECK, M. E.; DIETZ, V. Functional outcome following spinal cord injury: significance of motor-evoked potentials and ASIA scores. Arch Phys Med Rehabil, v. 79, p. 81-86, 1998.

[34] YANG, J. F. et al. Volitional muscle strength in the legs predicts changes in walking speed following locomotor training in people with chronic Spinal Cord Injury. Phys Ther, v. 91, n. 6, p. 931-943, 2011.

[35] HANSEN, N. L. et al. Reduction of common synaptic drive to ankle dorsiflexormotoneurons during walking in patients with spinal cord lesion. J Neurophysiol, v. 94, p. 934-942, 2005.

[36] Boonstra, T. W. (2013). The potential of corticomuscular and intermuscular coherence for research on human motor control. Frontiers in Human Neuroscience, 7, 855. http://doi.org/10.3389/fnhum.2013.00855

[37] HALLIDAY, D. M. et al. Functional coupling of motor units is modulated during walking in human subjects. J Neurophysiol, v. 89, p. 960–968, 2003.

[38] BARTHELEMY, D. et al. Impaired transmission in the corticospinal tract and gait disability in spinal cord injured persons. J Neurophysiol, v. 104, p. 1167–1176, 2010.

[39] HANSEN, N. L. et al. Synchronization of lower limb motor unit activity during walking in human subjects. J Neurophysiol, v. 86, p. 1266–1276, 2001.

[40] NORTON, J. A.; GORASSINI, M. A. Changes in cortically related intermuscular coherence accompanying improvements in locomotor skills in incomplete spinal cord injury. J Neurophysiol, v. 95, p. 2580–2589, 2006.

[41] SMITH, H. C. et al. Motor unit discharge characteristics during voluntary contraction in patients with incomplete spinal cord injury. Exp Physiol, v. 84, p. 1151–1160, 1999.

[42] CROS, D.; SOTO, O.; CHIAPPA, K. H. Transcranial magnetic stimulation during voluntary action: directional facilitation of outputs and relationships to force generation. Brain Res, v. 1185, p. 103–116, 2007.

[43] ZOGHI, M.; NORDSTROM, M. A. Progressive suppression of intracortical inhibition during graded isometric contraction of a hand muscle is not influenced by hand preference. Exp Brain Res, v. 177, n. 2, p. 266–274, 2007.

[44] WEIER, A. T.; PEARCE, A. J.; KIDGELL, D. J. Strength training reduces intracortical inhibition. Acta Physiol (Oxf), v. 206, n. 2, p. 109–119, 2012.

[45] BROUWER, B.; ASHBY, P. Corticospinal projections to lower limb motoneurons in man. Exp Brain Res, v. 89, p. 649–654, 1992.

[46] WIRTH, B.; VAN HEDEL, H. J.; CURT, A. Changes in corticospinal function and ankle motor control during recovery from incomplete spinal cord injury. J Neurotrauma, v. 25, p. 467–478, 2008.

[47] GOMEZ-SORIANO, J. et al. Voluntary ankle flexor activity and adaptive coactivation gain is decreased by spasticity during subacute spinal cord injury. Exp Neurol, v. 224, p. 507–516, 2010.

[48] WELCH, P. The use of fast Fourier transform for the estimation of power spectra: a method based on time averaging over short, modified periodograms. IEEE Transactions on Audio and Electroacoustics, v. 15, p. 70–73, 1967.

[49] CLARK, D. J. et al. Merging of healthy motor modules predicts reduced locomotor performance and muscle coordination complexity post-stroke. J Neurophysiol, v. 103, n. 2, p. 844-857, 2010.

[50] NEPTUNE, R. R.; MCGOWAN, C. P. Muscle contributions to whole-body sagittal plane angular momentum during walking. J Biomech, v. 44, n. 1, p. 6-12, 2011.

[51] Ilngle, D. (1968). The Co-ordination and Regulation of Movements. Papers translated from Russian and German. N. Bernstein. Pergamon, New York, 1967. xii + 196., illus. $8. Science, 159(3813), 415–416. Retrieved from http://science.sciencemag.org/content/159/3813/415.2.abstract.

[52] Santello M, Bianchi M, Gabiccini M, Ricciardi E, Salvietti G, Prattichizzo D, Ernst M, Moscatelli A, Jörntell H, Kappers AM, Kyriakopoulos K, Albu-Schäffer A, Castellini C, Bicchi A. Hand synergies: Integration of robotics and neuroscience for understanding the control of biological and artificial hands. Phys Life Rev. 2016 Feb 3. pii: S1571-0645(16)00026-9. doi: 10.1016/j.plrev.2016.02.001. [Epub ahead of print] Review. PubMed PMID: 26923030.

[53] ZEHR, E. P. et al. Neural regulation of rhythmic arm and leg movement is conserved across human locomotor tasks. J Physiol, v. 582, p. 209-227, 2007.

[54] WALL, J. C. et al. The timed get-up-and-go test revisited: measurement of the component tasks. J Rehabil Res Dev, v. 37, n. 1, p. 109-113, 2000.

[55] FORREST, G. F. et al. Are the 10 meter and 6 minute walk tests redundant in patients with spinal cord injury? PLoS One, v. 9, n. 5, 2014.

[56] SEDDON, H. W. J. Medical Research Council: Aids to the Exam of the Peripheral Nervous System. [S.l.]: London: Her Majesty's Stationery Office, 1976.

[57] HERMENS, H. J.; FRERIKS, B.; MERLETTI, R. European Recommendations for Surface ElectroMyoGraphy: Results of the SENIAM Project. Enschede, The Netherlands: Roessingh Research and Development, 1999.

[58] HUG, F. et al. Is interindividual variability of EMG patterns in trained cyclists related to different muscle synergies? J Appl Physiol, v. 108, n. 6, p. 1727-1736, 2010.

[59] LEE, D. D.; SEUNG, S. Learning the parts of objects by non-negative matrix factorization. Nature, v. 401, p. 788-791, 1999.

[60] TORRES-OVIEDO, G.; MACPHERSON, J. M.; TING, L. H. Muscle synergy organization is robust across a variety of postural perturbations. J Neurophysiol, v. 96, n. 3, p. 1530-1546, 2006.

[61] DOBKIN, B. et al. Weight-supported treadmill vs over-ground training for walking after acute incomplete SCI. Neurology, v. 66, n. 4, p. 484–493, 2006.

[62] XIE, J.; BOAKYE, M. Electrophysiological outcomes after spinal cord injury. Neurosurg Focus, v. 25, n. 5, p. E11, 2008.

[63] YANG, J. F.; MUSSELMAN, K. E. Training to achieve over ground walking after spinal cord injury: a review of who, what, when, and how. J Spinal Cord Med, v. 35, n. 5, p. 293-304, 2012.